Workbook to accompany

The Basic EMT:
Comprehensive
Prehospital
Patient Care

2003 edition

Norman E. McSwain, Jr., MD, FACS, NREMT-P
Professor of Surgery
Tulane University School of Medicine
New Orleans, Louisiana

James L. Paturas, EMT-P
West Haven, Connecticut

Catherine A. Parvensky Barwell, PHRN, MEd

MosbyJems

St. Louis Philadelphia London Sydney Toronto

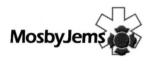

11830 Westline Industrial Drive
St. Louis, MO 63146

REVISED SECOND EDITION

Printed in the United States of America

International Standard Book Number: 0-323-02257-X

Publisher: Andrew Allen
Executive Editor: Claire Merrick
Developmental Editor: Laura Bayless
Project Manager: Gayle May
Designer: Judi Lange

03 04 05   FG /MV   9 8 7 6 5 4 3 2

Introduction

This workbook was written to help the EMT-B learn and understand the concepts presented in *The Basic EMT—Comprehensive Prehospital Patient Care, 2e*. The material is presented to allow you to progress at your own pace and monitor your progress and understanding by checking an answer key.

Each chapter of the workbook corresponds to a chapter in the textbook, which is identified as the *Reading Assignment*. Each chapter follows the same format and is divided into six components. The first section lists chapter *DOT Objectives*, which are those objectives identified by the U.S. Department of Transportation's 1994 *Emergency Medical Technician-Basic: National Standard Curriculum*. Where indicated, *Supplemental Objectives* are identified that involve information that is considered "supplemental" to the National Standard Curriculum. This material is included to expand on your basic knowledge of concepts as well as make the basic material more meaningful and easier to understand. Certification examinations, including State and National Registry, only test the information that is included in the National Standard Curriculum, so do not spend too much time focusing on supplemental material. Do review the material because it is valuable information. The objectives listed in the Workbook are the same as those listed in each corresponding chapter of the textbook.

There are three types of objectives identified in the National Standard Curriculum: cognitive, psychomotor, and affective. Cognitive objectives are those that involve knowledge and thinking skills. Psychomotor objectives involve hands on performance, and affective objectives involve feelings. Written examinations generally focus on cognitive objectives, and practical skills examinations focus on psychomotor skills. Affective skills sometimes develop over time. Appendix A is a sign-off form listing all DOT cognitive objectives that you should be able to perform on completion of the EMT-Basic course. Appendix B is a skills verification form that covers those skills identified in the psychomotor objectives of the National Standard Curriculum.

The second section of each chapter, *Key Terms*, involves key terms and definitions provided in the textbook chapter. This section is presented through a series of matching, short answer, and fill-in-the blank questions. The third section, *Key Concepts*, helps you learn the bulk of the material presented in the chapter. This section asks you to provide short answers, list items, compare and contrast concepts, and also includes some true/false questions.

The fourth section is a *Chapter Quiz*; this should be used as a self-assessment tool. These questions are provided in multiple-choice format with an occasional true/false question. Most certification examinations follow a multiple-choice format. These questions test information presented within that specific chapter of the textbook. By checking your answers with the answer key provided at the end of the chapter, you will get a better understanding of how you are progressing with the learning process.

The fifth section of each chapter is a *Case Scenario*. This section helps you put all the pieces together in a practical application. They require you to think and apply information learned not only in that chapter, but in previous chapters as well, in order to answer questions key to scene safety, roles and responsibilities, and patient care.

For chapters where practical skills demonstration is applicable, the last section of the chapter will include step-by-step *Skill Sheets*.

At the end of the workbook is a *Final Course Self-Evaluation*. This self-assessment tool is a 100-question multiple-choice test of all key material presented in the textbook and workbook. These questions focus only on the objectives of the National Standard Curriculum. You should take this test as a practice test prior to your final certification examination. Take it in one sitting and without looking up the answers. This will provide the most reliable indication as to how prepared you are for a certification exam. Then check your responses with the answer key. If you score 90% to 100% you are most likely ready. If you scored 80% to 90%, you are probably ready but may want to take one final review. If you scored 70% to 80%, you should do some more studying. Look at the questions you answered incorrectly to see if there is a pattern. If you missed many questions in one or two topics, go back and re-read those chapters and review the workbook chapters one more time. If you scored under 70%, you need to do some significant studying. Again, try to determine what sections you are missing the most questions on, and focus on those.

Additional information that you may find useful is included in the appendices. Appendix C is a list of acronyms and abbreviations commonly used by healthcare professionals. Appendix D is a chart of signs and symptoms, possible causes, and suggested emergency procedures to be followed for various illnesses and injuries. The list is not all inclusive, but it should serve as a starting point.

If you are not sure how to study or to take tests, read the following section. Studying and test taking are skills that require practice. Starting a course with the right skills may make all the difference in how much you take from the course and on how well you do.

Good luck in the course and on becoming the best EMT-Basic you can be.

Studying Strategies

The most effective means for preparing for an exam is to study throughout a training program. Waiting until exam week and "cramming" is not productive. Specific studying strategies to follow include:

- Use course objectives when studying. State and National exams are usually referenced to the National Standard Curriculum objectives for the EMT-Basic course. In this text, these objectives are "DOT Objectives." The supplemental material is "nice to know" but should not take time away from your learning the basic information.

- Complete reading assignments *before* a particular class session. This allows you to have a basic understanding, or at least recognize some of the terminology, so that it makes more sense during class.

- Attend class sessions and take notes based on the instructor's presentation. The instructor will most likely be identifying the material that is most important for you to know and understand.

- After a training session, reread assigned chapters and notes taken in class. Having attended class, the chapter will most likely make more sense the second time through. Again, focus on those areas your instructor identified as being most important. Take additional notes on this key information until you understand the material.

- Frequently review class notes throughout the course.

- Participate in multiple short study sessions rather than a few long ones. Take breaks when needed. Sometimes your body needs a rest. By spreading your study sessions throughout the week and throughout the course, there will be no need to "cram" for a test, so your body (and mind) should be well rested for exams.

- Complete practice quizzes, tests, and other aids. These are provided to help you throughout the course. They will help you determine how well you are progressing through the course and on what information you need additional help on.

- Pace study time in accordance with exam content percentages. Do not waste time studying insignificant information. This is often best gauged through the objectives since certification exams are usually based on the National Standard Curriculum objectives.

Preparing for Examinations

Certification examinations are often stressful for the EMT-Basic student. There are, however, various methods to help decrease the stress associated with examinations and to increase success rates associated with certification exams. It is important to remember that test taking is a skill that can be learned. Even though you may have a thorough knowledge of a particular content area, you may lack the ability to translate this knowledge in a testing situation. Therefore, learning test-taking skills can significantly improve your performance on examinations. The following information is presented to help you better prepare for examinations.

Exams

Written certification exams usually consist entirely of multiple-choice questions. These exams are graded based on the number of correct answers, not on the number of incorrect responses. Since there is no penalty for guessing, students should always enter a response. In multiple-choice questions the student usually has at least a 25% chance of a correct response, even if he or she has no idea of the correct answer.

A multiple-choice question is comprised of two parts: the stem (question) and the responses (choices). Responses include the correct answer and three or four plausible distractors.

Key points to remember when selecting the correct answer include:

- Read the stem without reading the responses.

- Understand what the question is asking.

- Determine a correct response to the question.

- Read all responses to select the one that is closest to the correct answer.

- Look for key words such as *not, first, never, except,* and *always.*

- Identify specific terms that would cause a different response such as infant versus adult CPR, chest pain that *radiates, cool, clammy skin, dyspnea,* etc.

- Before selecting a correct answer, read all possible responses.

- If the correct answer is not readily apparent, exclude those choices that are obviously incorrect. Most often students can exclude two of the four possible responses leaving a 50% chance of selecting the correct answer.

- If the option "all of the above" appears as a response, it is most likely the correct answer.

- Do not read into the question. If the question asks whether the administration of oxygen is indicated for a particular patient, do not read into the question and think "well yes, except if the patient....."

- Do not change a response unless you mis-read it the first time. Your first impulse is most often the correct choice.

- Do not spend too much time on a question. If the answer is not readily apparent, mark your answer sheet and move on. After answering the remaining questions, return to those marked and work out the answer.

- Fill in the answer sheet correctly. Use the proper tools as directed by test moderators (i.e., No. 2 pencils). Fill in circles completely and erase all stray marks.

- Check the test question numbers after every 10 answers to prevent a last-minute panic when it is discovered that the answer to question 89 was placed in the space for question 78 on the answer sheet.

To help alleviate test-taking anxiety:

- Get a full night's sleep before the exam.

- Before the exam, perform a few exercises to increase blood supply to the brain by increasing the status of the cardiovascular system.

- Eat normal meals before the exam but refrain from eating a heavy meal within 1 hour of the test.

- Layer clothing in order to maintain a comfortable personal climate regardless of classroom temperatures.

- Focus on the task at hand; sit away from distractors such as friends, noise, bad lighting, etc.

- Relax and take deep breaths before beginning the exam.

- Be prepared and be positive.

Good Luck!

Contents

Skill Sheets

The following skill sheets are referenced within the chapters of this Workbook:

Skill Sheet 1 – Patient Assessment/ Management Medical (Courtesy National Registry of Emergency Medical Technicians: EMT Basic Practical Examination Users Guide, Colombus, Ohio 1995.), 90

Skill Sheet 2 – Patient Assessment/Management Trauma (Courtesy National Registry of Emergency Medical Technicians: EMT Basic Practical Examination Users Guide, Columbus, Ohio, 1995.), 91

Skill Sheet 3 – Bleeding Control/Shock Management (Courtesy National Registry of Emergency Medical Technicians: EMT Basic Practical Examination Users Guide, Columbus, Ohio, 1995.), 104

Skill Sheet 4 – Pneumatic Antishock Garment (PASG) (Developed from the DOT EMT-Basic National Standard Curriculum, 1994.), 105

Skill Sheet 5 – Airway, Oxygen, and Ventilation Skills Upper Airway Adjuncts and Suction (Courtesy National Registry of Emergency Medical Technicians: EMT Basic Practical Examination Users Guide, Columbus, Ohio, 1995.), 118

Skill Sheet 6 – Mouth to Mask with Supplemental Oxygen (Courtesy National Registry of Emergency Medical Technicians: EMT Basic Practical Examination Users Guide, Columbus, Ohio, 1995.), 119

Skill Sheet 7 – Bag-valve-mask Apneic Patient (Courtesy National Registry of Emergency Medical Technicians: EMT Basic Practical Examination Users Guide, Columbus, Ohio, 1995.), 120

Skill Sheet 8 – Oxygen Administration (Courtesy National Registry of Emergency Medical Technicians: EMT Basic Practical Examination Users Guide, Columbus, Ohio, 1995.), 121

Skill Sheet 9 – Relief of FBAO—Responsive Adult or Child Victim Standing or Sitting (Developed from the American Heart Association's Guidelines 2000 for Cardiopulmonary Resuscitation and Emergency Cardiovascular Care.), 122

Skill Sheet 10 – Relief of FBAO—Adult Victim Found Unresponsive (Developed from the American Heart Association's Guidelines 2000 for Cardiopulmonary Resuscitation and Emergency Cardiovascular Care.), 123

Skill Sheet 11 – Relief of FBAO—Adult Victim Who Becomes Unresponsive (Developed from the American Heart Association's Guidelines 2000 for Cardiopulmonary Resuscitation and Emergency Cardiovascular Care.), 124

Skill Sheet 12 – Relief of FBAO—Child Victim Found Unresponsive (Developed from the American Heart Association's Guidelines 2000 for Cardiopulmonary Resuscitation and Emergency Cardiovascular Care.), 125

Skill Sheet 13 – Relief of FBAO—Child Victim Who Becomes Unresponsive (Developed from the American Heart Association's Guidelines 2000 for Cardiopulmonary Resuscitation and Emergency Cardiovascular Care.), 126

Skill Sheet 14 – Relief of FBAO—Infant Victim Who Becomes Unresponsive (Developed from the American Heart Association's Guidelines 2000 for Cardiopulmonary Resuscitation and Emergency Cardiovascular Care.), 127

Skill Sheet 15 – Relief of FBAO—Infant Victim Found Unresponsive (Developed from the American Heart Association's Guidelines 2000 for Cardiopulmonary Resuscitation and Emergency Cardiovascular Care.), 128

Reading Assignment: Chapter 1 pages 3–19.

DOT Objectives

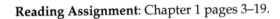

Upon successful completion of the EMT-Basic training program, the EMT-Basic should be able to do the following:

- Define Emergency Medical Services (EMS) System.
- Differentiate the roles and responsibilities of the EMT-Basic from those of other prehospital care providers.

Supplemental Objectives

- Define emergency medical care.
- Define the role that emergency medical services play in the public health community and the public safety community.
- Define emergency medical technician (EMT).
- Describe pertinent history, current events, and the future outlook for the EMT.
- Explain how emergency medical care relates to other components of the health care delivery system.
- Identify the role played by the United States Department of Transportation (DOT) in the training of the EMT.
- Identify common EMS system models.
- Describe the difference between an assessment-based approach to emergency care and a diagnosis-based approach.
- Explain the differing goals of initial and continuing education for the EMT.
- Identify the various components of EMT training.
- Identify the various certifying bodies for the EMT.
- Demonstrate a basic understanding of the types of health care that are available in the United States.
- Describe how changes in the health care system will affect the EMS system.
- Describe current challenges facing EMS systems.
- Identify current trends and likely future changes in EMS systems.

Key Terms

1. Match the following definitions with the appropriate type of care.

_E_ A form of health care insurance
_B_ Care provided for a persistent injury or disease with little change or slow progression
_F_ Care provided outside of the hospital
_A_ Short-term medical treatment for an injury or illness of rapid onset and short duration
_G_ Care provided to return a patient to normal form or function
_C_ Treatment provided to resolve a patient's illness or injury
_D_ Care provided to a patient outside of a licensed health care facility

A. Acute care
B. Chronic care
C. Definitive care
D. Home care
E. Managed care
F. Prehospital care
G. Restorative care

2. The traditional method of payment approach for health care is called _fee for service_

3. The type of response system that involves layers of care from basic and advanced emergency responders is called a(n) _tiered response ~~service~~ system_

4. Match the following definitions with the appropriate provider.

_C_ The most advanced level of prehospital provider
_D_ The emergency provider who usually arrives on the scene to provide basic life-saving skills until additional help arrives
_A_ An individual trained for approximately 110 hours in emergency care techniques
_B_ An individual trained in emergency procedures, IV therapy, and limited selection of medications

A. EMT-B
B. EMT-I
C. EMT-P
D. FR ?
   first responder

Content Review

1. List the four primary levels of emergency care providers throughout the United States, in order from the most basic to the most advanced.

1) _first responder_

2) _EMT-Basic_

3) _EMT-Intermediate_

4) _EMT-Paramedic_

2. What was the research paper that has been linked to the birth of the EMT called? ?

   Accidental Death and Disability: The Neglected Disease of Modern Society

3. The paper that was the foundation for setting standard minimum levels of training was published in _1966_.

4. The initial standardized EMT training program was introduced in _1969_.

5. The legislation passed by the federal government that specifically identified standardized training for prehospital personnel as an essential goal of the EMS system was called the _The Emergency Medical Services Systems Act_ and was passed in _1973_.

6. What organization has the overall responsibility for developing training programs?

   Department of Transportation + National Highway Traffic Safety Administration

7. States have adopted federal training for EMS personnel in order to received federal grant funds.
   - (A) True
   - B. False

8. Emergency care has been provided in the prehospital environment for hundreds of years.
   - (A) True
   - B. False

9. List the 10 standard components for evaluation of state EMS systems as identified by the National Highway Traffic and Safety Administration through the Technical Assistance Program.

   1) Regulation and policy
   2) Resource management
   3) Human Resources and training
   4) Transportation
   5) Facilities
   6) Communication
   7) Public information and education
   8) Medical direction
   9) Trauma systems
   10) Evaluation

10. Two nationally recognized levels of ALS providers are the _EMT-I_ and the _EMT-P_ _____.

11. List the six types of emergency service delivery models.

    1) Fire department
    2) Private ambulance
    3) Hospital - based Service
    4) Public Third Service
    5) Industrial
    6) Military

12. What are the three models for receiving funds to support EMS operations?

    1) Fee-for-service
    2) Subscription
    3) Subsidized

13. The current DOT EMT-Basic training course requires the student to participate in at least ___110___ hours of instruction.

14. What is the assessment-based approach to emergency medical care?

    a simple recognition of a patient's signs + symptoms to manage the problems or conditions a patient has

15. What are some methods for receiving continuing education?

    formal classrooms   case review sessions
    reading professional journal
    reviewing video tapes
    listening to audio tapes

16. A national certification for EMS personnel accepted by most states is offered by what organization?

    National Registry of EMTs

Chapter Quiz

1. The general term used to describe medical care that is provided to people who suddenly become seriously ill or injured is:
   A. Triage
   B. Definitive care
   C. Acute care services
   D. Emergency medical care

2. The process of determining the nature and extent of the patient's illness or injury is called:
   A. Stabilization
   B. Assessment
   C. Diagnosis
   D. Prognosis

3. At the national level, there are _____ levels of the EMT.
   A. 4
   B. 2
   C. 5
   D. 3

4. Responsibility for the development of training programs for prehospital providers is assigned to the:
   A. U.S. Department of Defense
   B. U.S. Department of Health Care
   C. U.S. Department of Transportation
   D. U.S. Department of Management and Finance

5. Legislation enacted in 1973 that set the stage for standardized training of prehospital personnel is called the:
   A. Emergency Medical Services Systems Act
   B. National Highway Traffic Safety Act
   C. Department of Transportation Act
   D. Medical Practice Act

6. A national, non-profit registration agency for prehospital providers that uses a written examination and a skills competency practical examination is the:
   A. National Academy of Health Sciences
   B. National Registry of Emergency Medical Technicians
   C. National Association of Emergency Medical Technicians
   D. American Medical Association

7. Financing or payment for EMS care is most often provided through:
   A. Insurance
   B. Fund Raisers
   C. Self-pay
   D. Subscription

8. The treatment provided to cure or solve the patient's current illness or injury is known as:
   A. Preventive care
   B. Postmortem care
   C. Definitive care
   D. Inpatient care

9. The acute care facility provides:
    A. Emergency and trauma care
    B. Critical intensive care
    C. Surgical intervention and diagnostic testing services
    D. All of the above

10. The type of care required when a patient continues to need health care intervention and does not improve is:
    A. Acute care
    B. Ambulatory care
    C. Preventative care
    D. Chronic care

11. Health care providers include:
    A. EMT-B
    B. EMT-P
    C. Physicians
    D. All of the above

12. EMTs provide:
    A. Initial assessment and stabilization
    B. Transport of the patient
    C. Physician-delegated activities
    D. All of the above

13. The turnover rate of prehospital personnel is _____ that of other industries.
    A. Equal to
    B. Higher than
    C. Lower than
    D. Not comparable to

14. To provide a quality, effective system of emergency medical care, which of the following must be in place?
    A. Laws
    B. Regulations
    C. Funding
    D. All of the above

15. Acute care is the medical treatment provided in response to a medical condition of sudden onset and short duration intended to stabilize the patient's condition prior to moving on to definitive care.
    A. True
    B. False

16. The EMS system model that involves layers of care is the:
    A. Dual response system
    B. Tiered response system
    C. Advanced support system
    D. Definitive care system

Case Scenario

• •

You are returning home from your first day of EMT class when you encounter the scene of a motor vehicle crash. You pull over to see if anyone needs assistance. You notice that there are two cars involved in the collision and that there are at least four patients involved: one person is trapped in the car. You ask if anyone called for help and someone had. You live in the area and know that the county has a "tiered response" system.

1. What personnel do you think will be sent to this scene?

2. Which of the 10 standard components of an EMS system will be used during the overall care of the patients involved in this emergency call (from initial incident through recovery)?

3. How would the care of the patients in this scenario differ in the year 2000 than that which they would have received in the early 1970s?

Answer Key

....

Key Terms
1. E, B, F, A, G, C, D
2. Fee-for-service
3. Tiered response system
4. C, D, A, B

Content Review
1. 1) First Responder; 2) EMT-Basic; 3) EMT-Intermediate; 4) EMT-Paramedic
2. Accidental Death and Disability: The Neglected Disease of Modern Society
3. 1966
4. 1969
5. EMS Systems Act (EMSS); 1973
6. DOT, National Highway Traffic Safety Administration (NHTSA)
7. True
8. True
9. 1) Regulation and policy; 2) resource management; 3) human resources and training; 4) transportation; 5) facilities; 6) communication; 7) public information and education; 8) medical direction; 9) trauma systems; 10) evaluation
10. EMT-Intermediate and EMT-Paramedic
11. 1) Fire department; 2) private ambulance; 3) hospital-based; 4) public third service; 5) individual; 6) military
12. 1) Fee-for-service; 2) subscription; 3) subsidized
13. 110 hours
14. The EMT is taught to quickly recognize important signs and symptoms and rapidly respond with appropriate emergency medical care rather than attempting to match signs and symptoms to arrive at a diagnosis
15. Attending formal classes; reading professional journals; reviewing videotapes; listening to audiotapes; attending case review sessions
16. National Registry of EMTs (NREMT)

Chapter Quiz

1. D	5. A	9. D	13. B
2. B	6. B	10. D	14. D
3. D	7. A	11. D	15. A
4. C	8. C	12. D	16. B

Case Scenario

1. Basic life support personnel including first responders and EMT-Basics or EMT-Intermediates, along with ALS personnel (EMT-Paramedic) to assist with the more critical patients. They may also send a rescue unit and law enforcement, if they are not already at the scene.

2. Resource management, human resources and training, transportation, facilities, communications, medical direction, and trauma systems.

3. Treatment is much more advanced with tiered response, faster response times, specialized rescue and advanced life support units using advanced emergency techniques. In the 1970s, emergency care was limited to transport by a funeral home director in the back of a hearse.

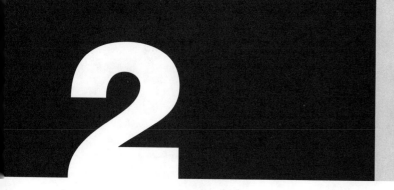

Reading Assignment: Chapter 2 pages 20–30.

DOT Objectives

Upon successful completion of the EMT-Basic training program, the EMT-Basic should be able to do the following:

- Define emergency medical services (EMS) systems.
- Differentiate among the roles and responsibilities of the emergency medical technician-basic (EMT-B) from other prehospital care providers.
- Describe the roles and responsibilities related to personal safety.
- Discuss the roles and responsibilities of the EMT-B toward the safety of the crew, patient, and bystanders.
- Define quality improvement and discuss the EMT-B's role in the process.

Supplemental Objectives

- Explain the various methods used to access the EMS system in differing communities.

Key Terms

1. The term that means a governing body has granted permission for an individual to perform certain tasks is _____.

2. The term that means that an agency or association attests to the accomplishments of a set of requirements by an individual is _____.

3. The network of services that provides emergency care to a community is called the _____ system.

4. The ongoing process of gathering information to improve the EMS system in order to deliver the highest level of service possible is called _____.

5. A formal plan with neighboring areas to ensure that help will be available when existing resources are overwhelmed is called a(n) _____.

Content Review

1. Identify three ways in which someone can access the EMS System.

   1)

   2)

   3)

2. The spoken word is referred to as _____ communication and actions of the EMT are _____ _____ communication.

3. Why is personal communication between the EMT and the patient important?

4. Identify characteristics that are important for the EMT to possess in order to ensure personal safety at the scene of an emergency.

5. Define patient assessment.

6. List five methods through which an EMT can obtain information during a patient assessment.

   1)

   2)

   3)

   4)

   5)

7. List 11 primary functions/responsibilities of the EMT.

    1)

    2)

    3)

    4)

    5)

    6)

    7)

    8)

    9)

    10)

    11)

8. Safely and efficiently delivering a patient to an appropriate destination is a major portion of the EMT's responsibility.
   A. True
   B. False

9. Identify three factors the EMT should consider when determining the most appropriate medical facility to transport a patient to.

    1)

    2)

    3)

10. Define patient advocacy.

11. List some of the professional attributes that an EMT should possess.

12. Moral standards that govern the conduct of a group of people are called _____.

13. Confidentiality means that information may not be released to a third party without a patient's consent.
    A. True
    B. False

14. Delivering a verbal or written report of patient's condition to a nurse at the receiving facility who will provide patient care, is not considered a third party release of information.
    A. True
    B. False

15. List three documents that provide the guiding principles for professional EMT services.

    1)

    2)

    3)

16. What is the goal of continuing education?

17. Identify some professional organizations available for EMTs.

18. What organization offers standardized testing and certification for EMTs and EMT-Paramedics?

Chapter Quiz

1. An EMT-B is an individual who possesses the knowledge to provide advanced life support care for the ill and injured.
   A. True
   B. False

2. The critical, first link in the chain of emergency care is the initiation of care by the:
   A. Emergency physician
   B. Allied health professional
   C. Informed and trained public
   D. State legislature

3. The EMT and all crew members must be prepared to perform their job at all times. Being prepared includes which of the following?
   A. Emotional and physical fitness
   B. Having an excellent working knowledge of all equipment and its location on the emergency vehicle
   C. Understanding of policies and procedures that define the EMS system
   D. All of the above

4. The EMT course teaches students to:
   A. Recognize life-threatening conditions
   B. Evaluate the status of the patient
   C. Provide appropriate treatment in a timely fashion
   D. All of the above

5. Prompt and effective treatment of a patient may include which of the following?
   A. Airway control
   B. Control of bleeding and traumatic injury management
   C. Cardiopulmonary resuscitation
   D. All of the above

6. An evaluation of the patient's illness or injury, as well as the location and availability of hospital resources, will assist the EMT in the selection of the:
   A. Most appropriate medical facility
   B. Most appropriate attending physician
   C. Need to take the patient to a prospective rehabilitation center
   D. Need for completing a prehospital care report

7. The EMT must represent the patient and act in the patient's best interest until that responsibility can be passed on to another provider in the health care system. In doing so, the EMT is functioning as a(n)
   A. Patient consultant
   B. Patient advocate
   C. Patient mentor
   D. Patient facilitator

8. The EMT's responsibilities include all of the following *except*:
   A. Ensuring that their uniform displays a professional image
   B. Maintaining licensure in other medical professions
   C. Demonstrating concern for personal safety
   D. Maintaining good physical and emotional stability

9. Providing a verbal and/or written report to a person who will be providing direct patient care is considered a:
   A. Third party release
   B. Component of patient assessment
   C. Transfer of care
   D. Continuum of patient confidentiality

10. The EMT should be familiar with certain documents concerning ethics and confidentiality. They include:
    A. The EMT Oath
    B. The NAEMT Code of Ethics
    C. The Oath of Geneva
    D. All of the above

11. The process by which a governmental body grants permission for the EMT to perform certain acts is known as:
    A. Licensure
    B. Certification
    C. Standards of care
    D. Principles of care

12. The process by which an agency or association grants a document that attests to the accomplishment of a set of requirements is known as:
    A. Standards of care
    B. Certification
    C. Licensure
    D. Reciprocity

13. Several national and state organizations are available for EMTs. The common goal of these organizations is to:
    A. Promote professionalism within the EMS service
    B. Write national consensus EMS standards
    C. Promote the professional status of ED personnel
    D. Increase revenue for national nonprofit organizations in the EMS system

14. Safely and efficiently delivering a patient to the hospital is a component of emergency treatment.
    A. True
    B. False

Case Scenario

You are at a "stand by" at a local charity event with your partner when you feel a tug on your pant leg. You look down to find a 4-year-old girl with sad eyes looking up at you. She says "I can't find my teddy."

1. What should you do? Why?

You find the child's teddy nearby and return her, and teddy, to her parents. You then notice a man staggering toward you. The man appears incoherent and, as you approach him, he begins swinging his arms and yelling "get away from me man" in an angry voice.

2. What should you do?

3. What should be the number one priority of an EMT when providing emergency care?

Answer Key

Key Terms
1. Licensure
2. Certification
3. Emergency Medical Services (EMS) system
4. Quality assurance
5. Mutual aid agreement

Content Review
1. 1) A special 7 digit phone number; 2) 911; 3) 911-enhanced
2. Verbal; non-verbal
3. Actions of the EMT are often the first communication between the patient and the EMT; if the patient perceives the EMT to be nervous, anxious, or excited, it may decrease the level of confidence he has in the EMT; if the EMT's actions are alarming to the patient, it may increase a patient's anxiety and worsen the patient's condition; patient's who are anxious are more challenging to treat.
4. Adequate sleep; confidence about skills; physical fitness; understanding of policies and procedures; knowledge of how to use all equipment on the ambulance.
5. The systematic collection of information about the patient.
6. 1) Observation; 2) physical assessment; 3) examination; 4) response to intervention; 5) an interview
7. 1) Preparedness; 2) response; 3) safety; 4) patient assessment; 5) prompt and efficient patient care; 6) lifting and moving patients; 7) safe and efficient transport; 8) transfer of a patient to a medical facility;

9) record keeping/data collection; 10) patient advocacy; 11) other related functions (restocking the ambulance, extrication, pub-ed, etc.)

8. True
9. 1) Evaluation of the extent of illness or injury the patient is experiencing; 2) the location and availability of hospital resources; 3) the need for a specialty hospital (trauma center, burn center, etc.)
10. Patient advocacy means the EMT must represent the patient and act in the patient's best interest until that responsibility can be passed on to another provider in the health care system.
11. Leadership; skills; compassion; honesty; physical fitness; emotional stability; clean and orderly attire
12. Ethics
13. True
14. True
15. 1) Oath of Geneva; 2) EMT Oath; 3) The EMT Code of Ethics
16. To increase and refresh the medical knowledge that an emergency care provider has.
17. National Association of EMTs; National Association of Search and Rescue; National Association of State EMS Directors; National Association of EMS Physicians; National Flight Paramedics Association; National Association of EMS Educators; American Academy of Medical Administrators; National Registry of EMTs
18. National Registry of EMTs (NREMT)

Chapter Quiz

1. B	6. A	11. A
2. C	7. B	12. B
3. D	8. B	13. A
4. D	9. C	14. A
5. D	10. D	

Case Scenario

1. Help the child look for her teddy while maintaining contact with your partner via a portable radio in case an emergency arises. Your role as an EMT involves more than just emergency care. You must also promote a positive and professional image to the community.
2. Move a safe distance away from the man, try to establish communication with the patient to determine what might be wrong, and request police assistance in the event the patient becomes violent.
3. Personal safety

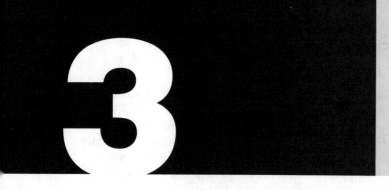

Medical/Legal Principles

Reading Assignment: Chapter 3 pages 31–41.

DOT Objectives

Upon successful completion of the EMT-Basic training program, the EMT-Basic should be able to do the following:

- Describe how an emergency medical technician (EMT) allows refusal of medical care and the interactions that must occur between the medical control physician and the EMT.
- Compare the functions of an EMT with those of a law enforcement officer at a crime scene.
- Define the EMT-Basic scope of practice.
- Define consent and discuss the methods of obtaining consent.
- Differentiate between expressed and implied consent.
- Explain the role of consent of minors in providing care.
- Discuss the implications for the EMT-Basic in patient refusal of transport.
- Discuss the issues of abandonment, negligence, assault and battery and their implications to the EMT-Basic.
- State the conditions necessary for the EMT-Basic to have a duty to act.
- Explain the importance, necessity, and legality of patient confidentiality.
- Discuss the considerations of the EMT-Basic in issues of organ retrieval.
- Differentiate the actions that an EMT-Basic should take to assist in the preservation of a crime scene.
- State the conditions that require an EMT-Basic to notify local law enforcement officials.

Supplemental Objectives

- Describe the rights of patients who make decisions regarding their medical care.
- Describe when a patient may not refuse medical care.
- Be able to correctly document the forensic aspects of a scene.

Key Terms

1. Failure to continue to care for a patient once care has been initiated is called _____.

2. A(n) _____ minor is one who has the legal right to consent to or refuse treatment regardless of his age.

3. A patient under the age of 18 years of age is called a(n) _____.

4. A patient is legally allowed to decline treatment based on an informed consent. This is called a(n) _____.

Content Review

1. Complete the following statement. If it is not written down, _____.

2. Before the EMT can provide care, he must obtain _____ from the patient.

3. A patient implies consent when he acts in a manner that suggests he accepts the treatment offered.
   A. True
   B. False

4. The _____ grants an exception regarding general rules of consent and allows the EMT to provide medical care to a patient in an emergent situation if the patient lacks the ability to understand the situation.

5. Identify five situations in which emergency consent would take effect.

   1)

   2)

   3)

   4)

   5)

6. What two steps must the EMT take before an individual can refuse medical care?

   1)

   2)

7. A minor has the same right to refuse care as an adult.
   A. True
   B. False

8. A parent can refuse treatment for their minor children regardless of the consequences of such refusal.
   A. True
   B. False

9. What should an EMT do if a parent is acting in a manner that jeopardizes the health of their child?

10. What is the "mature minor doctrine"?

11. Identify at least three situations that automatically provide a minor emancipation?

    1)

    2)

    3)

12. What four factors must exist for a patient to refuse prehospital medical treatment?

    1)

    2)

    3)

    4)

13. What four steps should the EMT take when the decision is made to treat a patient without consent?

    1)

    2)

    3)

    4)

14. When does a power of attorney come into play regarding health care matters?

15. Power of attorney overrides a patient's ability to make decisions, regardless of competency.
    A. True
    B. False

16. When responding to a crime scene, assuming the scene is safe, the EMT's primary responsibility is
    _____.

17. What steps should the EMT take when providing care at a crime scene?

Chapter Quiz

1. The EMT has legal responsibility to the:
   A. Patient
   B. Medical director
   C. Public
   D. All of the above

2. Providing emergency care when the patient does *not* consent to the treatment can result in charges against the EMT for:
   A. Assault
   B. Battery
   C. Liability for abuse
   D. All of the above

3. If the EMT touches a person without his or her consent, even if the EMT justifiably believes that the action is necessary to save the patient's life, he or she may be charged with:
   A. Battery
   B. Libel
   C. Slander
   D. Assault

4. To refuse care, the patient must be:
   A. Of legal age
   B. Mentally competent
   C. Conscious
   D. All of the above

5. The authority to restrain and transport patients against their will *generally* rests only with:
   A. A probate judge
   B. A police officer
   C. A spouse and/or significant other
   D. The EMS system Medical Director

6. Permission to treat minor children, even against the child's wishes, is *usually* granted under the jurisdiction of the:
   A. Child
   B. Parents or legal guardian
   C. Law enforcement officer
   D. Family court

7. Expressed consent means that:
   A. A patient can voluntarily express consent to be treated only if he or she is at least 18 years of age
   B. The patient must be informed via written documentation of the procedures and treatments to be administered
   C. The unconscious patient is requesting emergency care
   D. The consent must be informed

8. In which of the following situations would implied consent be applicable?
   A. A patient who is unconscious and bleeding profusely
   B. A patient who is describing his accident to bystanders
   C. A patient who nods in the affirmative when asked if he needs medical help
   D. A 14-year-old pregnant patient exhibiting extreme anxiety

9. Emancipated minors include those minors who are:
   A. Over the age of 16 years
   B. Freed from parental control
   C. Maintained and supported by only one parent
   D. Orphaned

10. All of the following statements are examples of abandonment *except*:
    A. The EMT initiates care and then leaves the patient
    B. The patient is left unattended for a brief period of time and his condition worsens
    C. The EMT fails to transfer information to the receiving facility regarding the patient
    D. The EMT responds to and completes an ambulance call

11. Duty to act:
    A. Implies a contractual or legal obligation to provide patient care
    B. Is formal, such as an ambulance service contracting to provide emergency care to the citizens of the community
    C. Is implied such as an EMT initiating treatment of the patient
    D. All of the above

12. A breach of duty can be shown by all of the following *except*:
    A. Offering evidence that the EMT did not conform to the standard of care by rendering inappropriate care
    B. Offering evidence that the EMT failed to act at all
    C. Offering evidence that the EMT acted beyond the scope of practice
    D. Offering evidence that the EMT acted as a reasonable EMT would in the same or similar circumstance

13. Which of the following statements regarding patient confidentiality is *true*?
    A. Confidentiality of patient information is only required when the patient requests such.
    B. Confidential information may include any history elicited through interview of the patient or their family.
    C. Assessment findings and treatment rendered are not confidential patient information.
    D. Medical information regarding a minor does not require a release.

14. The EMT's responsibilities at a crime scene include all of the following *except*:
    A. Providing emergency care of the patient only after ensuring that the crime scene is not disturbed
    B. Avoiding the disturbance of any item at the scene unless patient care requires it
    C. Observing and documenting anything unusual at the scene
    D. Avoiding cutting through holes in clothing that may be the result of gunshot wounds or stabbings

15. Common special situations which require the EMT to report to appropriate authorities include all of the following *except*:
    A. Abuse of children and the elderly
    B. Victims of domestic violence
    C. Crimes such as sexual assault
    D. Overdose by drug addicts

16. Which of the following elements must be proven in a successful negligence suit?
    A. A duty to act and a breach of the duty occurred
    B. A duty to act without a breach
    C. The patient experienced no injury but there was proximate cause
    D. The EMT breached the duty to act, but no injury occurred

Case Scenario

You receive an emergency call for a "possible cardiac arrest." En route, you witness a motor vehicle crash involving three cars.

1. What should you do?

2. What is the harm in stopping at the scene?

You arrive at the scene and are met by a woman who is hysterical, screaming that her son is in his room and is not moving. You enter his room and see a shotgun on the floor and a significant amount of blood on the floor. The scene appears safe.

3. What should you do?

You determine the patient has no pulse or ventilations. His pupils are dilated and skin is cold. There is a small wound on his forehead and a large exit wound in the back of his head. The wounds are not compatible with life, so you decide not to begin CPR.

4. What should you do?

5. What should you document for this call?

Answer Key

··

Key Terms
1. Abandonment
2. Emancipated
3. Minor
4. Refusal of care

Content Review
1. It did not happen
2. Consent
3. True
4. Emergency consent doctrine
5. 1) Unconsciousness/altered level of consciousness; 2) severe intoxication; 3) head injury; 4) psychological illness; 5) drug use
6. 1) Inform the patient of his or her condition, the treatment required, and the consequences of refusing treatment; 2) determine whether the patient has the mental capacity to understand his or her medical problem and the consequences of refusing treatment.
7. False
8. False
9. Call for consult with medical direction and support from law enforcement personnel
10. It allows minors to consent to medical care, providing he or she has the capacity to understand
11. Marriage; military service; pregnancy (in some states); or a court ruling
12. 1) The patient appears awake, alert, and oriented; 2) the patient is capable of understanding the nature and severity of the medical condition or injury; 3) the patient does not pose a suicidal risk; 4) the patient does not appear under the influence of intoxicants or has not suffered a medical problem or injury that affects his or her ability to understand the condition or injury
13. 1) Attempt to discuss the situation again with the patient and if he or she appears competent, obtain consent for treatment and transport; 2) explain to the patient the reasons he or she will receive treatment and the risks of not providing treatment; 3) ask medical control to attempt to locate the patient's closest relatives and inform them of the decision to treat, and transport despite the patient's refusal; 4) document the entire encounter for the record
14. When an ill patient loses mental competency and cannot understand information regarding the disease, injury, or illness that is affecting his or her ability to make informed decisions regarding medical treatment
15. False
16. Patient care
17. Do not disturb the scene unless necessary to render emergency care; if anything is moved, mentally note the initial location of potential evidence; document anything the EMT disturbs at the scene, as well as all pertinent information regarding the environment and type and location of potential evidence in an objective manner without personal opinions about the nature of the evidence.

Chapter Quiz

1. D	5. B	9. B	13. B
2. D	6. B	10. D	14. A
3. A	7. D	11. D	15. D
4. D	8. A	12. D	16. A

Case Scenario

1. Continue to your original call and inform dispatch of the crash and your observations of the scene so that they can send appropriate assistance.
2. You would be negligent in regard to the cardiac arrest call. Once dispatched to the initial call, you have a duty to act. By stopping at the scene, you would have breached that duty and, if the patient at the initial call then dies, you could be held liable.
3. 1) Call for law enforcement; 2) assess the patient to determine if he is in cardiac arrest; and 3) preserve the crime scene.
4. Do not start CPR, but rather follow local protocols (i.e., call the coroner, medical director, etc.)
5. Document how the scene looked on your arrival, anything the mother said to you, any items you may have moved, anything you noticed, or any actions you took at the scene. Note factual information only—do not speculate.

EMS Medical Director

Reading Assignment: Chapter 4 pages 45–52.

Supplemental Objectives

Upon successful completion of the EMT-Basic training program, the EMT-Basic should be able to do the following:

- Describe the roles and responsibilities of the emergency medical services (EMS) medical director.
- Identify three approaches to EMS medical direction.
- List the components of prospective medical direction.
- Identify the components of immediate medical direction.
- List the components of retrospective medical direction.
- Explain the importance of the relationship between the EMT and the medical director.
- Define the difference between protocols and standing orders.

Key Terms

1. Match the following definitions with the proper direction.

   _____ Another term for indirect medical direction
   _____ Activities the medical director provides while an emergency is taking place
   _____ Another term for on-line medical direction
   _____ A range of activities a medical director may be involved with before an emergency occurs
   _____ Clinical type of medical direction involving real-time direction of providers in the delivery of emergency care
   _____ Activities conducted by the physician after an emergency call is complete

   A. Direct medical direction
   B. Immediate medical control
   C. Off-line medical direction
   D. On-line medical direction
   E. Prospective medical direction
   F. Retrospective medical direction

2. The physician who oversees an EMS system is called a(n) _____.

3. Specially trained individuals trained to act as a physician's eyes, ears, and hands in the prehospital evaluation and management of an emergency patient are called _____.

4. Written instructions describing the step-by-step method to be used when dealing with a set of symptoms or conditions are called _____.

5. Written patient care instructions that authorize the EMT to take specific steps in patient assessment and care without the need for direct medical control are called _____.

Content Review

1. The delivery of health care in every state in the United States is governed in part by what law?

2. Describe the background that a physician providing medical direction should possess.

3. List the activities included in the administrative function of the medical director.

4. The administrative function of the medical director is known as _____ or _____.

5. List the activities included in the clinical aspect of the medical director's role.

6. Clinical medical direction is also known as _____ or _____ medical direction.

7. List the three components of medical direction.

    1)

    2)

    3)

8. The type of medical direction with which a medical director may be involved that takes place *before* an emergency occurs is called _____ medical direction.

9. List some of the activities the medical director may be involved with during prospective medical direction.

10. What is the purpose of protocols?

11. What are the goals of the approval process for protocols?

12. Identify the difference between protocols and standing orders?

13. What should the EMT do if a problem arises or he has a question about treatment for a patient?

14. All states require that the objectives set forth in the National Standard Curriculum, as developed by the U.S. DOT, be the minimal educational requirements for EMT-B training.
    A. True
    B. False

15. What is immediate medical direction?

16. The type of medical direction that is provided by a physician via radio or phone about patient care strategies is called _____ or _____ medical control.

17. EMTs function mostly under standing orders and only contact the physician for direct medical decision making, for an unusual occurrence, or to report a patient is being transported to the hospital.
    A. True
    B. False

18. Activities conducted by the physician *after* a call is complete is called _____ medical direction.

19. Another term for retrospective medical direction is _____.

20. An individual case review focuses on what five questions?

    1)

    2)

    3)

    4)

    5)

21. Identify the activities of a medical director that are included in retrospective medical direction.

Chapter Quiz

1. Prehospital emergency care providers are authorized to deliver health care through state laws or regulations.
   A. True
   B. False

2. All prehospital care providers, from First Responders to EMT-Paramedics function under the direct supervision of a medical director.
   A. True
   B. False

3. The three approaches to medical direction discussed in this chapter include all of the following *except*:
   A. Prospective medical direction
   B. Immediate medical direction
   C. Retrospective medical direction
   D. Proactive medical direction

4. The EMT-B National Standard Curriculum strongly recommends that even the most basic EMS service have a medical director.
   A. True
   B. False

5. _____ describe the entire evaluation and treatment process for a particular presenting symptom or chief complaint.
   A. Standing orders
   B. Protocols
   C. Guidelines
   D. Recommendations

6. Medical direction of EMS systems is standardized in all states.
   A. True
   B. False

7. Prospective medical direction includes the range of activities that a medical director may be involved with that occur _____ the time that the emergency occurs.
   A. Before
   B. After
   C. During
   D. Near

8. Immediate medical direction includes the range of activities that a medical director provides:
   A. While the emergency is actually taking place
   B. Before the emergency actually takes place
   C. After the emergency takes place
   D. Immediately after an emergency takes place

9. _____ describes the activities conducted by the physician after the call is complete.
   A. Prospective medical direction
   B. Immediate medical direction
   C. Retrospective medical direction
   D. Proactive medical direction

10. The EMS medical director must be involved in two different types of activities to accomplish the three approaches to medical direction. The first type of activities are administrative in nature and are known as:
    A. Off-line medical direction
    B. Indirect medical direction
    C. Direct medical direction
    D. A and B

11. Off-line medical direction includes activities such as:
    A. Writing protocols
    B. Reviewing EMT performance
    C. Administrative duties
    D. All of the above

12. On-line medical direction activities may include:
    A. Providing radio or telephone instructions to prehospital providers
    B. Direct observation of system and individual performance
    C. Responding to the scene and providing prehospital patient care (in some systems)
    D. All of the above

13. The physician who provides medical direction for an EMS system should possess all of the following characteristics *except*:
    A. Familiarity with the design and operation of prehospital EMS systems
    B. A state license as an EMT-Paramedic that certifies that the physician has completed an advanced level EMS course
    C. Experience in prehospital emergency care of the acutely ill or injured patient
    D. Knowledge of base-station radio control of prehospital emergency units

14. The prospective phase of EMS medical direction begins when:
    A. A community first makes the decision to provide EMS service
    B. A community identifies the type of EMS vehicles they want to purchase
    C. A community spells out the resources and limitations for system design
    D. All of the above

15. Protocol approval may come from a:
    A. State government agency
    B. Local government agency
    C. State medical organization
    D. All of the above

16. The goal of the protocol approval process is to ensure that:
    A. The medical community agrees with the proposed level of prehospital care
    B. The proposed level of care and protocols accurately reflect the standard of care in the community
    C. Community-wide medical personnel support the prehospital system
    D. All of the above

17. A list of basic equipment and supplies for an ambulance that identifies standard equipment necessary to provide adequate patient care at the basic, intermediate, and advanced levels has been identified by the:
    A. American Academy of Pediatric Surgeons
    B. American College of Family Practitioners
    C. American College of Surgeons/Committee on Trauma
    D. American College of Orthopedic Physicians

18. A list of basic equipment and supplies for an ambulance that identifies standard equipment necessary to provide adequate patient care has been identified by the:
    A. American Academy of Pediatric Surgeons
    B. American College of Family Practitioners/Committee on Emergencies
    C. American College of Surgeons/Committee on Trauma
    D. American College of Orthopedic Physicians

19. Retrospective medical direction is also known as:
    A. Quality assurance
    B. Prospective analysis
    C. Retrospective direction
    D. Retrospective critique

20. The EMS medical director should be involved in the routine review of the emergency medical calls handled by the EMS system. The purpose of this review is:
    A. To identify system-wide issues such as response time or skill problems that affect the system
    B. To identify individual providers who may have specific educational needs
    C. To compare the patient care report prepared by the EMT, as well as hospital records for the patient, if available, to determine the appropriateness of care given and areas in need of improvement
    D. All of the above

Case Scenario

● ●

You are on the scene of an industrial accident where the patient's hand was caught in a piece of machinery. The patient's arm is still in the machine and the patient is conscious, screaming, and in a significant amount of pain. You are uncertain of the proper steps to take. You contact the medical director via telephone and ask how to proceed.

1. What type of medical direction is this?

In the meantime, the patient begins to become less coherent. Although ALS and rescue personnel are on their way, you believe that the patient is beginning to show signs of shock. You ensure that power to the machine is turned off and attempt to free the patient. You begin to panic when you cannot free the patient. Your partner suggests that the machine be dismantled enough to take that part of the machine with the patient to the hospital.

You manage to dismantle part of the machine and transport the patient to the hospital with part of it still attached. En route, the patient loses consciousness. You decide to intubate the patient.

2. What are the different methods by which you may have been authorized to perform this procedure.

3. Later that month, the physician meets with you to discuss your actions at this call. You worry that he will take your license. Within which component of the EMS system would this action fall?

4. Under what component of medical direction does case reviews fall?

5. The medical director decides that your actions were not negligent, but that you may need additional training in some aspects of patient care. He sets out a schedule of weekly training sessions for you to complete. What is this type of training called?

Answer Key

● ●

Key Terms
1. C, B, A, E, D, F
2. Medical director
3. Physician extenders
4. Protocols
5. Standing orders

Content Review

1. Medical practice act
2. Familiarity with the design and operation of prehospital EMS systems; experience in prehospital emergency care of the acutely ill or injured patient; routine participation in base-station radio direction of prehospital emergency units; experience in emergency department management of acutely ill or injured patient; routine active participation in emergency department management of acutely ill or injured patients; active involvement in the training of basic and advanced life-support prehospital personnel; active involvement in the medical audit, review, and critique of basic and advanced life-support prehospital personnel; participation in the administrative and legislative process affecting the regional and/or state prehospital EMS system; active involvement in field patient care
3. Writing protocols and reviewing EMT performance
4. Off-line medical direction or indirect medical control
5. Providing radio or telephone instructions to prehospital providers; direct observation of the system; individual performance by responding to the scene; teaching in primary and ongoing EMS education; providing prehospital patient care
6. On-line or direct medical direction
7. 1) Prospective medical direction; 2) immediate medical direction; 3) retrospective medical direction
8. Prospective
9. Training of providers; identifying equipment to be used to treat patients; assisting with the selection of personnel; developing protocols used for patient care, ambulance dispatch, and ambulance placement strategy
10. They provide overall steps in patient care management to be undertaken by the EMT at every patient contact. They address each step of prehospital care to be provided for the medical conditions most likely to be encountered in the EMS system. They are the tools used by the medical director to clearly spell out how each patient should be evaluated and treated.
11. To ensure that the medical community agrees with the proposed level of prehospital care, the proposed level of care and protocols accurately reflect the standard of care in the community, and that the protocols provide community-wide medical support for the prehospital system.
12. Protocols describe the big picture and total treatment. Standing orders refer to a mechanism more limited range of actions (assessments and treatments) that the EMT can perform before contacting a physician.
13. Contact medical control for help.
14. True
15. The activities a medical director and designees provide while an emergency is taking place.
16. Direct or on-line
17. True
18. Retrospective
19. Quality assurance
20. 1) Was the prehospital field diagnosis the same as the emergency department diagnosis? 2) Was anything done in the field that should not have been done? 3) Was anything not done in the field that should have been done? 4) Was there an inappropriate delay in transporting the patient to the hospital? 5) Was the patient transported to the appropriate hospitals?
21. Case review; EMT counseling; education; and system review and revision

Chapter Quiz

1. A	6. B	11. D	16. D
2. B	7. A	12. D	17. C
3. D	8. A	13. B	18. C
4. A	9. C	14. D	19. A
5. B	10. D	15. D	20. D

Case Scenario
1. Direct or on-line medical direction
2. Protocols or standing orders, or from on-line medical direction by speaking directly with the physician
3. Quality review or continuous quality improvement
4. Retrospective medical direction
5. Continuing education

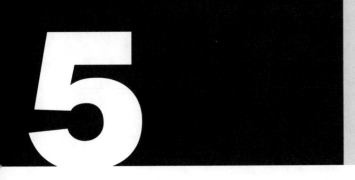

Well-Being of the EMT

Reading Assignment: Chapter 5 pages 53–73.

DOT Objectives

Upon successful completion of the EMT-Basic training program, the EMT-Basic should be able to do the following:

- Explain the importance of surveying the scene and determining scene safety.
- Discuss the importance of body substance isolation (BSI).
- List personal protective equipment and considerations necessary for special situations, including:
  —hazardous materials
  —crime scenes
  —rescue operations
  —violent scenes
- Discuss the possible reactions that the patient and family may exhibit when confronted with death and dying.
- List the steps that the emergency medical technician-basic (EMT-B) will take to approach a family confronted with death and dying.
- List the possible reactions that the EMT-B may experience when faced with trauma, illness, death, and dying.
- List the possible reactions that the family of the EMT-B may exhibit because of their indirect involvement with EMS.
- Recognize the signs and symptoms of critical incident stress, and discuss the benefits of debriefing.
- List the steps that the EMT-B should take to prevent, reduce, and alleviate stress.

Key Terms

1. The term for taking steps to prevent the spread of communicable diseases while handling material excreted from the body is _____.

2. Chemical substances that are toxic to humans are referred to as _____.

3. An internal response to an external factor such as work, family, or lifestyle changes, is called _____.

4. Strains and pressures caused by the stress a person places on himself from factors such as expectations, anxiety, and guilt are called _____ stressors.

5. An event or circumstance that overwhelms one or more person is a(n) _____ _____.

6. Stressors that are initiated by contact with other people are called _____ stressors.

Content Review

1. What scenes might an EMT-B be faced with that pose a threat to personal safety?

2. A violent scene should always be controlled by law enforcement personnel before the EMT-B provides patient care.
   A. True
   B. False

3. What should the EMT-B do if he or she is unsure if the perpetrator of a crime is still on the scene?

4. What should the EMT-B do if a scene becomes violent while providing patient care?

5. What clues should the EMT-B look for while assessing a scene or patient that may alert him or her to a violent or potentially violent scene?

6. Weather conditions, noise levels, and shift work are all examples of _____ _____ stressors.

7. Prior to entering a HazMat scene, specially trained personnel will don specialized protective equipment including:

8. What is the EMT's primary responsibility at a rescue scene?

9. What potential threats may exist at a rescue scene?

10. What protective clothing should an EMT-B wear at a rescue scene?

11. What should the EMT-B do if he or she is uncomfortable riding with a violent patient to the hospital?

12. The EMT-B has additional responsibilities at a crime scene. What are they?

13. What is the EMT-B's primary responsibility at a crime scene?

14. List the five stages of death and dying as identified by Dr. Elizabeth Kübler-Ross.

    1)

    2)

    3)

    4)

    5)

15. If multiple family members are injured in an accident and one dies, how should the EMT-B handle the scene? Why?

16. Match the following stages of death and dying with the appropriate description.

    _____ "Why me?"   A. Denial
    _____ "OK, I'm not afraid."   B. Anger
    _____ "Not me!"   C. Bargaining
    _____ "OK, but first let me ....." D. Depression
    _____ "OK, but I haven't ...."   E. Acceptance

17. An EMT-B is caring for a patient with mortal wounds. A loved one looks on screaming hysterically. What should the EMT-B do? Why?

18. An EMT-B is on the scene caring for a critical patient when a loved one arrives. What should the EMT-B do?

19. What are some of the physiological responses that the EMT-B may experience in response to a stressor?

20. The physiological response one experiences when faced with a sudden stressor is referred to as _____ or _____.

21. The physiological reaction that occurs en route to an emergency scene is a normal response.
    A. True
    B. False

22. What steps should the EMT-B take to prepare him- or herself en-route to an emergency call for help?

23. List some of the signs and symptoms an EMT-B may experience while responding to, or on the scene of, an emergency.

24. An EMT-B is on the scene of a murder/suicide. He feels very shaky and upset, and looks physically ill. What should he do?

25. The EMT-B should separate work from family, since it is very difficult for "outsiders" to understand EMS response.
    A. True
    B. False

26. If an EMT-B is feeling overwhelmed between work and personal and family life, what adjustments should he or she consider?

27. Positive or beneficial stress is called eustress.
    A. True
    B. False

28. Stress that gets out of control or has negative aspects is referred to as _____.

29. What are the three main categories or causes of stress?

    1)

    2)

    3)

30. Identify some environmental stressors.

31. Identify some personal stressors.

32. Identify some psychosocial stressors.

33. Stress that occurs over time, due to frequent ongoing stressors, is called _____ or _____ stress.

34. List some circumstances that may cause an EMT-B to experience an acute stressful reaction.

35. Define critical incident.

36. A critical incident might affect only one EMT-B or it might affect everyone at the scene.
    A. True
    B. False

37. Identify the serious condition involving illness, personality changes, and self-destructive behavior that can be caused by the suppression of emotions and thoughts after a traumatic event.

38. List the characteristics of PTSD.

39. What are the four categories of noting distress in an EMT-B?

    1)

    2)

    3)

    4)

40. List some of the *physical* signs of distress that require immediate corrective action.

41. List some of the *cognitive* signals of distress that require immediate corrective action.

42. List some of the *emotional* signals of distress that require immediate corrective action.

43. List some of the *behavioral* signals of distress that require immediate corrective action.

44. The build-up of distress until an individual is no longer productive is called _____.

45. When should defusings and debriefings be used?

46. When should a formal critical incident stress debriefing be conducted?

47. Who comprises a CISD team?

48. What criteria should lead one to consider holding a critical incident stress debriefing?

49. What is the purpose of CISD?

50. What dietary guidelines should the EMT-B follow to increase performance, stamina, and the ability to manage stress?

Chapter Quiz

....

1. EMTs face a greater chance of being injured or killed at work than do members of many other professions.
   A. True
   B. False

2. Distress is always caused by a significant event such as a major call, disaster, or multiple deaths.
   A. True
   B. False

3. All of the following steps are part of the scene survey *except*:
   A. Assess the scene for hazards
   B. Note the number of patients
   C. Note the mechanism of injury
   D. Decide if the patient's family requires notification

4. Continued scene security can be ensured by which of the following?
   A. Reassessing the ambulance or rescue vehicle's location
   B. Looking for hazards around the patient location
   C. Using specialized equipment such as turnout gear or breathing apparatus
   D. All of the above

5. You arrive on the location of a one vehicle crash. The female driver is restrained and still in the vehicle. You notice a diaper bag and baby bottle lying on the floor of the vehicle. Your next action would be to:
   A. Call for additional ambulances immediately
   B. Notify medical direction or dispatch to initiate disaster protocols
   C. Direct your partner to search for the infant
   D. Continue assessing your patient

6. Emergency medical technicians learn how to predict injuries best by noting the:
   A. Mechanism of injury
   B. Vehicle damage detail
   C. Type of vehicles involved
   D. Type(s) of weapons involved

7. After ensuring that the scene is safe, the EMT-B's primary responsibility is:
   A. Initiation of prehospital care reports
   B. Providing medical care to the patient
   C. Requesting rescue teams for extensive or heavy rescue
   D. Coordinating patient care with police officers

8. Violent scenes should always be controlled by law enforcement personnel before the EMT-B provides patient care because:
   A. Most EMT-Bs are not prepared to intervene in violent situations
   B. It is the EMT-B's responsibility to protect the patient by ensuring that no harm will come to him or her during the provision of emergency care
   C. Patient care cannot be not rendered if the perpetrator of the crime is still on the scene
   D. The EMT-B is not trained to recognize dangerous situations

9. "Why me?" expresses the emotion known as:
   A. Anger
   B. Denial
   C. Depression
   D. Paranoia

10. When facing a catastrophic illness or injury, some patients react initially by the process known as "bargaining." The person may:
    A. Bargain with God
    B. Bargain with their family
    C. Bargain with medical professionals
    D. All of the above

11. Family members should be allowed to stay with the patient in the patient compartment of the ambulance on the way to the hospital.
    A. True
    B. False

12. Some family members may want to touch or hold the body after death. Do not deny this request unless:
    A. It is a crime scene or it compromises your care or local protocol
    B. The family member appears too upset to deal with the situation
    C. The medical examiner or coroner arrives on the scene
    D. The family member appears mature enough to handle the situation

13. In stressful situations, epinephrine (adrenaline) and other chemicals are released to prepare the body to deal with the situation. Physiologic responses may include all of the following *except*:
    A. Respirations and blood pressure increase
    B. Muscles tighten and pupils dilate
    C. Glucose is released into the blood for immediate energy
    D. The heart rate decreases

14. The first stage in the dying process is usually:
    A. Anger
    B. Denial
    C. Bargaining
    D. Acceptance

15. While responding to or on the scene of an emergency, an EMT-B may experience signs and symptoms of the normal response to a stressful situation. These include:
    A. Upset stomach and dry mouth
    B. Nausea and vomiting
    C. Shivering or shakes and sweating
    D. All of the above

16. All of the following suggestions will assist the EMT in stress management *except*:
    A. Balancing life with work, recreation, family, and friends
    B. Recognizing that one's personality includes physical, mental, emotional, and spiritual needs
    C. Maintaining a positive attitude at all times
    D. Working out frustrations in which ever way works for that individual

17. In order to be termed a critical incident, an emergency call must affect more than one emergency responder.
    A. True
    B. False

18. The three main categories of stress include all of the following *except*:
    A. Psychosocial
    B. Personal
    C. Environmental
    D. Psychosomatic

19. When dealing with a dying patient, the EMT-B should:
    A. Be firm and control the situation
    B. Reassure the patient and family members, even if no hope exists
    C. Treat the patient with dignity and respect
    D. Distance himself from the situation

20. The EMT-B should try to eat only as many calories that are expended in a day.
    A. True
    B. False

Case Scenario

You and your partner are on the scene of a multi-vehicle crash involving four cars and 13 patients. You witness that two children have been ejected from the vehicle; one patient is trapped in a vehicle and is in cardiac arrest and his wife, who was also ejected from the vehicle has suffered significant injuries. The individual who ran through a red-light, thereby causing the crash appears intoxicated and uninjured. In total, there were four deaths, including the husband and two small children of one of the patients, and 12 injured patients.

1. What feelings might you have to deal with during this emergency call?

2. What physical reactions might you experience during this call?

3. How should you handle the scene where a patient is dead or dying?

4. At the conclusion of this incident, you and your peers are exhausted and have a lot of emotions concerning the event. How might you deal with the situation?

5. List 12 suggestions to stop stress from becoming distress during your EMS career.

   1)

   2)

   3)

   4)

   5)

   6)

   7)

   8)

   9)

   10)

   11)

   12)

6. Identify five characteristics that friends and family should look for that should alarm them to the fact that the EMT needs intervention.

   1)

   2)

   3)

   4)

   5)

7. You notice that in the days after the incident, your partner has difficulty making decisions and has angry outbursts. He stops talking to you and stops going out with you after work, something you have done for years. What should you do?

Answer Key

Key Terms
1. Body substance isolation
2. Hazardous materials
3. Stress
4. Personal
5. Critical incident stress
6. Psychosocial

Content Review
1. Hazardous materials; rescue scenes; violent scenes; crime scenes; and all scenes that possess exposure to communicable diseases
2. True
3. Wait for law enforcement personnel to determine the scene is safe for entry.
4. Retreat to a safe area until it is safe to re-enter. If possible, take the patient along.
5. Blood (location and amount); type and extent of injury; hidden weapons; potential weapons; family or bystander reactions
6. Environmental
7. A HazMat suit and self-contained breathing apparatus
8. Providing medical care to the patient.
9. Electricity, fire, explosion, and hazardous materials
10. Turnout gear, puncture-proof gloves, a helmet, and safety glasses or goggles
11. Request that a police officer accompany him and the patient to the hospital.
12. Do not disturb the scene unless required for medical care; take the same path in and out of the scene to avoid disturbing evidence; do not touch anything or remove anything from the scene unless required for patient care; avoid damaging bullet or knife holes in clothing by cutting through the holes when removing clothing; save all clothing removed during patient care; and assist the police officer when a statement is required or if called as a witness for court.
13. Patient care
14. 1) Denial; 2) anger; 3) bargaining; 4) depression; and 5) acceptance

15. Protect the other family members temporarily from the reality of the deceased loved one. Telling them may deprive the others of their will to survive and cause more harm. Simply state that "they are doing everything they possibly can" or something to that effect.
16. B, E, A, C, D
17. Get additional assistance to help care for the loved one. The EMT-B's first priority must be for the patient. The loved one, however, needs assistance because of possible emotional shock, and needs to be moved so that she does not interfere with the EMT-B's actions.
18. Don't delay transport; however, allow the loved one to say a quick good-bye. Allow them to express their love, address unfinished business, or say good-bye. Explain that the patient may be able to hear and understand, even though he or she appears unresponsive.
19. Heart rate, respirations, and blood pressure all increase; muscles tighten; pupils dilate; and glucose is released for immediate energy.
20. Fight or flight
21. True
22. Try to find out all he or she can about the situation including chief complaint, number of patients involved, type of injuries, and hazards that may be present.
23. Upset stomach; stomach cramps; dry mouth; diarrhea; nausea and vomiting; muscle aches; pounding heart; dizziness; shivering or shaking; sweating; and feeling clumsy
24. Alert his partner to the situation; step back and take a few deep breaths to try to calm down; if his reaction is interfering with patient care, he should inform his partner and remove himself from the scene.
25. True
26. Trading shifts or duty time to accommodate special times or events with family and friends; requesting a rotation, location, or duty assignment in a less busy area; requesting shifts that better coincide with the schedules of family and friends; requesting shift hours and rotations that allow for more time to relax with family and friends.
27. True
28. Distress
29. 1) Environmental; 2) personal; and 3) psychosocial
30. Demanding physical labor; lights, sirens, alarms, and noise; weather conditions and temperature extremes; angry, impatient bystanders and families; emergency driving and response; sharing quarters with other EMTs; long hours and shifts; overwork from high call volume
31. Anxiety about being responsible for a person's life; making life and death decisions; fear of making a serious error; dealing with dying patients and grieving family members; anxiety about being competent as an EMT-B; guilt of anger about mistakes or criticism
32. Agitated and combative patients; abusive parents of a young patient; patients under the influence of drugs or alcohol; patients from a violent domestic situations; death of a child or infant; hospital staff who do not listen to or respect the EMT-B; conflicts with supervisors, dispatchers, or medical directors; incompatibility with a partner
33. Chronic or cumulative
34. Responding to a serious illness or injury to a patient known by the EMT-B; serious injury or death of a co-worker; disaster; threat or attack on the EMT-B's life; involvement in a fatal collision while responding to another emergency call; witnessing child abuse, suicide, or homicide; or facing a scene of multiple mutilated bodies
35. Any event or circumstance that overwhelms the EMT's usual coping skills
36. True
37. Post traumatic stress disorder (PTSD)
38. The EMT-B has been exposed to a critical incident or disturbing event; the EMT-B avoids and blocks thinking about, talking about, or being reminded of the incident; despite attempts at avoidance, the EMT-B re-lives the incident in his or her thoughts, dreams, or real life; signs and symptoms of emotional, behavioral, mental, or physical change are noted that were not present before the incident; the signs and symptoms of dramatic change last longer than 1 month
39. 1) Physical; 2) cognitive; 3) emotional; and 4) behavioral

40. Chest pain; difficulty breathing; excessive blood pressure; collapse from exhaustion; cardiac arrhythmia; signs and symptoms of severe shock; dehydration; dizziness; excessive vomiting; or blood in the stool

41. Decreased alertness to surroundings; difficulty making decisions; hyper-alertness; general mental confusion; disorientation to person, place, or time; serious disruption in thinking; seriously slowed thinking; problems in naming familiar items; problems recognizing familiar people

42. Panic reactions; signs and symptoms of shock; phobic reactions; general loss of control; inappropriate emotions; wishing to die

43. Significant change in speech patterns; excessively angry outbursts; crying spells; antisocial acts (violence); extreme hypersensitivity

44. Burnout

45. For events that have extraordinary power to negatively affect emergency personnel. Overuse for routine events can dilute their power substantially.

46. Between 24 and 72 hours after a major incident.

47. Mental health professionals and peer support personnel from police, fire, EMS, disaster management, and other emergency oriented organizations.

48. Many individuals within a group appear to be distressed after a call; signals of distress appear to be severe; personnel demonstrate numerous behavioral changes; personnel make significant errors on calls occurring after the critical incident; personnel request help; the event is extraordinary; various agencies are showing the same reactions; signals of distress continue beyond 3 weeks

49. To accelerate the normal recovery process of emergency personnel after the experience of a critical incident. Thoughts and feelings are vented quickly in a supportive and non-threatening environment.

50. Avoid sugar, salt, white bread, alcohol, and caffeine; increase consumption of complex carbohydrates; decrease intake of fatty foods; watch intake of cholesterol; use polyunsaturated and monosaturated fats instead of saturated fats; decrease the use of refined sugars by 50%; decrease salt intake; if overweight, decrease food intake and increase exercises; increase consumption of fruits, vegetables, and whole grains; substitute low-fat and nonfat milk for whole milk; consume more fish and poultry; use multivitamin supplements; avoid crash diets

Chapter Quiz

1. A	6. A	11. A	16. D
2. B	7. B	12. A	17. B
3. D	8. A	13. D	18. D
4. D	9. A	14. B	19. C
5. C	10. D	15. D	20. A

Case Scenario

1. Anger, anxiety, fear, sadness, disbelief

2. Nausea, vomiting, increased respirations, muscle aches, dry mouth, sweating, diarrhea, pounding heart, shakes, feeling clumsy, dizziness

3. Remain calm, professional, and in control; clearly communicate what you are doing; allow family members to remain with the loved one; keep family members informed about what is happening; encourage family members to have a friend or neighbor drive them to the hospital; avoid negative or confidential statements about the patient's condition; be honest with the patient and family; do not falsely reassure the patient or family, but give some hope if possible; ensure patient privacy from onlookers and bystanders; make arrangements for family members to see the patient; treat the patient with dignity and respect; listen closely and empathetically and allow family members to express themselves without judgment; do not take anger or insults personally; if possible, stay with the body and family until police, the medical examiner, or coroner arrive.

4. Request CISD interventions such as participation in a debriefing; talk about your feelings.

5. 1) Balance life, including work, recreation, family, friends, etc.; 2) recognize that personality includes physical, mental, emotional, and spiritual needs; 3) maintain a positive attitude at all times; 4) maintain a healthy diet; 5) develop an exercise plan and follow it; 6) do not smoke; 7) avoid substance abuse, including alcohol and other drugs; 8) get 7 to 8 hours sleep every 24 hours; 9) be sure to get enough rest and relaxation; 10) develop hobbies to balance your life; 11) have a healthy sense of humor; 12) learn more about the human aspect of being an EMT-B

6. 1) The EMT has been exposed to a critical incident; 2) the EMT avoids thinking or talking about the incident; 3) despite attempts at avoidance, the EMT re-lives the incident; 4) signs of emotional, behavioral, mental, or physical change are noted that were not present before the incident; and 5) signs of dramatic change last longer than 1 month.

7. Try to get your partner to open up to you, and inform your supervisor that you think your partner is showing signs of extreme stress.

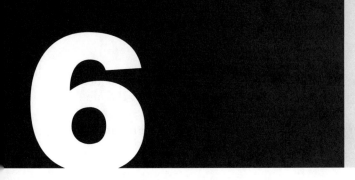

Infection Control

Reading Assignment: Chapter 6 pages 74–85.

DOT Objectives

Upon successful completion of the EMT-Basic training program, the EMT-Basic should be able to do the following:

- Discuss the importance of body substance isolation (BSI).
- Describe the steps that the EMT should take for personal protection from airborne and bloodborne pathogens.
- List the personal protective equipment necessary for exposure to bloodborne and airborne pathogens.

Supplemental Objectives

- Discuss common infectious diseases to which the EMT may be exposed.
- Discuss the Occupational Safety and Health Administration (OSHA) and Centers for Disease Control and Prevention (CDC) guidelines for bloodborne pathogens.

Key Terms

1. A disease that can be passed from one organism to another is termed a(n) _____
   _____.

2. Microorganisms that are present in, and transmitted through, body fluids are called _____
   _____.

3. A mask worn over the mouth and nose that decreases the spread of infection of airborne pathogens such as tuberculosis is a(n) _____.

4. A division of the U.S. Public Health service that is responsible for activities related to the control and prevention of the disease process is the _____.

5. The term for the precautions taken to prevent the transmission of substances excreted from the body is _____.

6. Microorganisms transmitted through infected droplets are called _____ pathogens.

7. The Division of the U.S. Department of Labor that is responsible for establishing and enforcing safety and health standards in the work place is the _____.

8. The plan an employer is required to develop in order to comply with legal standards and minimize the risk that employees will become exposed to a communicable disease is called a(n) _____ _____.

9. The introduction of a mixture of weakened or dead microorganisms into the body to produce immunity to a specific disease is called a(n) _____.

10. The term for the equipment used to decrease the risk that a rescuer will become infected with a communicable disease is _____.

Content Review

1. Which emergency situations place the EMT-B at the highest risk of being exposed to infected body substances?

2. List six steps the EMT-B must take to ensure that communicable diseases are not spread to family members, other patients, or health care workers.

   1)
   2)
   3)
   4)
   5)
   6)

3. Identify four types of microorganisms that may cause an infectious disease.

   1)
   2)
   3)
   4)

4. Identify communicable diseases that are potentially life-threatening to which the EMT-B may be exposed.

5. List six different methods by which communicable diseases are transmitted.

   1)
   2)
   3)
   4)
   5)
   6)

6. Pathogens that are transmitted when an EMT breathes the infected moisture when a patient exhales or coughs are called _____ pathogens.

7. Pathogens that are transmitted when an EMT comes in contact with substances secreted from the body are called _____ pathogens.

8. What type of pathogens place the EMT at the greatest risk of exposure to communicable diseases?
   _____

9. Identify three ways in which an EMT might become infected by a contaminated needle puncture.

   1)
   2)
   3)

10. The most severe infections are associated with which type of bites? _____

11. Identify contaminated materials that may be a source of infection for the EMT.

12. The period of time during which a patient is contagious is called the _____ period.

13. List four items required for inclusion in an employer's exposure control plan.

   1)
   2)
   3)
   4)

14. OSHA regulations place requirements on employers of EMS personnel. What are they?

15. Identify six topics that must be included in training sessions on exposure to communicable diseases.

    1)
    2)
    3)
    4)
    5)
    6)

16. How often must the employer provide training on communicable disease for its personnel?

17. How long must an employer maintain medical and training records?

18. When should the EMT wash his or her hands?

19. What should the EMT do if gloves are punctured during patient contact?

20. List five types of equipment that may protect the EMT from exposure to communicable diseases.

    1)
    2)
    3)
    4)
    5)

21. Identify acceptable types of eye protective equipment.

22. What is the most important aspect of protection against communicable diseases?

23. Identify when each of the following types of personal protection equipment should be worn.

    Gloves:

    Eye protection:

    Gowns:

    Face masks:

    Resuscitation equipment:

24. What vaccinations should the EMT obtain?

25. For each of the following tasks, identify which PPE the EMT should use.

	Gloves	Mask	Gown	Goggles
A. Bleeding control with spurting blood				
B. Bleeding control with minimal bleeding				
C. Emergency childbirth				
D. Oral/nasal suctioning				
E. Handling contaminated equipment				
F. Taking a patient's blood pressure				
G. Taking a patient's temperature				
H. Exposure to a patient with TB				

26. For each of the following, identify the mode of transmission.

Measles:
Mumps:
Rubella:
Chickenpox:
Meningitis:
Tuberculosis:
Hepatitis A:
Hepatitis B:
AIDS:
Genital herpes:

Chapter Quiz

1. Situations where there is a high risk of exposure to pathogens include:
   A. CPR and IV insertion
   B. Trauma and childbirth
   C. Open fractures and nosebleeds
   D. All of the above

2. Communicable diseases are transmitted by all of the following modes *except:*
   A. Direct contact and inhalation of droplets
   B. Contaminated needle puncture and bites
   C. Blood transfusions and contaminated materials
   D. Bronchial inhalers and BSI devices

3. A term frequently used to describe communicable diseases is:
   A. Infectious diseases
   B. Microorganisms
   C. Pathogens
   D. Immunizations

4. Topics that must be included in bloodborne pathogen training sessions include:
   A. An overview of the modes of transmission of bloodborne pathogens
   B. Principles regarding the control of risk and medical management of those who have been exposed
   C. Appropriate cleaning techniques for equipment and packaging techniques for specimens
   D. All of the above

5. EMTs are no longer susceptible to bloodborne pathogen exposure because of the special techniques used to prevent communicable diseases
   A. True
   B. False

6. The federal organization responsible for publishing the regulations designed to protect employees who are at risk for exposure to bloodborne pathogens is:
   A. Department of Human Resources
   B. OSHA
   C. CDC
   D. NHTSA

7. Examples of body fluids that should be considered dangerous include:
   A. Blood and urine
   B. Feces and tears
   C. Saliva and spinal fluid
   D. All of the above

8. Which of the following are examples of bloodborne pathogens?
   A. Viruses
   B. Bacteria
   C. Fungi
   D. All of the above

9. Which of the following communicable diseases is considered to be life threatening?
   A. Measles
   B. HIV
   C. Chickenpox
   D. Herpes

10. Organisms that cause infections are called:
    A. Pathogens
    B. Antigens
    C. Toxins
    D. Microbes

11. The time during which diseases are capable of being transmitted is called:
    A. Communicable period
    B. Exposure time
    C. Incubation period
    D. Infected period

12. An employer must provide training for its personnel at least how often?
    A. Monthly
    B. Quarterly
    C. Annually
    D. Twice yearly

13. Responsibilities of the EMT as it relates to ensuring a safe working environment include:
    A. Removal of gloves and jewelry and washing hands thoroughly after each patient contact
    B. Wiping down the vehicle floors, walls, and stretcher at least once daily
    C. Wiping down frequently used items such as radios, stethoscopes, monitors, and oxygen tanks
    D. All of the above

14. To clean properly after blood spillage, the EMT should clean the area with:
    A. 100% bleach
    B. A 1:10 mixture of bleach and water
    C. 100% sterile water
    D. Cold, soapy water

15. The most effective way to isolate EMS providers from potentially dangerous body substances is through:
    A. Immunizations
    B. Hand washing
    C. Using bactericidal lotion
    D. Wearing a mask

16. Which of the following statements regarding disposable gloves are *true*?
    A. Gloves should be used by all EMS personnel prior to initiating emergency care.
    B. Gloves are especially appropriate when the EMT may come into contact with body fluids.
    C. Gloves should fit tightly at the wrist.
    D. All of the above

17. If a patient is known or suspected of having tuberculosis, the EMT should:
    A. Wear a high-efficiency particulate air respirator
    B. Transport the patient in an internally ventilated ambulance
    C. Wear a surgical mask
    D. All of the above

18. Resuscitation equipment should be available to all EMS personnel to minimize the need for:
    A. CPR
    B. Mouth-to-mouth resuscitation
    C. Disposable items
    D. Disinfecting equipment

19. EMTs should ensure they are current on all recommended immunizations including all of the following *except:*
    A. HIV
    B. DPT (diptheria-pertussis-tetanus)
    C. Tetanus booster every 10 years
    D. MMR (measles, mumps, and rubella)

Case Scenario

You arrive at the scene of a bar fight where you find a 26-year-old male patient who has numerous cuts, scrapes, and bruises on his face, chest, arms, and abdomen. He also has a 2-inch laceration on his left cheek that is bleeding profusely. On further inspection, you note that there are needle tracks on the patient's arms and that his eyes are yellowish in color.

1. What warning signs should alert you to the need for BSI? Why?

2. What steps should you take to protect yourself, and others, from the dangers of this situation?

3. What BSI precautions should you take for this situation?

Answer Key

Key Terms
1. Communicable disease
2. Bloodborne pathogens
3. HEPA mask
4. Centers for Disease Control and Prevention (CDC)
5. Body substance isolation
6. Airborne
7. Occupational Safety and Health Administration (OSHA)
8. Exposure control plan
9. Vaccination
10. Personal protection equipment (PPE)

Content Review
1. CPR, IV line insertion, trauma, and childbirth.
2. 1) Understanding the importance of BSI; 2) understanding how common infectious diseases are spread; 3) knowing the risks associated with each disease; 4) knowing the basic pathophysiology of each disease as it applies to the prehospital environment; 5) knowing OSHA and CDC guidelines for dealing with bloodborne pathogens; 6) knowing methods for personal protection from bloodborrne and airborne pathogens.
3. 1) Bacteria; 2) viruses; 3) fungus; and 4) protozoa.
4. HIV/AIDS, new strains of TB; and hepatitis B and C.
5. 1) Direct contact; 2) inhalation of infected droplets; 3) contaminated needle puncture; 4) bites; 5) blood transfusions; 6) contaminated materials.

6. Airborne
7. Bloodborne
8. Bloodborne
9. 1) While working with another healthcare provider who administers an injection to a patient; 2) while "searching" a patient and being stuck with a patient's contaminated needle used for IV drug use; 3) when contaminated needles are not placed in the proper disposal containers.
10. Human
11. Handkerchiefs, washcloths, towels, linens, and used wound-dressing material
12. Communicable
13. 1) A list of the jobs and procedures in which exposure to bloodborne pathogens may occur; 2) a time-line and method by which the plan is to be implemented; 3) a plan outlining how exposure to incidents will be handled; 4) a plan for annual review and update to include any changes in the work place that may result in bloodborne pathogen exposure.
14. 1) Have an exposure control plan; 2) provide training for personnel that is free of charge; 3) provide protective equipment at no cost to employees; 4) provide hepatitis-B vaccinations and confidential medical evaluations and follow-up visits to the employee at no cost; 5) develop a written schedule to clean and decontaminate equipment and the work area after blood or other potentially infectious material has been exposed to the area; 6) devise procedures to handle regulated waste; 7) ensure that warning labels are secured to containers used to store or transport blood or other potentially infectious wastes; 8) maintain records on each employee who may be at risk of exposure and records that training has occurred as required
15. 1) An overview of all modes of transmission of bloodborne pathogens; 2) principles regarding the control of risk; 3) medical management of those who have been exposed; 4) appropriate equipment cleaning techniques; 5) appropriate packaging techniques for specimens; 6) methods of using personal protective equipment.
16. As soon as they are retained and at least annually thereafter.
17. Medical records must be retained for the duration of employment plus 30 years; training records must be kept for 3 years from the date the training occurred.
18. Before and after every patient encounter
19. Wash his or her hands and all other areas potentially touched by body fluids with hydrogen peroxide, Clorox, or other strong disinfectant that is effective against viruses, and follow local protocols.
20. 1) Eye protection; 2) gloves; 3) gowns; 4) face masks; 5) resuscitation equipment
21. Goggles, eyeglasses with removable side shields, and face shields
22. Handwashing
23. Gloves: prior to initiating any emergency care; especially when the EMT may come in contact with body fluids.
   Eye protection: when the potential exists for exposure of substances entering the eye or mucus membranes of the eyes.
   Gowns: when splashing to the skin or clothing is likely to occur, such as with field delivery of a baby or major trauma.
   Face masks: when contamination of the mucosal membranes, mouth, or nose is likely to occur.
   Resuscitation equipment: when mouth-to-mouth resuscitation is necessary.
24. HIB, DPT, MMR, polio, Hepatitis B, and tetanus
25. A. Gloves, gown, mask, and eyewear
   B. Gloves
   C. Gloves and gown (mask and eyewear if splashing is likely)
   D. Gloves (mask and eyewear if splashing is likely)
   E. Gloves (gown if splashing is likely)
   F. None
   G. None
   H. HEPA mask

26. Measles: airborne or secretions from mouth, nose, and eyes
    Mumps: airborne or contaminated materials
    Rubella: airborne or contaminated materials
    Chickenpox: airborne or direct contact with secretions from nose, mouth or pox
    Meningitis: airborne or direct contact with secretions from nose and mouth
    Tuberculosis: airborne
    Hepatitis A: ingestion of food or water contaminated by infected feces
    Hepatitis B: bloodborne, sexual contact or puncture with contaminated needle
    AIDS: bloodborne, sexual contact, being punctured with contaminated needle
    Genital herpes: sexual contact

Chapter Quiz

1. D	6. B	11. A	16. D
2. D	7. D	12. C	17. A
3. A	8. D	13. D	18. B
4. D	9. B	14. B	19. A
5. B	10. A	15. B	

Case Scenario

1. Blood indicates exposure to disease; the injuries indicate a potentially violent scene; needle tracks indicate possible drug use leading to a potential risk to serious communicable disease risks; the yellowish tint to the eyes is a sign of hepatitis.
2. Ensure scene safety; request law enforcement personnel; take BSI precautions to limit exposure.
3. Gloves and gown; a mask and eye shield should be used if there is the potential for the splattering of blood or body fluids.

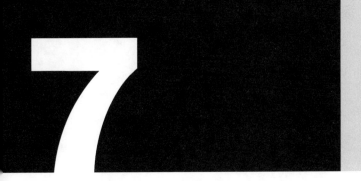

The Human Body

7

Reading Assignment: Chapter 7 pages 86–112.

DOT Objectives

Upon successful completion of the EMT-Basic training program, the EMT-Basic should be able to do the following:

- Identify the following directional terms: medial, lateral, proximal, distal, superior, inferior, anterior, posterior, midline, right and left, apices, midclavicular, bilateral, and midaxillary.
- Describe the structure and function of the following major body systems: respiratory, circulatory, musculoskeletal, integumentary, nervous, and endocrine.

Supplemental Objectives

- Describe the various components of medical terminology, including medical abbreviations.

Key Terms

1. Match the following definitions with the appropriate terms.

_____ Trunk of the body	A. Anterior
_____ Imaginary line running vertically	B. Bilateral
_____ Toward the midline	C. Distal
_____ Away from the midline	D. Dorsal
_____ Closer to the trunk	E. Inferior
_____ Farther from the trunk	F. Lateral
_____ Above	G. Medial
_____ Below	H. Midaxillary
_____ Imaginary line running vertically from middle of the armpit to the ankle	I. Midclavicular
_____ Toward the front	J. Midline
_____ Toward the rear	K. Palmar
_____ Imaginary line drawn vertically from the middle of the clavicle to the pelvis	L. Plantar
_____ Pertaining to both sides	M. Posterior
_____ Toward the back	N. Proximal
_____ Toward the front	O. Superior
_____ Relating to the palm	P. Torso
_____ Relating to the sole of the foot	Q. Ventral

2. Describe each of the following positions:

   Trendelenburg:
   Fowler:
   Supine:
   Prone:

3. Match the following areas of the skull with the appropriate definition.

   _____ Anterior section   A. Frontal
   _____ Posterior section   B. Parietal
   _____ Sides   C. Occipital
   _____ Top   D. Temporal

4. The only moveable bone in the face is the _____.

5. The cheek bones are called the _____ bones.

6. The upper jaw is called the _____.

7. The lower jaw bone is called the _____.

Content Review

∙∙

1. Identify the correct abbreviation for each of the following terms.

   A. Acute myocardial infarction   _____
   B. Arteriosclerotic heart disease   _____
   C. Blood pressure   _____
   D. Centigrade   _____
   E. Cancer   _____
   F. Cardiac care unit   _____
   G. Cerebrospinal fluid   _____
   H. Cerebrovascular accident   _____
   I. Congestive heart failure   _____
   J. Chronic obstructive pulmonary disease _____
   K. Diagnosis   _____
   L. Electrocardiogram   _____
   M. Fahrenheit   _____
   N. Fracture   _____
   O. Gastrointestinal   _____
   P. Gram   _____
   Q. Intensive care unit   _____
   R. Intravenous   _____
   S. Oxygen   _____
   T. Registered nurse   _____
   U. Treatment   _____

2. The skeleton is made up of _____ bones.

3. What is the function of cartilage?

4. The point at which bones connect to other bones are called _____.

5. What holds bones together? _____

6. Match the following types of joints with the appropriate descriptions.

   _____ Rotates on only one axis   A. Ball-and-socket joint
   _____ Moves in only one direction   B. Hinged joint
   _____ Contains bones that have minimal movement   C. Pivot joint
         for expansion and contraction only   D. Sutured joint
   _____ Moves freely in all directions

7. Identify each of the following types of joints.

   _____ Skull bones   A. Ball-and-socket
   _____ C1 - C2 vertebrae B. Hinged
   _____ Knee   C. Pivot
   _____ Shoulder   D. Sutured

8. Identify the following sections of the spinal column.

   Cervical
   Coccyx
   Lumbar
   Sacral
   Thoracic

A._____

B._____

C._____

D._____

E._____

9. The spinal column is composed of _____ vertebrae.

10. Identify how many vertebrae are in each section of the spinal column.

    Thoracic   _____
    Cervical   _____
    Coccyx   _____
    Lumbar   _____
    Sacral   _____

11. What is the function of the spinal column?

12. There are _____ pairs of ribs of which _____ are called floating ribs because they are not attached _____
    _____.

13. The thorax consists of _____.

14. The inferior portion of the sternum is called the _____.

15. Bones of the wrist are called _____.

16. Bones of the hand are called _____.

17. Bones of the fingers are called _____.

18. The forearm is comprised of the _____ and _____.

19. The medical term for the elbow is the _____.

20. The lower posterior portion of the hip is the _____.

21. The pelvis is comprised of what three bones?

22. Identify the following bones of the skeletal system.

    Cranium   Scapula
    Femur   Spinal column
    Fibula   Thorax
    Humerus   Tibia
    Radius   Ulna
    Sacrum

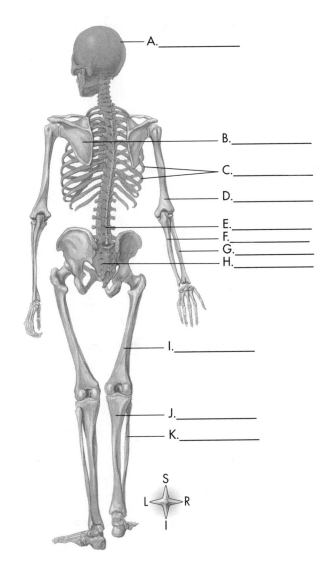

A._____

B._____

C._____

D._____

E._____
F._____
G._____
H._____

I._____

J._____
K._____

S
L ←✦→ R
I

23. The shin bone is called the _____.

24. The kneecap is called the _____.

25 The thigh bone is called the _____.

26. The lateral bone of the lower leg is the _____.

27. The ankle joint is made up of the _____ and _____.

28. What is the function of the muscular system?

29. What are the three types of muscles found in the body?

30. Voluntary muscles are also referred to as _____.

31. The major muscle mass of the body are the _____ muscles.

32. Involuntary muscles are also referred to as _____.

33. Identify the meaning of each of the following root words.
    Cardi   _____
    Osti   _____
    Gastr   _____
    Nephr   _____
    Phleb   _____
    Trache   _____
    Thorac   _____

34. Identify the meaning of each of the following prefixes.
    Ambi   _____
    Pre   _____
    Hypo   _____
    Epi   _____
    Inter   _____
    Post   _____

35. The nervous system has two divisions, the _____ and the _____ _____.

36. The central nervous system is made up of two types of nerves, the _____ and _____ _____.

37. Sensory nerves carry messages from _____ to _____.

38. Motor nerves carry messages from _____ to _____.

39. The central nervous system is composed of the _____ and _____.

40. The three main components of the brain are the: _____, _____ and _____.

41. The _____ controls basic functions such as breathing and other involuntary bodily functions.

42. The largest organ of the body is the _____.

43. The skin is also referred to as the _____ system.

44. What four functions does the skin serve?
    1)

    2)

    3)

    4)

45. The three layers of the skin, in order from top to bottom, are the _____, _____ and _____.

46. The _____ system secretes hormones.

47. Identify the major organs contained in each of the abdominal quadrants:

    LUQ:

    RUQ:

    LLQ:

    RLQ:

48. The abdominal cavity is lined by a thin membrane called the _____.

49. Identify the following components of the digestive system.

Appendix	Liver
Ascending colon	Pancreas
Descending colon	Spleen
Duodenum	Stomach
Gall bladder	Transverse colon

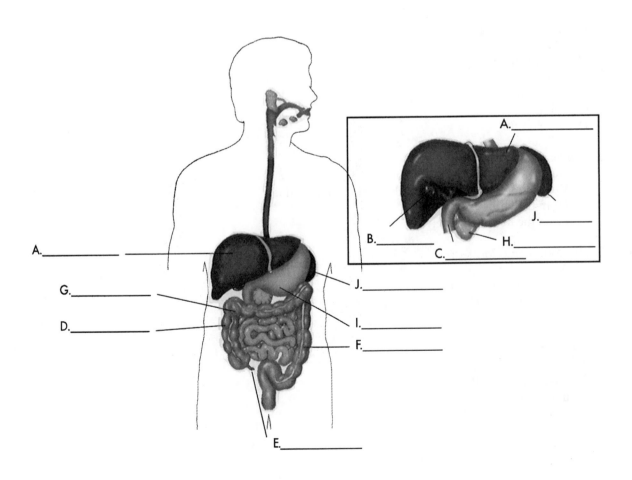

Chapter Quiz

• •

1. The term anatomical position refers to the patient:
   A. Standing upright and facing forward
   B. Standing with his arms down at the side
   C. Standing with his palms facing forward
   D. All of the above are correct

2. The heart is medial to the:
   A. Pelvis
   B. Left arm
   C. Femur
   D. Mouth

3. The elbow is:
   A. Distal to the wrist
   B. Lateral to the shoulder
   C. Proximal to the wrist
   D. Proximal to the shoulder

4. The heart is superior to the:
   A. Clavicles
   B. Skull
   C. Pelvis
   D. Scapula

5. The heart is inferior to the:
   A. Patella
   B. Cranium
   C. Pelvis
   D. Diaphragm

6. The midaxillary line runs:
   A. Horizontally through the shoulders
   B. Vertically from the middle of the armpit to the ankle
   C. From the chest to the back
   D. From the nose to the pelvis

7. The abdomen is located:
   A. Anterior to the spine
   B. Posterior to the heart
   C. Inferior to the pelvis
   D. Lateral to the chest

8. Clavicles are:
   A. Superior to the heart
   B. Posterior to the liver
   C. Inferior to the pelvis
   D. Lateral to the chest

9. The term meaning toward the back is:
    A. Ventral
    B. Superior
    C. Bactral
    D. Dorsal

10. Plantar refers to the:
    A. Palm of the hand
    B. Sole of the feet
    C. Dorsal side of the foot
    D. Medial side of the wrist

11. Prone refers to:
    A. Lying face up
    B. Lying face down
    C. Sitting up
    D. Lying on the side

12. Supine refers to:
    A. Lying face up
    B. Lying face down
    C. Sitting up
    D. Lying on the side

13. A patient in a Fowler's position on the stretcher would indicate he was:
    A. Lying face up
    B. Lying face down
    C. Sitting up
    D. Lying on his side

14. The musculoskeletal system:
    A. Is the framework for the body
    B. Protects vital internal organs
    C. Provides for body movement
    D. All of the above

15. Joints are the points at which:
    A. Tendons connect to other tendons
    B. Ligaments connect to other ligaments
    C. Bones connect to other bones
    D. Cartilage connects to bone

16. The four areas of the skull are the frontal, occipital, temporal, and parietal, and they are located _____ respectively.
    A. Anterior, posterior, sides, and top
    B. Posterior, sides, anterior, and top
    C. Posterior, anterior, sides, and top
    D. Anterior, sides, posterior, and top

17. The number of vertebrae per section of the spinal column, in order from top to bottom is:
    A. 7, 12, 5, 5, and 4
    B. 5, 12, 7, 5, and 4
    C. 7, 12, 4, 5, and 5
    D. 5, 12, 7, 4, and 1

18. The major organs and blood vessels contained within the thorax are the:
    A. Heart, lungs, diaphragm, aorta, and superior and inferior vena cavae
    B. Heart, lungs, kidneys, aorta, superior and inferior vena cavae
    C. Heart, lungs, kidneys, aorta, and superior and inferior aorta
    D. Heart, lungs, cerebellum, aorta, and superior and inferior vena cavae

19. Each upper extremity consists of the:
    A. Shoulder and arm
    B. Elbow and forearm
    C. Wrist and hand
    D. All of the above

20. The pelvis rests at the inferior section of the torso and is made up of the:
    A. Iliac crest
    B. Ischium
    C. Pubic symphysis
    D. All of the above

21. The bone of the thigh is called the:
    A. Tibia
    B. Fibula
    C. Femur
    D. Patella

22. Voluntary muscles are also referred to as:
    A. Unconscious muscles
    B. Smooth muscles
    C. Myocardial muscles
    D. Skeletal muscles

23. Involuntary muscles are also referred to as:
    A. Instinctive muscles
    B. Smooth muscles
    C. Myocardial muscles
    D. Skeletal muscles

24. Cardiac muscle is unique because it can:
    A. Be controlled voluntarily
    B. Generate its own contractions
    C. Tolerate interruption of blood supply
    D. Regenerate after cell and tissue damage

25. The vocal cords are contained within the:
    A. Air passages
    B. Larynx
    C. Trachea
    D. Thyroid cartilage

26. Which of the following muscles of the heart contract?
    A. Endocardium
    B. Pericardium
    C. Myocardium
    D. Epicardium

27. The heart is supplied with oxygenated blood by the:
    A. Coronary arteries
    B. Superior vena cavae
    C. Inferior vena cava
    D. Descending aorta

28. The _____ system evaluates internal and external stimuli and directs body functions in response to these stimuli.
    A. Integumentary
    B. Nervous
    C. Cardiovascular
    D. Muscular

29. Involuntary functions such as respiration, circulation, and digestion, are carried out by the _____ _____ system.
    A. Endocrine
    B. Autonomic
    C. Cardiovascular
    D. Integumentary

30. The outermost layer of the skin is the:
    A. Dermis
    B. Epidermis
    C. Fascia
    D. Adipose

31. The circulatory system delivers hormones to the largest tissue where they:
    A. Regulate growth and produce energy
    B. Maintain fluid balance and respond to stress
    C. Manage reproductive functions
    D. All of the above

32. Two major hormones are:
    A. Adrenaline and insulin
    B. Epinephrine and hemoglobin
    C. Insulin and heparin
    D. Glucose and insulin

33. The abdominal cavity is lined by a thin membrane called the:
    A. Peritoneum
    B. Pericardium
    C. Endocardium
    D. Perineum

34. The kidneys lie behind the abdominal cavity in what is referred to as the:
    A. Retroperitoneal space
    B. Peritoneum
    C. Umbilicus inferior
    D. Mesenteric arterious

Case Scenario

You are on the scene of a patient who was struck by a car. He is lying on his back and is not responding. You note a large (2-inch) laceration on the back of his head, a 1-inch cut on the inside of his right upper leg, and a scrape above his left eyebrow. His left leg is deformed with a bone protruding from just below the knee.

1. What major body systems may be involved as a result of these injuries?

2. What organs may be involved as a result of these injuries?

3. What bones may be involved as a result of these injuries?

4. Using appropriate terminology, describe the location of the patient's injuries.

Answer Key

Key Terms
1. P, J, G, F, N, C, O, E, H, A, M, I, B, D, Q, K, L
2. Trendelenburg: Feet up, head down
   Fowler: Sitting up
   Supine: Lying face up
   Prone: Lying face down
3. A, C, D, B
4. Mandible
5. Zygomatic
6. Maxilla
7. Mandible

Content Review

1. AMI
   ASHD
   BP
   C
   CA
   CCU
   CSF
   CVA
   CHF
   COPD
   Dx
   ECG
   F
   Fx
   GI
   Gm
   ICU
   IV
   O_2
   RN
   Rx
2. 206
3. To lubricate and cushion the joint
4. Joints
5. Ligaments
6. C, B, D, A
7. D, C, B, A
8. Cervical
   Thoracic
   Lumbar
   Sacral
   Coccyx
9. 33
10. Thoracic: 12
    Cervical: 7
    Coccyx: 1
    Lumbar: 5
    Sacral: 5
11. It forms a flexible backbone that supports the torso and head and protects the spinal cord.
12. 12; 2; anteriorly
13. Ribs, sternum, and 12 thoracic vertebrae
14. Xiphoid process
15. Carpals
16. Metacarpals
17. Phalanges
18. Radius and ulna
19. Olecranon
20. Ischium
21. Iliac crest, pubis, and ischium

22. A. Cranium
    B. Scapula
    C. Thorax
    D. Humerus
    E. Spinal Column
    F. Ulna
    G. Radius
    H. Sacrum
    I. Femur
    J. Tibia
    K. Fibula
23. Tibia
24. Patella
25. Femur
26. Fibula
27. Medial, lateral malleolus
28. It works with the skeletal system to protect the body, give it structure, and provide for movement.
29. Voluntary, involuntary, and cardiac
30. Skeletal muscles
31. Voluntary
32. Smooth muscles
33. Heart
    Bone
    Stomach
    Kidney
    Vein
    Trachea
    Chest
34. Both
    Before
    Under or below
    Upon
    Between
    After
35. Central nervous system; peripheral nervous system
36. Sensory and motor
37. The body; the CNS
38. The CNS; the body
39. Brain; spinal cord
40. Brainstem, cerebrum, and cerebellum
41. Brainstem
42. Skin
43. Integumentary
44. 1) Keeps out harmful microorganisms; 2) helps regulate body temperature; 3) prevents water loss; 4) allows for the transmission of sensations through motor nerves and the CNS
45. Epidermis, dermis, and subcutaneous layer
46. Endocrine
47. LUQ: stomach, spleen, part of the liver, and part of the colon
    RUQ: liver, gall bladder, and part of the colon
    LLQ: part of the colon
    RLQ: the appendix and part of the colon
48. Peritoneum

49. A. Liver
    B. Gallbladder
    C. Duodenum
    D. Ascending colon
    E. Appendix
    F. Descending colon
    G. Transverse colon
    H. Pancreas
    I. Stomach
    J. Spleen

Chapter Quiz

1. D	8. A	15. C	22. D	29. B
2. B	9. D	16. A	23. B	30. B
3. C	10. B	17. A	24. B	31. D
4. C	11. B	18. A	25. B	32. A
5. B	12. A	19. D	26. C	33. A
6. B	13. C	20. D	27. A	34. A
7. A	14. D	21. C	28. B	

Case Scenario

1. Musculoskeletal, integumentary, and nervous systems
2. The brain and skin.
3. Cranium (occipital and frontal lobes), femur, and tibia
4. Upon your arrival you find a patient unresponsive in a *supine* position. There is a 2-inch laceration on the *posterior* portion of his cranium and a 1-inch laceration on the *medial* portion of his right thigh and a scrape *superior* to his left eyebrow. There is also deformity to his left leg with a bone protruding *inferior* to (or *distal* to) the patella.

8

Assessment

Reading Assignment: Chapter 8 pages 113–149.

DOT Objectives

• •

Upon successful completion of the EMT-Basic training program, the EMT-Basic should be able to do the following:

- Summarize the reasons for forming a general impression of the patient.
- Discuss methods of assessing altered mental status.
- Discuss methods of assessing and managing the airway (medical and trauma patients).
- Describe methods used for assessing and managing difficulty breathing.
- Describe the methods used to obtain a pulse.
- Discuss the need for assessing the patient for external bleeding.
- Describe normal and abnormal findings when assessing skin (color, temperature, condition, capillary refill time).
- Explain the reason for prioritizing a patient for care and transportation.
- Describe the areas included in the rapid trauma assessment, and discuss what should be evaluated.
- Describe when the rapid assessment may be altered in order to provide patient care.
- Discuss the reason for performing a focused history and physical examination.
- Discuss the components of the detailed physical examination and how it is performed.
- Distinguish between the detailed physical examination that is performed on a trauma patient and that performed on a medical patient.
- Discuss the reasons for repeating the initial assessment as part of the on-going assessment.
- State the reasons for management of the cervical spine once the patient has been determined to be a trauma patient.
- Describe the methods used for assessing whether a patient is breathing.
- State what care should be provided to the patient with adequate breathing.
- State what care should be provided to the patient without adequate breathing.
- Differentiate between a patient with adequate breathing and a patient without adequate breathing.
- Differentiate among methods of assessing breathing.
- Compare the methods of providing airway care.
- Differentiate among methods of obtaining a pulse.
- Demonstrate the techniques for assessing mental status.
- Demonstrate the techniques for assessing the airway.
- Demonstrate the techniques for assessing whether the patient is breathing.
- Demonstrate the techniques for assessing whether the patient has a pulse.
- Demonstrate the techniques for assessing the patient for external bleeding.
- Demonstrate the techniques for assessing the patient's skin color, temperature, condition, and capillary refill.
- Demonstrate the ability to prioritize patients.

- Discuss the reasons for reconsideration concerning the mechanism of injury.
- State the reasons for performing a rapid trauma assessment.
- Recite examples and explain why patients should receive a rapid trauma assessment.
- Demonstrate the rapid trauma assessment that should be used to assess a patient based on mechanism of injury.
- Describe the unique needs for assessing an individual with a specific chief complaint with no known history.
- Differentiate between the history and physical examination that are performed for responsive patients with no known prior history and those that are performed for responsive patients with a known history.
- Describe the needs for assessing an individual who is unresponsive.
- Differentiate between the assessment that is performed for a patient who is unresponsive or has an altered state of consciousness and the assessment that is performed for other medical patients.
- Demonstrate the patient assessment skills that should be used to assist a patient who is responsive with no known history.
- Demonstrate the patient assessment skills that should be used to assist a patient who is unresponsive or has an altered mental status.
- State the areas of the body that are evaluated during the detailed physical examination.
- Explain what additional care should be provided while performing the detailed physical examination.
- Describe the components of the on-going assessment.
- Describe trending of assessment components.
- Demonstrate the skills involved in performing the on-going assessment.

Key Terms

....

1. Match each of the following terms to their appropriate definition.

_____ Looking at body parts during patient assessment
_____ An abnormal accumulation of fluid in tissues
_____ Damage to the dermis from shearing forces; a scrape
_____ To examine by feeling
_____ A crackling sensation felt when air escapes from the lungs into surrounding tissue
_____ Discoloration of the skin from blood leaking into surrounding tissue
_____ A sign of respiratory distress marked by inward pulling of the skin with inspiration
_____ A break in the skin from a forceful impact with a sharp instrument
_____ To listen through a stethoscope
_____ A state of adequate supply of oxygen and nutrients to tissues

A. Abrasion
B. Auscultate
C. Contusion
D. Crepitus
E. Edema
F. Inspection
G. Laceration
H. Palpate
I. Perfusion
J. Retraction

2. During patient assessment, a _____ is something that the EMT-B observes, such as a bruise or diaphoretic skin.

3. During patient assessment, a _____ is something that the patient tells the EMT-B, such as complaining of nausea or pain.

4. The term for making something smaller, such as when pupils react to light, is called _____ _____.

5. Pupils react to darkness by getting bigger. This is called _____.

6. The pressure in the heart measured when the heart muscle is contracting is called the _____ _____ pressure.

7. The process of sorting patients to determine who requires immediate treatment or transport is called _____.

8. Match each of the following terms to their appropriate definition.

_____ The number of respirations in 1 minute
_____ The intervals between heart beats
_____ The difference between systolic and diastolic blood pressures
_____ The wave of blood moving through vessels as the heart beats
_____ An observable indication of illness or injury
_____ The lower reading of a blood pressure
_____ A strong pulse
_____ Measurement of a blood pressure by feeling for a pulse
_____ A subjective indication of illness or injury
_____ Shrinking of pupils
_____ A weak pulse
_____ The upper reading of a blood pressure
_____ To get larger
_____ Measurement of a blood pressure with a stethoscope
_____ Acronym for assessing a patient's condition
_____ Acronym to describe a patient's responsiveness
_____ The depth and ease with which a patient breathes
_____ The amount of air exchanged with each breath

A. Pulse pressure
B. Respiratory depth
C. Diastolic
D. Ventilatory rate
E. Auscultation
F. Thready
G. Pulse
H. Systolic
I. Constrict
J. Pulse rhythm
K. AVPU
L. Bounding
M. Symptom
N. Palpation
O. Dilate
P. SAMPLE
Q. Ventilatory character
R. Sign

Content Review

1. Why is a patient assessment so important?

2. What three things should the EMT-B consider in order to determine if he or she can make an unsafe scene safe?

1)

2)

3)

3. An EMT is providing care for a patient when the scene suddenly becomes unsafe. What should he or she do?

4. What is the minimum BSI precautions for any emergency response?

5. What is the mechanism of injury, and why is it important?

6. For each of the following, identify what types of injury the EMT-B might expect to find.

    A. A minor motor vehicle crash with no damage to the vehicle

    _____

    B. A front end collision with significant vehicle damage

    _____

    C. Side impact collision with a patient wearing a seat belt

    _____

    D. A patient ejected from a car

    _____

    E. A patient falls 10 feet from a roof and lands on his knees

    _____

7. Identify five ways in which the EMT-B can obtain information regarding the mechanism of injury or the nature of injury.

    1)

    2)

    3)

    4)

    5)

8. What is the initial assessment?

9. What senses should the EMT-B use while assessing a patient?

10. What are the five steps of the initial assessment?

    1)

    2)

    3)

    4)

    5)

11. During the initial assessment, when should a life-threatening problem be corrected?

12. An EMT-B approaches a patient who is crying. What can he tell about the patient's airway?

13. An EMT-B encounters a patient with an airway obstruction. Repeated attempts at clearing the obstruction are unsuccessful. What should the EMT do?

14. Breathing rates that generally constitute warning signs of breathing difficulty are those less than _____ or greater than _____ breaths per minute.

15. An EMT-B is assessing a patient and finds a pulse at the ankle. What does this tell the EMT?

16. An EMT-B can palpate a carotid and femoral pulse but cannot palpate the radial pulse. What does this tell the EMT?

17. Determining a blood pressure reading is one of the most important aspects of the initial assessment.
    A. True
    B. False

18. What does the mnemonic OPQRST stand for? When is it used?

    O:
    P:
    Q:
    R:
    S:
    T:

19. List the steps of the rapid focused history and physical examination of a trauma patient.

20. A rapid focused history and physical examination of a medical patient places much more emphasis on a _____ to determine what is wrong with the patient.

21. List the components of the rapid focused history and physical examination the EMT-B must complete during the assessment of a medical patient.

22. What is the purpose of a rapid history and physical examination?

23. Why is it important to watch a patient's facial expression and eyes when performing a history and examination?

24. For each of the following areas, identify what key items the EMT-B should look for when completing the rapid focused history and physical examination of a medical patient.

    Neck:
    Chest:
    Abdomen:
    Pelvis:
    Extremities:
    Back:

25. The detailed physical examination should always be initiated at the scene, prior to transport of the patient.
    A. True
    B. False

26. There are two methods by which an EMT can assess a patient's blood pressure. What are they?

    1)

    2)

27. What does the mnemonic AVPU stand for? What is it used to describe?

    A:
    V:
    P:
    U:

28. A heart rate less than _____ beats per minute would be termed bradycardia.

29. A heart rate greater than _____ beats per minute would be termed tachycardia.

30. The upper number of a blood pressure is the _____ reading and the lower number is the _____ reading.

31. Where can a pulse be felt?

32. List the normal values for pulse rates of the following.

    Newborn:
    Infant:
    Child:
    Adult:

33. An adult heart rate greater than _____ beats per minute is considered fast and called _____ _____.

34. If an adult's pulse rate falls below _____ beats per minute it is considered slow which is called _____ _____.

35. How do you determine the pulse rate of an adult patient?

36. How do you determine the pulse rate if the pulse is irregular?

37. How do you determine the pulse rate of a child?

38. An unusually strong pulse is termed _____.

39. A weak pulse is termed _____.

40. If the intervals between pulse beats are not constant, they are termed _____.

41. The number of ventilations in 1 minute is called the _____.

42. Identify the normal ventilatory rates for the following:

    Infant:
    Adult:

43. When little air is exchanged and there is little chest wall movement, ventilations are termed _____ _____.

44. If the patient has to exert a lot of effort to take each breath, ventilations are described as _____ _____.

45. A blood pressure is measured in _____.

46. The pressure that occurs when the left ventricle is relaxed and refilling with blood is called the _____ _____ pressure.

47. The pressure created by the contraction of the left ventricle is the _____ pressure.

48. The difference between the systolic and diastolic pressure is called the _____.

49. An average blood pressure for an adult patient is _____.

50. What is the rule of thumb for estimating a normal blood pressure for an adult patient?

51. A woman's systolic pressure is usually _____ mm Hg _____ than a male's.

52. Blood pressure in children is usually lower until approximately _____ years of age.

53. The diastolic pressure for men and women averages _____ mm Hg.

54. To quickly assess a patient's systolic pressure, assess pulses in specific areas of the body. Identify the systolic pressures if pulses are felt in the following areas.

    Carotid:
    Femoral:
    Radial:

55. There are 2 methods for assessing a blood pressure. _____ is more accurate than measuring by _____.

56. The systolic pressure reading is usually _____ mm Hg lower than the same reading obtained by palpation.

57. For each of the following conditions, indicate the skin color and condition the EMT would expect to find.

    Normal skin:
    Fever:
    Shock:

58. Identify the following pupils as:

    _____ Normal
    _____ Unequal
    _____ Dilated
    _____ Constricted

    A.

    B.

    C.

    D.

59. From the following diagram, place the appropriate letter indicating the pulse points used for assessment.

    _____ Brachial
    _____ Carotid
    _____ Dorsalis pedis
    _____ Femoral
    _____ Popliteal
    _____ Radial
    _____ Right common iliac

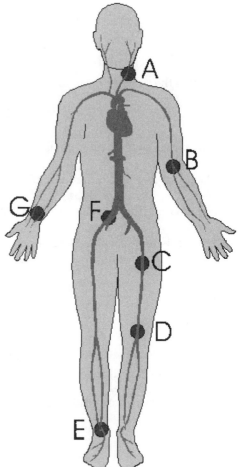

60. What does the mnemonic SAMPLE stand for? When is it used?

S:
A:
M:
P:
L:
E:

Chapter Quiz
· ·

1. The correct order for performing the first three steps of patient assessment is:
   A. Initial assessment, scene size-up, ongoing assessment
   B. Scene size-up, initial assessment, detailed physical examination
   C. Scene size-up, initial assessment, rapid, focused history and physical examination
   D. Initial assessment, rapid, focused history and physical examination, scene size-up

2. To quickly determine the patient's level of consciousness or responsiveness, the EMT should use the mnemonic:
   A. APGAR
   B. SAMPLE
   C. AVPU
   D. OPQRST

3. When assessing the mental status of an adult patient, you note that the patient does not respond until you apply a painful stimulus. This patient's level of consciousness is best indicated by the letter:
   A. A
   B. V
   C. P
   D. U

4. To check the level of consciousness in a 6-month-old infant who appears drowsy, the EMT should:
   A. Pinch the arms
   B. Perform a sternal rub
   C. Gently pat the baby on his head
   D. Tap the bottom of the feet

5. If the EMT determines that the patient is a priority or that attempted life-saving interventions are not working, he or she should quickly finish the patient assessment and interventions and then transport the patient.
   A. True
   B. False

6. Airway problems require immediate interventions. If an intervention does not work:
   A. Reevaluate the general impression
   B. Consider prompt transportation
   C. Employ triage
   D. Contact the medical director

7. Initial assessment of a 16-year-old diabetic patient reveals adequate breathing. Based on this finding, the EMT should:
   A. Immediately transport the patient
   B. Observe the patient while continuing the initial assessment
   C. Assist ventilations with a BVM
   D. Ventilate the patient without supplemental oxygen

8. The airway of the adult patient without traumatic injury should be opened by the rescuer placing one hand on the forehead and the other hand:
   A. On the larynx
   B. Under the chin
   C. Above the neck
   D. Under the neck

9. If major external bleeding is evident, the EMT should initially control the bleeding with:
   A. Direct pressure
   B. Pressure point
   C. Pressure dressing
   D. Tourniquet

10. Internal bleeding and poor perfusion are suspected based on:
    A. The mechanism of injury
    B. The nature of the illness
    C. Assessment findings
    D. All of the above

11. Cool, clammy extremities may indicate:
    A. Poor perfusion
    B. Hypothermia
    C. Hyperthermia
    D. Hypertension

12. The purpose of the ongoing assessment is to:
    A. Reassess the patient for changes that may require new interventions
    B. Look for omissions and evaluate the effectiveness of earlier interventions
    C. Reassess earlier significant findings
    D. All of the above

13. Critical patients should be reassessed every:
    A. 3 minutes
    B. 5 minutes
    C. 10 minutes
    D. 15 minutes

14. Which of the following is a sign of a patient's illness or injury?
    A. Hemorrhaging
    B. Pain
    C. Nausea
    D. Weakness

15. Which of the following is a symptom of a patient's illness or injury?
    A. Noisy ventilations
    B. Chest pain
    C. Deformity
    D. External bleeding

16. The pulse can be felt wherever a(n) _____ lies close to the skin and can be pressed against any underlying firm tissue.
    A. Vein
    B. Artery
    C. Capillary
    D. Aorta

17. Pulses are most often assessed in the _____ artery in the wrist at the base of the thumb or in the _____ artery on either side of the front of the neck.
    A. Carotid; brachial
    B. Carotid; femoral
    C. Radial; carotid
    D. Femoral; carotid

18. The normal pulse rate for an adult at rest is _____ beats per minute.
    A. 60 to 80
    B. 60 to 100
    C. 100 to 120
    D. 112 to 140

19. If an adult's pulse rate falls below 60 beats per minute, it is called:
    A. Bradycardia
    B. Tachycardia
    C. Dysrhythmia
    D. Arrhythmia

20. An extremely strong pulse is described as being:
    A. Heavy
    B. Bounding
    C. Normal
    D. Thready

21. When the pulse wave feels weak and feeble, the pulse is said to be:
    A. Irregular
    B. Bounding
    C. Thin
    D. Thready

22. Heart beats that are not delivered at constant intervals are described as a(n) _____ pulse.
    A. Inconsistent
    B. Irregular
    C. Thready
    D. Weak

23. When assessing a pulse on a child, count for _____ seconds.
    A. 15
    B. 30
    C. 60
    D. 120

24. The normal ventilatory rate for an adult is _____ breaths per minute.
    A. 10 to 16
    B. 12 to 20
    C. 10 to 30
    D. 16 to 28

25. Respiratory _____ most often refers to the amount of air that is exchanged with each breath.
    A. Quality
    B. Quantity
    C. Rate
    D. Depth

26. If a patient must exert effort to take each breath, ventilations are described as:
    A. Shallow
    B. Labored
    C. Weak
    D. Stridored

27. The pressure exerted on the walls of the arteries as blood is forced through the circulatory system by the contraction of the heart is called the:
    A. Pulse pressure
    B. Diastolic pressure
    C. Systolic pressure
    D. Ventricular pressure

28. Under normal conditions, the most accurate method for assessing blood pressure is:
    A. Percussion
    B. Auscultation
    C. Palpation
    D. Automation

29. Pale skin may indicate:
    A. Shock
    B. Heart attack
    C. Emotional distress
    D. All of the above

30. Cyanosis may indicate poor oxygenation in the blood and is most often described as _____ discoloration of the skin.
    A. Bluish
    B. Yellowish
    C. Reddish
    D. Greenish

31. A red skin color may be caused by:
    A. High blood pressure
    B. Low-grade fever
    C. Extensive blood loss
    D. Liver disease

32. Skin temperature is assessed by touching the patient's skin with the _____ of the hand.
    A. Side
    B. Back
    C. Front
    D. Palm

33. Normally, the patient's pupils will _____ when exposed to bright light.
    A. Dilate
    B. Constrict
    C. Become unequal
    D. Not react

Case Scenario

You are dispatched to a residence for a patient having difficulty breathing. En route to the scene, dispatch informs you that the call came from a 6-year-old boy described as the patient's son. He stated that his mother is lying on the floor and that he can't wake her.

1. From the information given you at dispatch, what is your general impression of the call?

2. How should you prepare for this call?

3. When should you and your partner begin putting a plan of action together?

4. What would be your plan of action for handling this call?

Skill Sheet #1

PATIENT ASSESSMENT/MANAGEMENT – MEDICAL

Start Time: _____

Stop Time: _____   **Date:** _____

Candidate's Name: _____

Evaluator's Name: _____

		Points Possible	Points Awarded
Takes, or verbalizes, body substance isolation precautions		1	
SCENE SIZE-UP			
Determines the scene is safe		1	
Determines the mechanism of injury/nature of illness		1	
Determines the number of patients		1	
Requests additional help if necessary		1	
Considers stabilization of spine		1	
INITIAL ASSESSMENT			
Verbalizes general impression of the patient		1	
Determines responsiveness/level of consciousness		1	
Determines chief complaint/apparent life threats		1	
Assesses airway and breathing	Assessment	1	
	Initiates appropriate oxygen therapy	1	
	Assures adequate ventilation	1	
Assesses circulation	Assesses/controls major bleeding	1	
	Assesses pulse	1	
	Assesses skin (color, temperature and condition)	1	
Identifies priority patients/makes transport decision		1	
FOCUSED HISTORY AND PHYSICAL EXAMINATION/RAPID ASSESSMENT			
Signs and symptoms (*Assess history of present illness*)		1	

Respiratory	Cardiac	Altered Mental Status	Allergic Reaction	Poisoning/ Overdoes	Environmental Emergency	Obstetrics	Behavioral
*Onset? *Provokes? *Quality? *Radiates? *Severity? *Time? *Interventions?	*Onset? *Provokes? *Quality? *Radiates? *Severity? *Time? *Interventions?	*Description of the episode. *Onset? *Duration? *Associated Symptoms? *Evidence of Trauma? *Interventions? *Seizures? *Fever	*History of allergies? *What were you exposed to? *How were you exposed? *Effects? *Progression? *Interventions?	*Substance? *When did you ingest/become exposed? *How much did you ingest? *Over what time period? *Interventions *Estimated weight?	*Source? *Environment? *Duration? *Loss of consciousness? *Effects – general or local?	*Are you pregnant? *How long have you been pregnant? *Pain or contractions? *Bleeding or discharge? *Do you feel the need to push? *Last menstrual period?	*How do you feel? *Determine suicidal tendencies. *Is the patient a threat to self or others? *Is there a medical problem? *Interventions?

		Points Possible	Points Awarded
Allergies		1	
Medications		1	
Past pertinent history		1	
Last oral intake		1	
Event leading to present illness (rule out trauma)		1	
Performs focused physical examination (assesses affected body part/system or, if indicated, completes rapid assessment)		1	
Vitals (obtains baseline vital signs)		1	
Interventions (obtains medical direction or verbalizes standing order for medication interventions and verbalizes proper additional intervention/treatment)		1	
Transport (re-evaluates the transport decision)		1	
Verbalizes the consideration for completing a detailed physical examination		1	
ONGOING ASSESSMENT (verbalized)			
Repeats initial assessment		1	
Repeats vital signs		1	
Repeats focused assessment regarding patient complaint or injuries		1	
	Total:	30	

Critical Criteria

_____ Did not take, or verbalize, body substance isolation precautions when necessary
_____ Did not determine scene safety
_____ Did not obtain medical direction or verbalize standing orders for medical interventions
_____ Did not provide high concentration of oxygen
_____ Did not find or manage problems associated with airway, breathing, hemorrhage or shock (hypoperfusion)
_____ Did not differentiate patient's need for transportation versus continued assessment at the scene
_____ Did detailed or focused history/physical examination before assessing the airway, breathing and circulation
_____ Did not ask questions about the present illness
_____ Administered a dangerous or inappropriate intervention

Skill Sheet #2

● ●

PATIENT ASSESSMENT/MANAGEMENT – TRAUMA

Start Time: _____

Stop Time: _____ **Date:** _____

Candidate's Name: _____

Evaluator's Name: _____

		Points Possible	Points Awarded
Takes, or verbalizes, body substance isolation precautions		1	
SCENE SIZE-UP			
Determines the scene is safe		1	
Determines the mechanism of injury		1	
Determines the number of patients		1	
Requests additional help if necessary		1	
Considers stabilization of spine		1	
INITIAL ASSESSMENT			
Verbalizes general impression of the patient		1	
Determines responsiveness/level of consciousness		1	
Determines chief complaint/apparent life threats		1	
Assesses airway and breathing	Assessment	1	
	Initiates appropriate oxygen therapy	1	
	Assures adequate ventilation	1	
	Injury management	1	
Assesses circulation	Assesses/controls major bleeding	1	
	Assesses pulse	1	
	Assesses skin (color, temperature and condition)	1	
Identifies priority patients/makes transport decision		1	
FOCUSED HISTORY AND PHYSICAL EXAMINATION/RAPID TRAUMA ASSESSMENT			
Selects appropriate assessment (focused or rapid assessment)		1	
Obtains, or directs assistance to obtain, baseline vital signs		1	
Obtains S.A.M.P.L.E history		1	
DETAILED PHYSICAL EXAMINATION			
Assesses the head	Inspects and palpates the scalp and ears	1	
	Assesses the eyes	1	
	Assesses the facial areas including oral and nasal areas	1	
Assesses the neck	Inspects and palpates the neck	1	
	Assesses for JVD	1	
	Assesses for trachael deviation	2	
Assesses the chest	Inspects	1	
	Palpates	1	
	Auscultates	1	
Assesses the abdomen/pelvis	Assesses the abdomen	1	
	Assesses the pelvis	1	
	Verbalizes assessment of genitalia/perineum as needed	1	
Assesses the extremities	1 point for each extremity includes inspection, palpation, and assessment of motor, sensory and circulatory function	4	
Assesses the posterior	Assesses thorax	1	
	Assesses lumbar	1	
Manages secondary injuries and wounds appropriately 1 point for appropriate management of the secondary injury/wound		1	
Verbalizes re-assessment of the vital signs		1	
	Total:	40	

Critical Criteria

_____ Did not take, or verbalize, body substance isolation precautions

_____ Did not determine scene safety

_____ Did not assess for spinal protection

_____ Did not provide for spinal protection when indicated

_____ Did not provide high concentration of oxygen

_____ Did not find, or manage, problems associated with airway, breathing, hemorrhage or shock (hypoperfusion)

_____ Did not differentiate patient's need for transportation versus continued assessment at the scene

_____ Did other detailed physical examination before assessing the airway, breathing and circulation

_____ Did not transport patient within (10) minute time limit

Answer Key

Key Terms

1. F, E, A, H, D, C, J, G, B, I
2. Sign
3. Symptom
4. Constriction
5. Dilation
6. Systolic
7. Triage
8. D, J, A, G, R, C, L, N, M, I, F, H, O, E, P, K, Q, B

Content Review

1. The patient assessment determines what patient management is necessary. If done incorrectly and incorrect results obtained, management of the patient may be incorrect and the patient's outcome poor.
2. 1) Does the EMT have the necessary training and/or experience to handle the unsafe scene?
   2) Does the EMT have the necessary equipment required to manage the unsafe situation?
   3) Does the EMT have the necessary trained personnel to manage the unsafe scene?
3. Stop, leave the scene, and wait for it to become safe again. If possible without compromising the safety of himself or others, the EMT-B should try to take the patient to a safe area in order to provide emergency care.
4. Latex gloves
5. The mechanism of injury describes how the energy of motion is transferred to an individual resulting in injury. It is estimated that identifying the mechanism of injury allows the EMT to predict up to 90% of the potential injuries a patient will experience.
6. A. No or minor injuries to the patient
   B. Significant injury to the patient's head, chest, neck, and/or abdomen
   C. Injury to the ribs (flail chest, pulmonary contusion, pneumothorax), pelvis; ruptured liver or spleen, cervical injury, spinal cord injury, head injury, clavicular injury if arm was sticking out
   D. Spinal injury, internal injuries, fractures (depending on the area landed on)
   E. Injury to the femur, pelvis, and lower spine
7. 1) The patient; 2) observations from the scene; 3) family members; 4) bystanders; 5) other emergency responders.
8. The rapid evaluation of a patient's major body systems to identify life-threatening problems, initiate interventions, identify priority patient, and determine whether immediate transport is necessary.
9. Eyes (seeing); hands (feeling); ears (hearing); nose (smelling)
10. 1) A = airway; 2) B = breathing or ventilation; 3) C = circulation or perfusion; 4) D = disability (AVPU); 5) E = expose patient for rapid focused exam and detailed examination.
11. As soon as it is detected.
12. The airway is open and functional
13. Prepare the patient for immediate transport and consider possible ALS rendezvous en route.
14. 12; 20
15. The circulatory system is working well enough to supply the most distant parts of the body.
16. The body may have begun shunting blood from the extremities to more central parts of the body, indicating poor perfusion due to possible circulatory system problems (heart, vascular system, or blood volume), or there may be an injury to the arm causing compression of the blood vessels.
17. False
18. O: onset (when did it start); P: provocation (what makes it worse); Q: quality (how does it feel); R: radiation (does it move); S: severity (how mad does it feel); T: time (how long has it hurt). It is used to further evaluate a patient's chief complaint.

19. Determining the mechanism of injury; examination of the head, neck, chest abdomen, pelvis, extremities, and back; accurate assessment of vital signs.
20. Patient history
21. Assessment of vital signs; facial expression and eyes; examination of neck, chest, abdomen, pelvis, extremities, and back
22. To find life-threatening problems and provide appropriate interventions.
23. It reflects the patient's level of interest and interactions with the environment, thereby providing clues about the severity of a patient's illness.
24. Neck: distended neck veins, swelling, tightening of neck muscles (during respirations)
    Chest: uneven movement, evidence of labored breathing (retractions or abdominal breathing)
    Abdomen: distention, tenderness, firmness, lumps, pregnancy (if female patient)
    Pelvis: if in labor, check perineum for evidence of imminent delivery
    Extremities: skin (cool, clammy = poor circulation), movement, edema (swelling)
    Back: edema, pain, movement
25. False
26. 1) Auscultation; 2) palpation
27. A: alert; V: verbal; P: painful; U: unresponsive. It describes a patient's level of responsiveness.
28. 60
29. 100
30. Systolic; diastolic
31. Wherever an artery lies close to the skin and can be pressed against firm tissue such as bone or cartilage
32. Newborn: 130 to 140; infant: 100 to 120; child: 80 to 100; adult: 60 to 100
33. 100; tachycardia
34. 60; bradycardia
35. Count the number of beats for 30 seconds and multiply by 2. If experienced, count for 15 seconds and multiply by 4.
36. Count the number of beats for 60 seconds.
37. Count the number of beats for 60 seconds.
38. Bounding
39. Thready
40. Irregular
41. Ventilatory rate
42. Infant: 25 to 30 breaths per minute
    Adult:12 to 20 breaths per minute
43. Shallow
44. Labored
45. mm Hg
46. Diastolic
47. Systolic
48. Pulse pressure
49. 120/80 mm Hg
50. 100 + Age = Systolic pressure to 150 mm Hg
51. 8 to 10; lower
52. 14
53. 60 to 90
54. Carotid: 60 mm Hg
    Femoral: 70 mm Hg
    Radial: 80 mm Hg
55. Auscultation; palpation
56. 10
57. Normal skin: pink, warm, and dry
    Fever: flushed, very hot, and dry
    Shock: pale, cold and moist

58. D, C, A, B
59. A. carotid
    B. brachial
    C. femoral
    D. popliteal
    E. dorsalis pedis
    F. right common iliac
    G. radial
60. S: signs and symptoms; A: allergies; M: medications; P: pertinent past medical history; L: last oral intake; E: events leading to current illness or injury

Chapter Quiz

1. C	7. B	13. B	19. A	24. B	29. D
2. C	8. B	14. A	20. B	25. D	30. A
3. C	9. A	15. B	21. D	26. B	31. A
4. D	10. D	16. B	22. B	27. C	32. B
5. B	11. A	17. C	23. C	28. B	33. B
6. B	12. D	18. B			

Case Scenario

1. The patient could be suffering from any number of medical conditions or from an injury that caused her to become unconscious.

2. Prepare for the worst (CPR); know that the son will be concerned and may need emotional support.

3. Immediately

4. Establish scene safety; assess the patient and correct any life-threatening problems; perform CPR/AED if necessary; look at the scene for any clues to the situation; interview the son and anyone else around for clues to the problem; look for any prescription bottles that might indicate a significant medical condition; perform a rapid assessment; call for assistance as appropriate; transport per local protocol, performing detailed and on going assessments while en route to the hospital.

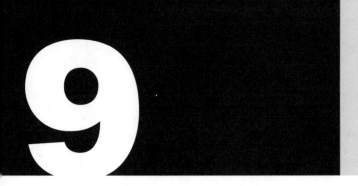

9

Management of Shock

Reading Assignment: Chapter 9 pages 150–176.

DOT Objectives

Upon successful completion of the EMT-Basic training program, the EMT-Basic should be able to do the following:

- Describe the structure and function of the circulatory system and its most important structures: the heart, arteries, veins, and capillaries.
- Identify and demonstrate methods of emergency medical care for internal and external bleeding.
- Explain the relationship between body substance isolation and bleeding, and identify the measures that must be taken by the EMT-Basic for self-protection and patient protection.
- Identify the relationship between airway management and the trauma patient.
- Identify the relationship between mechanism of injury and causes of internal bleeding.
- Identify the signs and symptoms of internal bleeding.
- State the principles of treatment for the patient with signs and symptoms of shock.
- Differentiate between arterial and venous bleeding.
- List the signs and symptoms of shock (hypoperfusion).
- Demonstrate direct pressure as a method of emergency medical care of external bleeding.
- Demonstrate the use of diffuse pressure as a method of emergency medical care of external bleeding.
- Demonstrate the use of pressure points and tourniquets as a method of emergency medical care of external bleeding.
- Demonstrate the care of the patient exhibiting signs and symptoms of internal bleeding.
- Demonstrate the care of the patient exhibiting signs and symptoms of shock (hypoperfusion).

Supplemental Objectives

- Describe the difference of the systemic and circulatory systems.
- Define cardiac output and stroke volume.
- Describe and differentiate between aerobic and anaerobic metabolism.
- Describe the Fick principle.
- List the indications and contraindications for PASG use.
- Identify the importance of checking the pulse at various locations to assess the patient.
- Describe the relationship of cellular energy production in shock.

Key Terms

••

1. Match each of the following terms to their appropriate definitions.

     _____ In the presence of oxygen
     _____ The time it takes for a patient's skin color to return to
          normal after the nailbed has been pressed
     _____ Abnormally low blood pressure
     _____ Away from the core
     _____ Chemical reactions that take place within an organism
          to maintain life
     _____ In the absence of oxygen
     _____ A state of adequate supply of oxygen and nutrients
          to the tissues
     _____ Central part
     _____ A protein that binds to oxygen in red blood cells
          and gives RBCs their color
     _____ The total amount of blood pumped in 1 minute
     _____ Key or critical
     _____ Severe loss of blood
     _____ Expansion of blood vessels
     _____ Contraction of blood vessels

   A. Aerobic
   B. Anaerobic
   C. Capillary refill
   D. Cardiac output
   E. Cardinal
   F. Core
   G. Hemoglobin
   H. Hemorrhage
   I. Hypotension
   J. Metabolism
   K. Perfusion
   L. Periphery
   M. Vasoconstriction
   N. Vasodilation

2. A state of inadequate supply of oxygen and nutrients to tissues is called _____.

3. An injury that is evident immediately to the human eye, usually involving a sharp object or high-velocity weapon is called _____ trauma.

4. A device used to externally vasoconstrict blood vessels to move blood from the periphery to the core of the body is a(n) _____.

5. Failure of the circulatory system to perfuse tissue is called _____.

Content Review

••

1. The position sometimes used to treat shock is the _____ position.

2. The production of energy using oxygen as its driving force is called _____ _____.

3. The term for the production of energy without oxygen is _____.

4. _____ metabolism produces 18 times more energy than _____ metabolism.

5. Explain the significance of anaerobic metabolism.

6. How is anaerobic metabolism stopped?

7. The body is comprised of approximately _____ % fluid.

8. What determines the color of blood?

9. Blood in arteries is what color of red?

10. The average adult blood volume is approximately _____ mL or almost _____ quarts of blood.

11. The average total blood volume for a 1-year-old child is _____ mL.

12. The three organs that can survive for only 6 to 8 minutes using anaerobic metabolism before cells start to die are the _____, _____, and _____.

13. Why does skin become cold in the early stage of shock?

14. What are the three primary causes of shock?
    1)
    2)
    3)

15. What are the three reasons pump failure occurs?
    1)
    2)
    3)

16. What are the five types of true shock?

    1)
    2)
    3)
    4)
    5)

17. The type of "shock" that does not result from decreased perfusion nor cause anaerobic metabolism and is therefore not shock in the true definition is _____ shock also known as _____ _____ shock.

18. A trauma patient who is conscious and breathing on his own should receive how much oxygen?

19. What should you do for a patient who is not breathing on his own?

20. The sudden loss of _____ mL of blood in the adult produces uncompensated shock and is considered severe.

21. The loss of blood over an extended period of time is not as serious as rapid blood loss because it does not create hypoperfusion problems for the patient.
    A. True
    B. False

22. A sudden loss of _____ mL of blood in a child is considered severe.

23. A sudden loss of _____ mL of blood in an infant is considered severe.

24. List the signs of shock.

25. List some symptoms of shock.

26. Which of the following is a late sign of shock?
    A. Increased respirations
    B. Cyanosis
    C. Altered LOC
    D. Decreased blood pressure

27. In adults, _____ % total blood volume must be lost before a decrease in BP occurs.

28. What are the initial steps for management of shock?

29. Identify and give an example of each of the three general categories of shock.

    1)
    2)
    3)

30. General principles of shock management include:

    S:
    H:
    O:
    C:
    K:

31. What is the best treatment for a patient with internal bleeding?

32. In what position should a patient in shock be transported? _____

33. When are PASG helpful?

34. When might PASG be detrimental?

35. When are PASG contraindicated?

36. It is better to transport a patient to a trauma facility further away from the scene than to a closer hospital that is not prepared to definitively treat a traumatic injury.
    A. True
    B. False

Chapter Quiz

• •

1. Aerobic metabolism is the first stage of death.
   A. True
   B. False

2. The kidney and liver can tolerate _____ minutes of ischemia before organ death occurs.
   A. 6 to 8
   B. 30 to 45
   C. 45 to 90
   D. 120 to 180

3. Which type of shock is very seldom seen in the field?
   A. Anaphylactic
   B. Psychogenic
   C. Cardiogenic
   D. Septic

4. A type of shock by which death can occur within minutes is:
   A. Anaphylactic
   B. Psychogenic
   C. Hypovolemic
   D. Septic

5. Prolonged dehydration, such as with diarrhea or vomiting, can cause which type of shock?
   A. Anaphylactic
   B. Neurogenic
   C. Cardiogenic
   D. Hypovolemic

6. Which of the following types of shock usually results in quick recovery?
   A. Anaphylactic
   B. Neurogenic
   C. Psychogenic
   D. Cardiogenic

7. Blood pressure measurement is one of the most important factors in the assessment and identification of shock.
   A. True
   B. False

8. Vasodilation of blood vessels to the lower extremities would result in a(n) _____ blood pressure.
   A. Lowered
   B. Higher
   C. Unchanged
   D. All of the above

9. Neurogenic shock results from:
   A. Vasodilation
   B. Hypovolemia
   C. Vasoconstriction
   D. Hypervolemia

10. During shock, the body attempts to survive by moving blood to the:
    A. Abdomen and heart from the legs, arms, lungs, and brain
    B. Legs and lungs from the heart, abdomen, and brain
    C. Heart and lungs from the legs, arms, and abdomen
    D. Abdomen and brain from the heart, lungs, legs, and arms

11. Signs of shock include:
    A. Rapid and weak pulse and pale skin
    B. Cold and clammy skin and cyanosis
    C. Increased respiratory rate and decreased level of consciousness
    D. All of the above

12. What is typically considered to be a severe sudden loss of blood in a child?
    A. 50 mL
    B. 100 mL
    C. 250 mL
    D. 500 mL

13. Symptoms of shock include:
    A. Mental confusion and feeling of weakness
    B. Feeling of impending doom and nausea
    C. Vomiting, headache, and thirst
    D. All of the above

14. The initial steps for management of shock include:
    A. Establishing and maintaining a patent airway
    B. Administering high-flow oxygen and bleeding control
    C. Managing hypotension and immediate transport
    D. All of the above

15. A trauma patient that is conscious and breathing on his own should be provided with oxygen via a:
    A. Nonrebreather mask at 15 L/minute flow
    B. Nonrebreather mask at 5 L/minute flow
    C. BVM at 15 L/minute flow
    D. Nasal cannula at 5 L/minute flow

16. What is generally considered to be a severe sudden loss of blood in an infant?
    A. 50 mL
    B. 100 mL
    C. 150 mL
    D. 250 mL

17. Even though the Trendelenburg position uses gravity to assist in core perfusion, it increases pressure on the diaphragm and moves the abdominal organs against the diaphragm, making ventilations more labored and difficult for the patient in crisis.
    A. True
    B. False

18. Indications for use of the PASG include:
    A. Severe hypertension
    B. Profoundly low blood pressure
    C. Pulmonary edema
    D. All of the above

19. Which of the following are contraindications for the use of the PASG?
    A. Objects impaled in a site that would be covered
    B. Pregnancy
    C. Pulmonary edema
    D. All of the above

20. Medical direction is ultimately responsible for the selection of the most appropriate treatment facility for a patient.
    A. True
    B. False

21. Steps for managing shock include which of the following?
    A. Establishing a patent airway
    B. Administering low-flow oxygen
    C. Placing the patient in a prone position
    D. Giving fluids by mouth

22. The cardinal sign of shock is:
    A. Hypertension
    B. Hypoperfusion
    C. Hypotension
    D. Perfusion

23. Metabolism that occurs in the presence of oxygen is best described as:
    A. Acidic
    B. Aerobic
    C. Anaerobic
    D. Apneic

Case Scenario

You are on the scene of a patient who fell approximately 15 feet from a roof. He is lying on his stomach (the way in which he landed) and is not responding. You note blood coming from his mouth. His right leg is deformed and he has numerous abrasions. With spinal precautions, you carefully turn the patient to examine his abdomen and note rigidity and a contusion on the RUQ of his abdomen. Ventilations are asymmetrical. He has a bone protruding from his left thigh. Vital signs are as follows: BP = 90/60 mm Hg; pulse = 110 and weak; ventilations = 32 and shallow with no breath sounds heard on the right side.

1. What major body systems may be involved as a result of these injuries?

2. What organs may be involved as a result of these injuries?

3. What bones may be involved as a result of these injuries?

4. What injuries would you suspect this patient has suffered?

5. When should you perform a detailed examination on this patient?

Skill Sheet #3

• •

BLEEDING CONTROL/SHOCK MANAGEMENT

Start Time: _____

Stop Time: _____   **Date:** _____

Candidate's Name: _____

Evaluator's Name: _____

	Points Possible	Points Awarded
Takes, or verbalizes, body substance isolation precautions	1	
Applies direct pressure to the wound	1	
Elevates the extremity	1	
Note: The examiner must now inform the candidate that the wound continues to bleed.		
Applies an additional dressing to the wound	1	
Note: The examiner must now inform the candidate that the wound still continues to bleed. The second dressing does not control the bleeding.		
Locates and applies pressure to appropriate arterial pressure point	1	
Note: The examiner must now inform the candidate that the bleeding is controlled.		
Bandages the wound	1	
Note: The examiner must now inform the candidate the patient is now showing signs and symptoms indicative of hypoperfusion.		
Properly positions the patient	1	
Applies high-concentration oxygen	1	
Initiates steps to prevent heat loss from the patient	1	
Indicates the need for immediate transportation	1	
Total:	10	

Critical Criteria

_____ Did not take, or verbalize, body substance isolation precautions

_____ Did not apply a high concentration of oxygen

_____ Applied a tourniquet before attempting other methods of bleeding control

_____ Did not control hemorrhage in a timely manner

_____ Did not indicate a need for immediate transportation

Skill Sheet #4

· ·

PNEUMATIC ANTISHOCK GARMENT (PASG)

Start Time: _____

Stop Time: _____   **Date:** _____

Candidate's Name: _____

Evaluator's Name: _____

	Points Possible	Points Awarded
Takes, or verbalizes, body substance isolation precautions	1	
Determines that the criteria for use of PASG are met	1	
Removes clothing or ensures that no sharp objects will come in contact with PASG	1	
Assesses areas that will be covered by PASG (abdomen, pelvis, lower extremities)	4	
Secures PASG around patient in a manner that does not compromise integrity of the spine and does not cause respiratory compromise	1	
Ensures top of garment is positioned below level of lowest rib	1	
Wraps left leg of garment around patient's left leg and secures in place	1	
Wraps right leg of garment around patient's right leg and secures in place	1	
Wraps abdominal section and secures in place	1	
Attaches hoses	1	
Assesses vital signs	1	
Inflates garment using foot pump per local protocol	1	
Verbalizes when to stop inflation sequence	1	
Closes appropriate valves; disconnects hoses	2	
Reassesses vital signs	1	
Total:	19	

Critical Criteria

_____ Did not take, or verbalize, body substance isolation precautions

_____ Inflated abdominal section of PASG before lower extremities

_____ Positioned PASG above level of lowest rib

_____ Accidental deflation of PASG occurred after inflation

_____ Did not assess patient's vital signs before inflation of PASG

_____ Did not assess patient's vital signs after inflation of PASG

_____ Did not assess areas covered by the PASG (abdomen, pelvis, or lower extremities)

_____ Applied the garment in a manner that compromised the integrity of the spinal column, resulted in respiratory compromise, or other potential injury to the patient

Answer Key

Key Terms
1. A, C, I, L, J, B, K, F, G, D, E, H, N, M
2. Hypoperfusion
3. Penetrating
4. Pneumatic antishock garment (PASG)
5. Shock

Content Review
1. Trendelenburg
2. Aerobic metabolism
3. Anaerobic metabolism
4. Aerobic; anaerobic
5. Prolonged anaerobic metabolism produces cell death. Death of a critical mass of cells within an organ produces organ death. Death of critical organs produces patient death.
6. By making sure the body delivers enough oxygen to cells so they can produce energy for the body.
7. 60
8. The amount of oxygen the blood carries
9. Bright red
10. 5000; 5
11. 800
12. Heart; brain; lungs
13. The body redirects the blood from the periphery to the core
14. 1) Pump failure; 2) container failure; and 3) volume failure.
15. 1) A decrease in the ability of the heart muscle to contract; 2) disturbances in heart rate and rhythm (dysrhythmias); 3) a decrease in the ability to receive blood and to pump blood.
16. 1) Hypovolemic; 2) cardiogenic; 3) psychogenic; 4) septic; and 5) anaphylactic.
17. Spinal; neurogenic
18. 15 L/min flow via a nonrebreather mask
19. Administer support ventilations with a BVM with oxygen reservoir at a rate of 15 L/min
20. 2000 (2 L)
21. True
22. 500
23. 150
24. Increased ventilations (20 to 30/min); rapid, weak pulse; pale or cyanotic skin; cold and clammy or diaphoretic skin; decreased level of consciousness; decreased blood pressure; increased ventilations; increased capillary refill time; evidence of major blood volume
25. headache, confusion, feeling of weakness, feeling of impending doom, nausea
26. D
27. 25
28. Establish a patent airway; administer high-concentration oxygen; control bleeding; manage hypotension; transport
29. 1) Medical—from dehydration (diarrhea, vomiting, or GI hemorrhage); 2) cardiac — from cardiac failure; 3) trauma — from external or internal hemorrhage due to a traumatic injury

30. S: Secure the airway.
    H: Heat conservation in the body to decrease energy production (keep the patient warm).
    O: Oxygenation of RBCs to replace tissue deficit (give the patient high-flow O_2).
    C: Core perfusion improvement by elevation of lower extremities.
    K: Keep field time as short as possible by transporting quickly to an appropriate medical facility.
31. High-concentration oxygen and rapid transport to a trauma center
32. Trendelenburg
33. For patients requiring control of blood loss, management of pelvic instability, and during prolonged transport times
34. Patients with penetrating thoracic trauma or with short transport times
35. For patients with pulmonary edema, traumatic diaphragmatic herniation, or known hemorrhage above the diaphragm
36. True

Chapter Quiz

1. B	6. C	11. D	16. C	21. A
2. C	7. B	12. D	17. A	22. B
3. D	8. A	13. D	18. B	23. B
4. A	9. A	14. D	19. D	
5. D	10. C	15. A	20. A	

Case Scenario

1. Musculoskeletal, integumentary, nervous, cardiovascular, and respiratory systems
2. Brain, skin, liver, and lungs
3. Ribs and right femur
4. Possible internal hemorrhage, chest injury, fractured femur, possible c-spine injury, and concussion
5. This patient is in shock and should receive only an initial assessment and then the rapid focused physical examination on the scene. A detailed examination would occur en route to the hospital, if time permits and the patient does not require life-saving skills en route. Performing life-saving skills and on-going assessment will take precedence. However, if time and conditions permit, the detailed examination should be completed en route to the hospital.

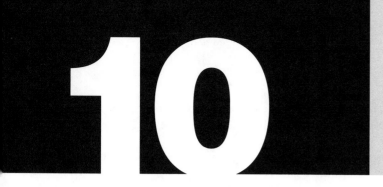

Airway Management and Ventilation

Reading Assignment: Chapter 10 pages 177–211.

DOT Objectives

Upon successful completion of the EMT-Basic training program, the EMT-Basic should be able to do the following:

- Identify major respiratory structures and relate these structures to the function of the respiratory system.
- Identify indications for and proper use of common airway equipment, including the pocket mask, bag-valve-mask device, nasopharyngeal and oropharyngeal airway.
- Describe techniques for opening and protecting the airway, including the head-tilt chin-lift, jaw thrust, and Sellick maneuvers.
- Describe the importance of suctioning equipment, and demonstrate proper suctioning techniques.
- List the signs of adequate breathing.
- List the signs of inadequate breathing.
- Relate mechanisms of injury to opening the airway.
- Describe the steps in performing the skill of artificially ventilating a patient with a bag-valve- mask while using the jaw thrust.
- List the parts of a bag-valve-mask system
- Describe the steps in performing the skill of artificially ventilating a patient with a bag-valve- mask for one and two rescuers.
- Describe the signs of adequate assisted ventilation using the bag-valve-mask.
- Describe the signs of inadequate assisted ventilation using the bag-valve-mask.
- Define and describe the steps in providing mouth-to-mouth assisted ventilation with body substance isolation (barrier shields).
- Define and describe the assembly of a bag-valve-mask unit.
- Define and describe how to artificially ventilate a patient using a stoma.
- Define and describe how to insert an oropharyngeal (oral) airway.
- Define and describe how to insert a nasopharyngeal (nasal) airway.
- Define and describe the correct operation of oxygen tanks and regulators.
- Define and describe the use of a nonrebreather face mask and state the oxygen flow requirements needed for its use.
- Define and describe the use of a nasal cannula and state the flow requirements needed for its use.
- Define and describe how to artificially ventilate the infant and child patient.
- Define and describe oxygen administration for the infant and child patient.

Supplemental Objectives

- Explain why assisted ventilation and airway management skills take priority over most other basic life-support skills.
- Assess whether a patient is breathing adequately, and appropriately manage a patient who needs ventilatory assistance.
- Explain the rationale for giving a high-inspired oxygen concentration to patients who need it, even if there is a possibility of depression of ventilatory drive.

Key Terms

1. Match the following terms with their definitions.

_____ Fine breath sounds simulated by rubbing hair between the fingers	A. Agonal ventilations
_____ Low-pitched bubbling sounds produced by fluid in the lower airways	B. Apnea
_____ Complete lack of ventilations	C. Aspiration
_____ Sweating skin	D. Crackles
_____ A collection of air in the pleural space	E. Diaphoretic
_____ A incision made into the trachea through the neck below the vocal cords to gain access to the airway	F. Dyspnea
_____ Occasional, gasping breaths just before death	G. Hemopneumothorax
_____ Accumulation of blood and fluid in the pleural cavity	H. Hemothorax
_____ The amount of air inhaled in 1 minute	I. Hyperventilation
_____ A sign of respiratory distress marked by inward pulling of skin above the clavicles with inspiration	J. Hypoventilation
_____ A maneuver designed to prevent passive aspiration during artificial ventilation	K. Minute ventilation
_____ The accidental inhalation of fluid or other particles in the lower airway	L. Pneumothorax
_____ High-pitched sounds heard when air moves through constricted airways	M. Rales
_____ Shortness of breath or difficulty breathing	N. Retractions
_____ A process of increasing minute ventilations above normal	O. Sellick maneuver
_____ Collection of blood and air in the pleural space	P. Tracheostomy
_____ Lowered minute ventilation	Q. Wheezing

2. Widening of the nostrils that occurs during inhalation in patients with respiratory distress is called
_____.

3. The area in the lungs that contains air that is inhaled but does not reach the alveoli for exchange, usually about 150 mL in volume, is called _____.

4. The thin membrane that covers the lungs and lines the thoracic cavity is called the _____
_____.

5. The muscles located between the ribs that lift the ribs upward and outward during inhalation are the _____ muscles.

6. A potential space between the two layers surrounding the lungs is called the _____ _____.

7. A maneuver that opens the airway of an unconscious patient where spinal injury is not suspected is the _____.

8. The division of the lower end of the trachea into the two main stem bronchi is called the _____ _____.

9. The dome-shaped muscle that separates the thoracic cavity from the abdominal cavity is the _____.

10. The bony structure made of ribs, muscle, and cartilage that protects the lungs and vital organs is called the _____ cavity.

11. The volume of air inhaled with each breath is called the _____.

12. An artificially created opening between two passages or between a cavity or passage and the body's surface is called a(n) _____.

Content Review

1. Identify the following components of the thoracic cavity.

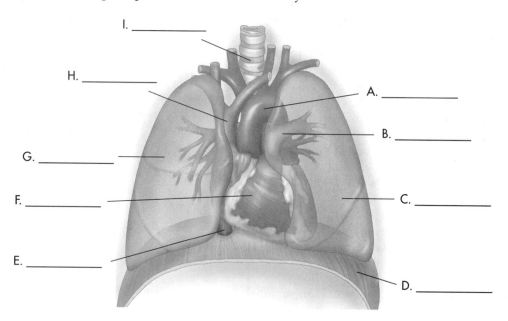

I. _____

H. _____

A. _____

B. _____

G. _____

F. _____

C. _____

E. _____

D. _____

2. Identify the following components of the upper airway.

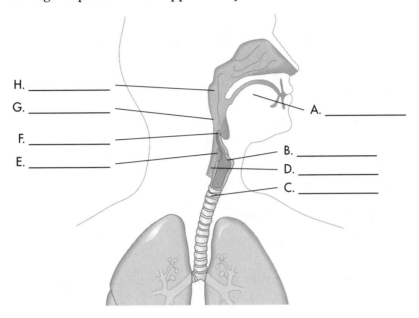

H. _____

G. _____

F. _____

E. _____

A. _____

B. _____

D. _____

C. _____

3. What are the two main functions of the respiratory system?
   1)
   2)

4. The structure that prevents food and liquid from entering the trachea during swallowing is the

   _____.

5. Foreign bodies aspirated into the trachea are more likely to enter the _____ mainstem bronchus than the _____.

6. The small air sacs surrounding capillaries, where the exchange of O_2 for CO_2 takes place, are called

   _____.

7. The lower airway begins at the _____ and extends to the _____

   _____.

8. The upper airway extends from the _____ and the _____

   _____.

9. The lowest (most inferior) part of the pharynx is the _____, where the tongue often collapses, causing an obstruction.

10. The _____ lung has three lobes and the _____ lung has two lobes.

11. What anatomical features make infants and children more susceptible to airway obstruction by foreign bodies and swelling?

12. What are the four primary factors on which the EMT-B should focus when assessing breathing?
   1)
   2)
   3)
   4)

13. The breath sound heard when fluid is collected in the smaller airways, often heard in patients with pneumonia and other infections in the lung, are called _____.

14. The breath sounds heard when areas of collapsed alveoli expand with inhalation or when fluid collects in smaller airways, often referred to as fine crackles, are called _____.

15. Absent breath sounds are a sign of _____.

16. In adults, the tidal volume is normally about _____ mL per breath.

17. The space that stores inhaled air that does not get to the alveoli for gas exchange but rather remains in the upper and lower airways is called the _____ and normally contains approximately _____ mL of air.

18. How is the minute ventilation determined?

19. If a patient is breathing 16 times per minute with a tidal volume of 400 mL per breath, the minute ventilation is _____ mL or _____ L per minute.

20. The most obvious symptom of inadequate breathing is _____.

21. Widening of the nostrils with inspiration, in an attempt to increase the volume of breaths, often seen in infants and children, is called _____.

22. List some of the signs and symptoms that indicate respiratory compromise.

23. The occasional gasping breaths that occur just before death, usually with little or no movement, are called _____.

24. A complete lack of ventilatory effort is called _____.

25. A device used to determine the oxygenation of the tissues of the fingers and toes, as an indicator of the amount of oxygen saturation in the blood, is a(n) _____.

26. Identify the maximum percentage of oxygen delivered by each of the following devices using the optimized oxygen flow rate:
    A. Nasal cannula   _____
    B. Nonrebreather mask   _____
    C. Bag-valve mask without supplemental O_2 _____
    D. BVM with supplemental oxygen   _____
    E BVM with a reservoir   _____

27. What technique should the EMT-B use to open the airway of a patient with a suspected cervical spine injury?

28. What should the EMT-B do if an unconscious patient has dentures?

29. Which type of catheter should be used to suction the mouth and oropharynx of infants, children, and unresponsive adults?

30. When should a soft catheter be used for suctioning?

31. How do you measure a soft catheter?

32. Suction is applied while _____ the catheter for a maximum of _____ seconds.

33. Identify the components of a bag-valve-mask on the following diagram.

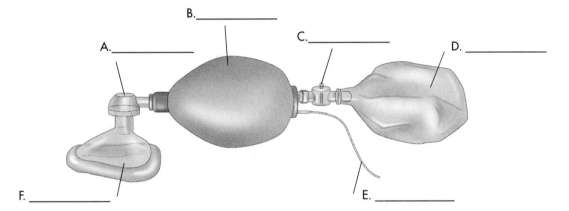

B. _____

A. _____

C. _____

D. _____

F. _____

E. _____

34. To secure the airway of an unresponsive patient, the EMT-B should use a(n) _____
_____.

35. List the steps of inserting an oral airway.

36. How is the proper sized oral airway selected?

37. When is a nasal airway used?

38. How is the correct size of a nasal airway selected?

39. List the steps for inserting a nasal airway.

40. What is the most effective method of artificial ventilation for a single EMT-B?

41. Without supplemental oxygen, a patient receives _____ % oxygen concentration via mouth- to-mask ventilation.

42. Patients with a decreased level of consciousness and ventilatory rate less than _____ or greater than _____ may require assisted ventilations to improve oxygenation.

43. A full oxygen cylinder contains approximately _____ psi.

44. The maximum flow rate for a nasal cannula is _____ L/minute.

45. A patient with COPD should never be given more than 4 L/minute of oxygen via a nasal cannula.
    A. True
    B. False

46. What is the best method of providing high concentration supplemental oxygen to a spontaneously breathing prehospital patient?

Chapter Quiz

1. The lowest (most inferior) part of the pharynx is called the:
   A. Hypopharynx
   B. Lungs
   C. Oropharynx
   D. Nasopharynx

2. The most common cause of an obstructed airway in an unconscious patient is the:
   A. Saliva
   B. Mucous
   C. Tongue
   D. Teeth

3. A leaf-shaped structure located just above the larynx that prevents food and liquids from entering the trachea during swallowing is called the:
   A. Epiglottis
   B. Oropharynx
   C. Carina
   D. Tongue

4. The division where the trachea divides into the left and right mainstem bronchi is called the:
   A. Carina
   B. Larynx
   C. Adam's apple
   D. Thyroid cartilage

5. The term used to describe the accidental inhalation of liquids or solids into the lower airway is _____
   _____.
   A. Regurgitation
   B. Asphyxiation
   C. Aspiration
   D. Exsanguination

6. The small air sacs with thin walls surrounded by capillaries are called:
   A. Alveoli
   B. Protein
   C. RBCs
   D. Venules

7. Nasal airways are less likely to stimulate the gag reflex than are oral airways.
   A. True
   B. False

8. The head-tilt chin-lift maneuver is used to open the airway in patients without a suspected spinal injury.
   A. True
   B. False

9. To perform a jaw thrust maneuver, the EMT kneels behind the patient, and while maintaining cervical immobilization, the EMT thrusts the jaw:
   A. Forward
   B. Downward
   C. Backward
   D. Sideways

10. A patient requires suctioning whenever:
    A. Other attempts to clear the airway fail
    B. A gurgling sound is heard during breathing
    C. Fluid is seen in the airway of an unconscious patient
    D. All of the above

11. Suction is applied while withdrawing the catheter for a maximum of _____ seconds.
    A. 10
    B. 15
    C. 30
    D. 25

12. The proper size oropharyngeal airway is selected by measuring from the:
    A. Corner of the mouth to the angle of the jaw
    B. Corner of the eye to the tip of the nose
    C. Corner of the ear to the tip of the chin
    D. All of the above

13. The proper size nasopharyngeal airway is selected by measuring from the:
    A. Tip of the nose to the tip of the ear
    B. Corner of the eye to the tip of the nose
    C. Corner of the ear to the tip of the chin
    D. All of the above

14. Mouth-to-mask ventilation is the most effective method of artificial ventilation for a single rescuer.
    A. True
    B. False

15. Increasing minute ventilation above normal is called:
    A. Hyperventilation
    B. Hypoventilation
    C. Hypertension
    D. Ventilation escalation

16. The pressure of a full cylinder of oxygen is approximately _____ psi.
    A. 1000
    B. 2000
    C. 3000
    D. 4000

17. The appropriate BVM for prehospital care use consists of all of the following *except:*
    A. Face mask
    B. One-way valve
    C. Self-inflating bag and oxygen reservoir
    D. Working pop-off valve

18. Because of the difficulty of maintaining an airtight seal while squeezing the bag, a single EMT should perform mouth-to-mask ventilation before using the BVM alone.
    A. True
    B. False

19. When opening an infant's airway and administering oxygen, the neck should be kept in a _____ _____ position.
    A. Extended
    B. Hyperextended
    C. Neutral
    D. Hyperflexed

20. Any cylinder that contains oxygen is _____ in color.
    A. Red
    B. Green
    C. Brown
    D. Black

21. The maximum flow rate with the nasal cannula is:
    A. 5 to 6 L/min
    B. 8 to 10 L/min
    C. 2 to 4 L/min
    D. 10 to 12 L/min

22. Patients with acute respiratory distress should be given high concentrations of oxygen with a nonrebreather mask, even if they have a history of chronic obstructive pulmonary disease.
    A. True
    B. False

23. With a flow rate of 15 L/min, a nonrebreather mask can deliver up to _____ % oxygen.
    A. 40
    B. 50
    C. 60
    D. 90

24. The symptom shortness of breath is called:
    A. Eupnea
    B. Orthopnea
    C. Tachypnea
    D. Dyspnea

Case Scenario

You are called to the scene of a 68-year-old female patient who is unresponsive, lying in bed, and attached to oxygen at 4 L/minute via a nasal cannula. On auscultation of lung sounds, you note rales bilaterally. The patient's ventilations are 38 and shallow, her skin is pale, and her lips cyanotic. The patient's daughter informs you that the patient has a history of COPD.

1. How would you treat this patient?

2. You have an oral airway in place when the patient begins to gag. What should you do?

Skill Sheet #5

• •

AIRWAY, OXYGEN AND VENTILATION SKILLS
UPPER AIRWAY ADJUNCTS AND SUCTION

Start Time: _____

Stop Time: _____   **Date:** _____

Candidate's Name: _____

Evaluator's Name: _____

OROPHARYNGEAL AIRWAY	Points Possible	Points Awarded
Takes, or verbalizes, body substance isolation precautions	1	
Selects appropriately sized airway	1	
Measures airway	1	
Inserts airway without pushing the tongue posteriorly	1	
Note: The examiner must advise the candidate that the patient is gagging and becoming conscious		
Removes the oropharyngeal airway	1	

SUCTION

Note: The examiner must advise the candidate to suction the patient's airway		
Turns on/prepares suction device	1	
Assures presence of mechanical suction	1	
Inserts the suction tip without suction	1	
Applies suction to the oropharynx/nasopharynx	1	

NASOPHARYNGEAL AIRWAY

Note: The examiner must advise the candidate to insert a nasopharyngeal airway		
Selects appropriately sized airway	1	
Measures airway	1	
Verbalizes lubrication of the nasal airway	1	
Fully inserts the airway with the bevel facing toward the septum	1	
Total:	13	

Critical Criteria

_____ Did not take, or verbalize, body substance isolation precautions

_____ Did not obtain a patent airway with the oropharyngeal airway

_____ Did not obtain a patent airway with the nasopharyngeal airway

_____ Did not demonstrate an acceptable suction technique

_____ Inserted any adjunct in a manner dangerous to the patient

Skill Sheet #6

....

MOUTH TO MASK WITH SUPPLEMENTAL OXYGEN

Start Time: _____

Stop Time: _____ **Date:** _____

Candidate's Name: _____

Evaluator's Name: _____

	Points Possible	Points Awarded
Takes, or verbalizes, body substance isolation precautions	1	
Connects one-way valve to mask	1	
Opens patient's airway or confirms patient's airway is open (manually or with adjunct)	1	
Establishes and maintains a proper mask to face seal	1	
Ventilates the patient at the proper volume and rate *(800-1200 mL per breath/10-20 breaths per minute)*	1	
Connects the mask to high concentration of oxygen	1	
Adjusts flow rate to at least 15 L/minute	1	
Continues ventilation of the patient at the proper volume and rate *(800-1200 mL per breath/10-20 breaths per minute)*	1	
Note: The examiner must witness ventilations for at least 30 seconds		
Total:	8	

Critical Criteria

_____ Did not take, or verbalize, body substance isolation precautions

_____ Did not adjust liter flow to at least 15 L/minute

_____ Did not provide proper volume per breath
(more than 2 ventilations per minute were below 800 mL)

_____ Did not ventilate the patient at a rate of 10 to 20 breaths per minute

_____ Did not allow for complete exhalation

skill sheet #7

BAG-VALVE-MASK
APNEIC PATIENT

Start Time: _____

Stop Time: _____   **Date:** _____

Candidate's Name: _____

Evaluator's Name: _____

	Points Possible	Points Awarded
Takes, or verbalizes, body substance isolation precautions	1	
Voices opening the airway	1	
Voices inserting an airway adjunct	1	
Selects appropriately sized mask	1	
Creates a proper mask-to-face seal	1	
Ventilates patient at no less than 800 mL volume *The examiner must witness for at least 30 seconds*	1	
Connects reservoir and oxygen	1	
Adjusts liter flow to 15 L/minute or greater	1	
The examiner indicates arrival of a second EMT. The second EMT is instructed to ventilate the patient while the candidate controls the mask and the airway.		
Voices re-opening the airway	1	
Creates a proper mask-to-face seal	1	
Instructs assistant to resume ventilation at proper volume per breath *(The examiner must witness for at least 30 seconds)*	1	
Total:	11	

Critical Criteria

_____ Did not take, or verbalize, body substance isolation precautions

_____ Did not immediately ventilate the patient

_____ Interrupted ventilations for more than 20 seconds

_____ Did not provide a high concentration of oxygen

_____ Did not provide, or direct assistant to provide, proper volume/breath
  (more than 2 ventilations per minute are below 800 mL)

_____ Did not allow adequate exhalation

Skill Sheet #8

. . . .

OXYGEN ADMINISTRATION

Start Time: _____

Stop Time: _____   **Date:** _____

Candidate's Name: _____

Evaluator's Name: _____

	Points Possible	Points Awarded
Takes, or verbalizes, body substance isolation precautions	1	
Assembles the regulator to the tank	1	
Opens the tank	1	
Checks for leaks	1	
Checks tank pressure	1	
Attaches non-rebreather mask to oxygen	1	
Prefills reservoir	1	
Adjusts liter flow to 12 L/minute or greater	1	
Applies and adjusts the mask to the patient's face	1	
Note: The examiner must advise the candidate that the patient is not tolerating the non-rebreather mask. The medical director has ordered you to apply a nasal cannula to the patient.		
Attaches nasal cannula to oxygen	1	
Adjusts liter flow to L/minute or less	1	
Applies nasal cannula to the patient		
Note: The examiner must advise the candidate to discontinue oxygen therapy.		
Removes the nasal cannula from the patient	1	
Shuts off the regulator	1	
Relieves the pressure within the regulator	1	
Total:	15	

Critical Criteria

_____ Did not take, or verbalize, body substance isolation precautions

_____ Did not assemble the tank and regulator without leaks

_____ Did not prefill the reservoir bag

_____ Did not adjust the device to the correct liter flow for the non-rebreather mask (12 L/minute or greater)

_____ Did not adjust the device to the correct liter flow for the nasal cannula (6 L/minute or less)\

Skill Sheet #9

RELIEF OF FOREIGN BODY AIRWAY OBSTRUCTION (FBAO)
Responsive Adult or Child Victim Standing or Sitting

Start Time: _____

Stop Time: _____   **Date:** _____

Candidate's Name: _____

Evaluator's Name: _____

	Points Possible	Points Awarded
Takes or verbalizes body substance isolation precautions	1	
Determines if the victim is choking and obtains consent to intervene	1	
Stands behind the victim, wraps arms around the victim's waist, and makes a fist with one hand	1	
Places the thumb side of the fist against the victim's abdomen, in the midline slightly above the navel and well below the tip of the xiphoid process	1	
Grasps the fist with the other hand and presses the fist into the victim's abdomen with a quick inward and upward thrust	1	
Repeats the thrusts until the object is expelled from the airway or the victim becomes unresponsive	1	
Each new thrust is a separate and distinct movement administered with the intent of relieving the obstruction	1	
Repeats the sequence of attempts (and reattempts) to ventilate, Heimlich maneuver, and tongue-jaw lift and finger sweep until the obstruction is cleared or advanced procedures are available to establish a patent airway	1	
If the FBAO is not removed, follows the procedures for FBAO in an unconscious victim	1	
If the FBAO is removed and the airway is cleared, checks breathing	1	
If the victim is not breathing, provides rescue breaths; then checks for signs of circulation (pulse check and evidence of breathing, coughing, or movement); if there are no signs of circulation, begins chest compression.	1	
If the victim is breathing or resumes effective breathing, places victim in recovery position	1	
Total:	12	

Critical Criteria

_____ Did not take, or verbalize, body substance isolation precautions

_____ Did not determine if victim was choking and obtain consent

_____ Incorrect hand placement

_____ Did not follow the correct sequence

_____ Did not perform the Heimlich maneuver until the FBAO was relieved or the victim became unresponsive

_____ Did not assess breathing or circulation after relieving the FBAO

_____ Did not provide rescue breathing or CPR as necessary after relieving the FBAO

Skill Sheet #10
● ●

RELIEF OF FOREIGN BODY AIRWAY OBSTRUCTION (FBAO)
Adult Victim Found Unresponsive

Start Time: _____

Stop Time: _____   Date: _____

Candidate's Name: _____

Evaluator's Name: _____

	Points Possible	Points Awarded
Takes or verbalizes body substance isolation precautions	1	
Establishes unresponsiveness	1	
Opens the airway and attempts to provide rescue breaths	1	
If unable to make the chest rise, repositions the victim's head (reopens the airway) and tries to ventilate again	1	
If the victim cannot be ventilated even after attempt to reposition the airway, straddles the victim's knees and performs the Heimlich maneuver (up to 5 times)	1	
After 5 abdominal thrusts, opens the victim's airway using a tongue-jaw lift and performs a finger sweep to remove the object	1	
Repeats the sequence of attempts (and reattempts) to ventilate, Heimlich maneuver, and tongue-jaw lift and finger sweep until the obstruction is cleared or advanced procedures are available to establish a patent airway	1	
If the FBAO is removed and the airway is cleared, checks breathing	1	
If the victim is not breathing, provides rescue breaths; then checks for signs of circulation (pulse check and evidence of breathing, coughing, or movement); if there are no signs of circulation, begins chest compression	1	
If the victim is breathing or resumes effective breathing, places victim in recovery position	1	
Total:	10	

Critical Criteria

_____ Did not take, or verbalize, body substance isolation precautions

_____ Did not establish unresponsiveness

_____ Did not open the victim's airway

_____ Did not establish that the victim was not breathing

_____ Did not attempt to provide rescue breaths

_____ Did not reposition the victim's airway and reattempt to provide rescue breaths

_____ Did not perform the Heimlich maneuver (up to 5 times)

_____ Did not follow the correct sequence

_____ Did not repeat the sequence of attempts (and reattempts) to ventilate, Heimlich maneuver, and tongue-jaw lift and finger sweep until the obstruction was cleared

_____ Did not assess breathing or circulation after relieving the FBAO

_____ Did not provide rescue breathing or CPR as necessary after relieving the FBAO

skill sheet #11

•••

RELIEF OF FOREIGN BODY AIRWAY OBSTRUCTION (FBAO)
Adult Victim Who Becomes Unresponsive

Start Time: _____

Stop Time: _____ Date: _____

Candidate's Name: _____

Evaluator's Name: _____

	Points Possible	Points Awarded
Takes or verbalizes body substance isolation precautions	1	
Establishes unresponsiveness	1	
Performs a tongue-jaw lift, followed by a finger sweep to remove the object	1	
Opens the airway and attempts to ventilate	1	
If unable to make the victim's chest rise, repositions the victim's head and tries to ventilate again	1	
If the chest does not rise with attempted breaths even after repositioning the airway, straddles the victim's thighs and performs the Heimlich maneuver (up to 5 times)	1	
After 5 abdominal thrusts, opens the victim's airway using a tongue-jaw lift and performs a finger sweep to remove the object	1	
Repeats the sequence of attempts (and reattempts) to ventilate, Heimlich maneuver, and tongue-jaw lift and finger sweep until the obstruction is cleared or advanced procedures are available to establish a patent airway	1	
If the FBAO is removed and the airway is cleared, checks breathing	1	
If the victim is not breathing, provides rescue breaths; then checks for signs of circulation (pulse check and evidence of breathing, coughing, or movement); if there are no signs of circulation, begins chest compression	1	
If the victim is breathing or resumes effective breathing, places victim in recovery position	1	
Total:	11	

Critical Criteria

_____ Did not take, or verbalize, body substance isolation precautions

_____ Did not establish unresponsiveness

_____ Did not open the victim's airway

_____ Did not establish that the victim was not breathing

_____ Did not attempt to provide rescue breaths

_____ Did not reposition the victim's airway and reattempt to provide rescue breaths

_____ Did not perform the Heimlich maneuver (up to 5 times)

_____ Did not repeat the sequence of attempts (and reattempts) to ventilate, Heimlich maneuver, and tongue-jaw lift and finger sweep until the obstruction was cleared

_____ Did not assess breathing or circulation after relieving the FBAO

_____ Did not provide rescue breathing or CPR as necessary after relieving the FBAO

Skill Sheet #12

RELIEF OF FOREIGN BODY AIRWAY OBSTRUCTION (FBAO)
Child Victim Found Unresponsive

Start Time: _____

Stop Time: _____   **Date:** _____

Candidate's Name: _____

Evaluator's Name: _____

	Points Possible	Points Awarded
Takes or verbalizes body substance isolation precautions	1	
Establishes unresponsiveness	1	
Opens the airway and attempts to provide rescue breaths	1	
If unable to make the chest rise, repositions the victim's head (reopens the airway) and tries to ventilate again	1	
If the victim cannot be ventilated even after an attempt to reposition the airway, straddles the victim's knees and performs the Heimlich maneuver (up to 5 times)	1	
After 5 abdominal thrusts, opens the victim's airway using a tongue-jaw lift and looks for an object in the pharynx; if an object is visible, performs a finger sweep to remove the object; *DOES NOT* perform a blind finger sweep	1	
Repeats the sequence of attempts (and reattempts) to ventilate, Heimlich maneuver, and tongue-jaw lift, visualize, and finger sweep if appropriate, until the obstruction is cleared or advanced procedures are available to establish a patent airway	1	
If the FBAO is removed and the airway is cleared, checks breathing	1	
If the victim is not breathing, provides rescue breaths; then checks for signs of circulation (pulse check and evidence of breathing, coughing, or movement); if there are no signs of circulation, begins chest compression	1	
If the victim is breathing or resumes effective breathing, places victim in recovery position	1	
Total:	10	

Critical Criteria

_____ Did not take, or verbalize, body substance isolation precautions
_____ Did not establish unresponsiveness
_____ Did not open the victim's airway
_____ Did not establish that the victim was not breathing
_____ Did not attempt to provide rescue breaths
_____ Did not reposition the victims airway and reattempts to provide rescue breaths
_____ Did not perform the Heimlich maneuver
_____ Performed a blind finger sweep
_____ Did not look for an object in the pharynx after abdominal thrusts but before attempting ventilation
_____ Did not follow the correct sequence
_____ Did not assess breathing or circulation after relieving the FBAO
_____ Did not provide rescue breathing or CPR as necessary after relieving the FBAO

Skill Sheet #13

● ●

RELIEF OF FOREIGN BODY AIRWAY OBSTRUCTION (FBAO)
Child Victim Who Becomes Unresponsive

Start Time: _____

Stop Time: _____   **Date:** _____

Candidate's Name: _____

Evaluator's Name: _____

	Points Possible	Points Awarded
Takes or verbalizes body substance isolation precautions	1	
Performs a tongue-jaw lift and looks for an object in the pharynx; if an object is visible, removes it using a finger sweep; *DOES NOT* perform a blind finger sweep	1	
Opens the airway and attempts to ventilate	1	
If unable to make the victim's chest rise, repositions the victim's head and tries to ventilate again	1	
If the chest does not rise with attempted breaths, even after repositioning the airway, straddles the victim's hips and performs the Heimlich maneuver (up to 5 times)	1	
After 5 abdominal thrusts, opens the victim's airway using a tongue-jaw lift and looks for an object in the pharynx; if visible, removes it with a finger sweep	1	
Repeats the sequences of attempts (and reattempts) to ventilate, Heimlich maneuver, and tongue-jaw lift, visualize, and finger sweep, if appropriate, until the obstruction is cleared or advanced procedures are available to establish a patent airway	1	
If the FBAO is removed and the airway is cleared, checks breathing	1	
If the victim is not breathing, provides rescue breaths; then checks for signs of circulation (pulse check and evidence of breathing, coughing, or movement); if there are no signs of circulation, begins chest compression	1	
If the victim is breathing or resumes effective breathing, places victim in recovery position	1	
Total:	11	

Critical Criteria

_____ Did not take, or verbalize, body substance isolation precautions

_____ Did not open victim's airway

_____ Did not visualize for an object before the attempting ventilation

_____ Incorrect hand placement

_____ Did not follow the correct sequence

_____ Performed a blind finger sweep

_____ Did not assess breathing or circulation after relieving the FBAO

_____ Did not provide rescue breathing or CPR as necessary after relieving the FBAO

Skill Sheet #14

RELIEF OF FOREIGN BODY AIRWAY OBSTRUCTION (FBAO)
Infant Victim Who Becomes Unresponsive

Start Time: _____

Stop Time: _____   **Date:** _____

Candidate's Name: _____

Evaluator's Name: _____

	Points Possible	Points Awarded
Takes or verbalizes body substance isolation precautions	1	
Performs a tongue-jaw lift and looks for an object in the pharynx; if an object is visible, removes it using a finger sweep; *DOES NOT* perform a blind finger sweep	1	
Opens the airway and attempts to ventilate	1	
If unable to make the victim's chest rise, repositions the victim's head and tries to ventilate again	1	
If the chest does not rise with attempted breaths, even after repositioning the airway, performs the sequence of up to 5 back blows and up to 5 chest thrusts	1	
Opens the victim's airway using a tongue-jaw lift and looks for an object in the pharynx; if object is visible, removes it	1	
Attempts to ventilate	1	
Repeats the sequences of attempts (and reattempts) to ventilate, up to 5 back blows, up to 5 chest thrusts, open the airway, visualize for an object and finger sweep if appropriate, and attempts to ventilate until the obstruction is cleared or advanced procedures are available to establish a patent airway	1	
If the FBAO is removed and the airway is cleared, checks breathing	1	
If the victim is not breathing, provides rescue breaths; then checks for signs of circulation (pulse check and evidence of breathing, coughing, or movement); if there are no signs of circulation, begins chest compression	1	
If the victim is breathing or resumes effective breathing, places victim in recovery position	1	
Total:	11	

Critical Criteria

_____ Did not take, or verbalize, body substance isolation precautions
_____ Incorrect hand placement
_____ Performed a blind finger sweep
_____ Did not open the victim's airway
_____ Did not perform a tongue-jaw lift and visualize for an object before attempting to ventilate
_____ Did not follow the correct sequence
_____ Did not perform the Heimlich maneuver until FBAO was relieved or the victim became unresponsive
_____ Did not assess breathing or circulation after relieving the FBAO
_____ Did not provide rescue breathing or CPR as necessary after relieving the FBAO

Skill Sheet #15

RELIEF OF FOREIGN BODY AIRWAY OBSTRUCTION (FBAO)
Infant Victim Found Unresponsive

Start Time: _____

Stop Time: _____　　**Date:** _____

Candidate's Name: _____

Evaluator's Name: _____

	Points Possible	Points Awarded
Takes or verbalizes body substance isolation precautions	1	
Establishes unresponsiveness	1	
Opens the airway and attempts to ventilate	1	
If unable to make the victim's chest rise, repositions the victim's head and tries to ventilate again	1	
If the chest does not rise with attempted breaths, even after repositioning the airway, performs the sequence of up to 5 back blows and up to 5 chest thrusts	1	
Opens the victim's airway using a tongue-jaw lift and looks for an object in the pharynx; if the object is visible, removes it	1	
Repeats the sequences of attempts (and reattempts) to ventilate, up to 5 back blows, up to 5 chest thrusts, open the airway, visualize for an object and finger sweep if appropriate, and attempts to ventilate until the obstruction is cleared or advanced procedures are available to establish a patent airway	1	
If the FBAO is removed and the airway is cleared, checks breathing	1	
If the victim is breathing, checks for signs of circulation (pulse check and evidence of breathing, coughing, or movement); if there are no signs of circulation, begins chest compression	1	
If the victim is not breathing, provides rescue breaths	1	
If the victim is breathing and has a pulse, places victim in recovery position	1	
Total:	11	

Critical Criteria

_____ Did not take, or verbalize, body substance isolation precautions

_____ Incorrect hand placement

_____ Performed a blind finger sweep

_____ Did not open the victim's airway

_____ Did not assess for breathing

_____ Did not follow the correct sequence

_____ Did not perform a tongue-jaw lift and visualize for an object before attempting to ventilate

_____ Did not assess breathing or circulation after relieving the FBAO

_____ Did not provide rescue breathing or CPR as necessary after relieving the FBAO

Answer Key

●●●

Key Terms

1. M, D, B, E, L, P, A, H, K, N, O, C, Q, F, I, G, J
2. Nasal flaring
3. Dead space
4. Pleura
5. Intercostal
6. Pleural space
7. Head-tilt chin-lift
8. Carina
9. Diaphragm
10. Thoracic
11. Tidal volume
12. Stoma

Content Review

1. A. Aorta
   B. Pulmonary artery
   C. Left lung
   D. Diaphragm
   E. Inferior vena cava
   F. Heart
   G. Right lung
   H. Superior vena cava
   I. Trachea
2. A. Tongue
   B. Larynx
   C. Trachea
   D. Esophagus
   E. Hypopharynx
   F. Epiglottis
   G. Oropharynx
   H. Nasopharynx
3. 1) It supplies oxygen to the blood, which then carries the oxygen to the body tissues and off loads the oxygen into the cells; and 2) it gets rid of the CO_2 brought back to the lungs by the blood.
4. Epiglottis
5. Right; left
6. Alveoli
7. Cricoid cartilage; lungs
8. Mouth and nose; larynx
9. Hypopharynx
10. Right; left
11. Smaller airways and a proportionally larger tongue
12. 1) Rate; 2) rhythm; 3) quality; and 4) depth.
13. Crackles
14. Rales
15. Lung collapse
16. 500
17. Dead space; 150
18. Tidal volume × ventilatory rate for 1 minute

19. 6400; 6.4
20. Shortness of breath
21. Nasal flaring
22. Shortness of breath; posture (sitting upright and breathing through the mouth instead of the nose); speaking in short sentences; increased ventilatory rate; slow or irregular breathing; nasal flaring; retractions; cool, pale, diaphoretic skin; cyanosis
23. Agonal ventilations
24. Apnea
25. Pulse oximeter
26. A. 45%
    B. 85%
    C. 21%
    D. 40%
    E. 95%
27. Jaw-thrust maneuver
28. Leave them in place unless they are loose or causing airway compromise
29. Rigid
30. To suction the nose, nasopharynx, and other areas that cannot be suctioned with a rigid catheter.
31. From the tip of the patient's nose to the tip of the ear.
32. Withdrawing, 15
33. A. Non-rebreathing valve
    B. Self-inflating bag
    C. Oxygen reservoir valve
    D. Reservoir
    E. High-flow oxygen supply
    F. Face mask
34. Oropharyngeal airway
35. Select the appropriate size airway. Insert upside down and rotate 180 degrees so the flange rests on the patient's teeth (or use a tongue depressor to push the tongue down and forward during insertion).
36. Measure from the corner of the mouth to the angle of the jaw
37. When a patient cannot tolerate an oral airway (gag reflex, facial injury, etc.)
38. Measure from the tip of the patient's nose to the tip of the ear.
39. Select the proper size airway. Lubricate the airway with water-soluble lubricant. Insert the tube into a nostril and advance it posteriorly with the bevel toward the base of the nose or nasal septum.
40. Mouth-to-mask ventilation
41. 16
42. 12; 20
43. 2000
44. 5 to 6
45. False
46. Nonrebreather mask

Chapter Quiz

1. A	6. A	11. B	16. B	21. A
2. C	7. A	12. A	17. D	22. A
3. A	8. A	13. A	18. A	23. D
4. A	9. A	14. A	19. C	24. D
5. C	10. D	15. A	20. B	

Case Scenario

1. Perform an initial assessment; administer high-concentration oxygen immediately; and insert an oral airway. If the patient has a gag reflex, change to a nasal airway. Be prepared to suction as necessary and transport to the closest appropriate facility. Perform a detailed and on-going assessment en route to the hospital.

2. Remove the airway, reassess the patient, and insert a nasal airway, if indicated.

Reading Assignment: Chapter 11 pages 212–234.

DOT Objectives

Upon successful completion of the EMT-Basic training program, providing inclusion of this lesson within the student's course based on Medical Direction, the EMT-Basic should be able to do the following:

- Describe and identify the anatomical structures involved in performing endotracheal intubation in the adult, infant, and child.
- Describe and demonstrate the techniques used for endotracheal intubation in the infant, child, and adult, which include choosing an appropriate-size endotracheal tube, inserting a stylet, using both curved and straight blades for intubation, securing the endotracheal tube, and demonstrating endotracheal suctioning.
- Recognize the complications of advanced airway management, including the consequences of unrecognized esophageal intubation.
- Differentiate between the airway anatomy of the infant, child, and adult.
- Explain the pathophysiology of airway compromise.
- Describe the proper use of airway adjuncts.
- Review the use of oxygen therapy in airway management .
- Describe the indications, contraindications, and technique for insertion of nasal gastric tubes.
- Describe how to perform the Sellick maneuver (cricoid pressure).
- Describe the indications for advanced airway management.
- List the equipment required for orotracheal intubation.
- List complications associated with advanced airway management.
- Describe the skill of orotracheal intubation in the adult patient.
- Describe the skill of orotracheal intubation in the infant and child patient.
- Describe the skill of confirming endotracheal tube placement.
- Describe the skill of securing the endotracheal tube.
- Demonstrate how to perform the Sellick maneuver (cricoid pressure).
- Demonstrate the skill of orotracheal intubation in the adult patient.
- Demonstrate the skill of orotracheal intubation in the infant and child patient.
- Demonstrate the skill of confirming endotracheal tube placement in the adult patient.
- Demonstrate the skill of confirming endotracheal tube placement in the infant and child patient.
- Demonstrate the skill of securing the endotracheal tube in the infant and child patient.

Supplemental Objectives

- Recognize and respect the feelings of the patient and family regarding advanced directives as they apply to endotracheal intubation.
- Describe and demonstrate the skill of confirming endotracheal tube placement, including the use of end-tidal carbon dioxide detection or other detection techniques.
- Explain and recognize the pathophysiology of airway compromise, including the indications and rationale for airway management by EMT-Bs.

Key Terms

1. The area between the umbilicus and the xiphoid process is called the _____.

2. The process of hyperventilating a patient with 100% oxygen prior to attempting endotracheal intubation is called _____.

3. A metal rod inserted into the endotracheal tube to provide stiffness for intubation is called a(n) _____.

4. The structure made of soft tissue that hangs from the roof of the mouth is called the _____.

5. The preferred patient position for ET intubation is the _____ position.

6. The small structure that serves as the posterior attachments for the vocal cords and is located behind the glottic opening on each side of the larynx is the _____.

7. An oxygen-powered device designed to provide artificial ventilation for intubated patients is a(n) _____.

8. The instrument used to visualize the vocal cords for endotracheal tube insertion is called a(n) _____.

9. A tube placed through the nose and esophagus into the stomach is called a _____ tube.

10. Intubation in which the tube is passed through the nose and into the trachea is called _____ intubation.

11. A tube placed through the mouth and esophagus into the stomach is called a(n) _____ tube.

12. The term referring to the relative stiffness of the lungs is _____.

13. A tube placed in the trachea to prevent aspiration and improve oxygenation is a(n) _____.

14. The small balloon that prevents aspiration around an ET tube is called a(n) _____.

Content Review

1. The opening between the vocal cords through which an ET tube is passed is the _____ _____.

2. Identify the following components of the respiratory system.

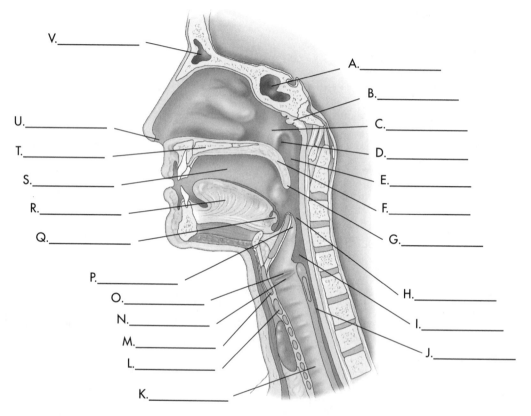

Cricoid cartilage   Internal naris   Oropharynx   Tongue
Epiglottis   Laryngopharynx   Pharyngeal tonsil   True vocal cord
Esophagus   Lingual tonsil   Soft palate   Trachea
External naris   Nasopharynx   Sphenoidal sinus   Uvula
Frontal sinus   Opening of auditory tube   Thyroid cartilage   Vestibular fold
Hard palate   Oral cavity

3. As compliance increases, the lungs become more difficult to artificially ventilate.
   A. True
   B. False

4. Ventilation takes priority over intubation.
   A. True
   B. False

5. The _____ protects the opening of the trachea from aspiration of liquids and foreign material.

6. Identify the following structures within the mouth.
   Lip
   Soft palate
   Uvula
   Hard palate
   Tongue

   A._____ _____

   B._____

   C._____

   D._____

   E._____

7. Identify the following components of the larynx as seen during endotracheal intubation.
   Base of tongue
   Epiglottis
   Trachea
   Vocal cords

   A._____

   B._____

   C._____

   D._____

8. The valley formed between the tongue and epiglottis is called the _____.

9. Unrecognized _____ is a fatal complication of endotracheal intubation.

10. What are the anatomical differences between adults and infants/children relative to the structures of the upper airway?

11. The most common cause of an airway obstruction in an unconscious patient is _____
    _____.

12. What are common causes of airway obstruction?

13. What are the criteria indicating the need for endotracheal intubation?

14. _____ is a method of definitive airway control.

15. What is the quickest way to correct hypoxia?

16. Nasotracheal intubation is only performed on patients who are breathing.
    A. True
    B. False

17. Nasotracheal intubation is easier to perform than endotracheal intubation.
    A. True
    B. False

18. List the potential complications of endotracheal intubation.

19. A single attempt at ET intubation should be limited to _____ seconds.

20. A single EMT should not attempt to intubate a patient more than _____ time(s).

21. The priority of care for an apneic patient is _____.

22. Extubation can occur without complete removal of the ET tube.
    A. True
    B. False

23. How can endotracheal tube placement be confirmed?

24. Breath sounds that are heard on the right side but not on the left side after intubation are indicative of what complication?

25. What is the procedure to correct mainstem intubation?

26. What are the appropriate BSI precautions for intubation?

27. Describe the difference between the two types of laryngoscope blades.

28. Endotracheal tube sizes are based on external diameters.
    A. True
    B. False

29. Endotracheal tube sizes are available in increments of _____ mm.

30. Adult female patients generally require what size ET tube?

31. Adult male patients generally require what size ET tube?

32. The ET tube cuff holds approximately how much air?

33. The ET tube cuff should be inflated until _____.

34. What should the EMT do if he or she hears air leaking around an endotracheal tube despite instilling 10 ml of air into the cuff?

35. A small baloon near the adapter end of an endotracheal tube that verifies inflation of the ET tube cuff, is called the _____.

36. Using the markings on the tube, in most adult patients, proper endotracheal tube position is confirmed between _____ and _____ cm.

37. What is the correct procedure for entrotracheal tube intubation?

38. Identify the correct procedure for NG tube insertion.

39. How can NG tube placement be confirmed?

40. How is the correct size of an NG tube determined?

41. Gurgling breath sounds over the epigastrium after ET tube insertion is most likely indicative of what complication?

42. Complete the following mnemonic regarding ET tube placement confirmation.

    R:
    I:
    S:
    E:

43. Which type of laryngoscope blade is usually preferred for intubating infants? Why?

44. Which type of laryngoscope blade is usually preferred for intubating older children? Why?

45. Identify the cm length from midtrachea to teeth for endotracheal tube insertion for the following ages.

    _____ 6 months to 1 year   _____ 6 to 10 years
    _____ 2 years   _____ 10 to 12 years
    _____ 4 to 6 years

46. What is the formula for selecting the appropriate endotracheal tube size for children?

47. What size ET tube is usually used for newborns and small infants?

48. Identify possible complications of suctioning through an ET tube.

49. What are the indications for endotracheal suctioning?

Chapter Quiz

1. The mouth and nose are the beginning of the upper airway. The base of the tongue extends down to the:
   A. Epiglottis
   B. Carina
   C. Pharynx
   D. Vallecula

2. The _____ is used as a landmark during endotracheal intubation.
   A. Turbinate
   B. Carina
   C. Pharynx
   D. Vallecula

3. The _____ protect the opening of the trachea from aspiration of liquids and foreign material.
   A. Front teeth
   B. Vocal cords
   C. Chordae tendineae
   D. Nasal turbinates

4. The combination of a proportionally larger tongue and a smaller larynx makes the vocal cords appear more _____ in infants and children than in adults.
   A. Posterior
   B. Anterior
   C. Inferior
   D. Superior

5. The most common cause of an obstructed airway in an unconscious patient is the:
   A. Teeth
   B. Mucous
   C. Tongue
   D. Epiglottis

6. Causes of airway obstruction include:
   A. Respiratory secretions
   B. Gastric contents and foreign bodies
   C. Blood and teeth
   D. All of the above

7. Prior to intubation, a patient must always be ventilated with BLS techniques.
   A. True
   B. False

8. The immediate concern with a patient who has poor or absent ventilations is:
   A. Hypoxia
   B. Anemia
   C. Tachypnea
   D. Asphyxia

9. Endotracheal intubation is indicated when any of the following criteria exist *except:*
   A. The patient is unresponsive to painful stimuli.
   B. The patient has a gag reflex.
   C. The patient is unable to protect the airway.
   D. The patient is in cardiac arrest.

10. The _____ is the instrument used to visualize the vocal cords for endotracheal tube placement.
    A. Microscope
    B. Laparoscope
    C. Otoscope
    D. Laryngoscope

11. The straight blade is designed to lift the _____ directly during endotracheal intubation.
    A. Trachea
    B. Carina
    C. Epiglottis
    D. Vocal cords

12. A stylet is used to:
    A. Provide firmness to the endotracheal tube during insertion
    B. Act as a guide for the laryngoscope blade
    C. Insert the nasopharyngeal airway
    D. Target the carina

13. When choosing the appropriate size endotracheal tube, the EMT should remember the emergency rule that states:
    A. A 7.5 mm tube fits most adults
    B. A 4 mm tube fits most adults
    C. A 10 mm tube fits most males
    D. A 7 mm tube fits a small child

14. A curved blade is often preferred for intubating infants because of better tongue displacement and vocal cord visualization.
    A. True
    B. False

15. An uncuffed endotracheal tube is used in children less than _____ years old.
    A. 10
    B. 12
    C. 16
    D. 8

16. The most critical and potentially fatal complication of endotracheal intubation is:
    A. Trauma to the pharynx
    B. Esophageal intubation
    C. Trauma to the lips and teeth
    D. Hyperventilation

17. To avoid inadequate oxygenation due to prolonged unsuccessful attempts at intubation, the EMT should limit any single attempt to _____ seconds.
    A. 30
    B. 60
    C. 45
    D. 15

18. The priority of care for an apneic patient is ventilation, not intubation.
    A. True
    B. False

19. Once the ET tube is properly positioned, it must be properly secured in place to avoid accidental:
    A. Extubation
    B. Hyperperfusion
    C. Hyperventilation
    D. Hypotension

20. The only true way of confirming that the endotracheal tube enters the trachea is by:
    A. Visualizing the tube as it passes through the pharynx
    B. Listening to lung sounds on the right
    C. Visualizing the tube as it passes between the vocal cords
    D. Ausculating over the epicardium

21. A nasogastric tube is used for:
    A. Stomach decompression
    B. Medication administration
    C. Nutrition and/or gastric lavage
    D. All of the above

22. An absolute contraindication for NG tube placement is:
    A. The presence of major facial trauma
    B. The possibility of a gastric ulcer
    C. The presence of major abdominal injury
    D. An open pneumothorax

23. To insert an NG tube, the patient is placed in a _____ position with the head turned to the _____ side.
    A. Prone; right
    B. Supine; left
    C. Prone; left
    D. Supine; right

24. The Sellick maneuver involves applying pressure to the:
    A Cricoid cartilage
    B. Hyoid cartilage
    C. Pleural cartilage
    D. Vocal cords

25. Methods frequently used to check ET tube placement include all of the following *except:*
    A. Carbon dioxide detectors
    B. Observing chest rise and fall
    C. Listen to right and left apex
    D. Auscultate over the epicardium

Case Scenario

You respond to the scene of a reported cardiac arrest. On your arrival you find a male patient approximately 50 years old in confirmed cardiac arrest with CPR in progress by first responders. They are using a BVM with supplemental oxygen attached.

A quick assessment and history reveals that the patient has been in cardiac arrest for approximately 4 minutes. The arrest was witnessed by family members and CPR was started immediately. First responders have been on the scene for approximately 1 minute. There is no past medical history of significance. The patient was moving furniture when he complained to his wife of chest pain and went to sit down. He then collapsed on the floor.

1. What significant anatomy of the patient's airway is used to successfully accomplish intubation?

2. What are the steps involved in endotracheal intubation of this patient?

3. How can you confirm that you have inserted the ET tube correctly?

4. What are the indications for the placement of a nasogastric tube in this patient?

5. What are the correct steps in placing the NG tube?

Skill Sheet #16

NASOGASTRIC TUBE INSERTION

Start Time: _____

Stop Time: _____   **Date:** _____

Candidate's Name: _____

Evaluator's Name: _____

	Points Possible	Points Awarded
Takes, or verbalizes, body substance isolation precautions	1	
Identifies/selects the proper equipment for the procedure	1	
Connects the rigid suction catheter to suction and turns the unit on	1	
Measures the tube from the tip of the nose, around the ear, to below the xiphoid process	1	
Marks the tube with a piece of tape at the level of the tip of the nose	1	
Lubricates the distal end of the tube with water-soluble lubricant	1	
Note: The examiner states, "Trauma is not suspected in this patient situation."		
Places the patient supine with the head turned to the left side	1	
Gently inserts the tube into one nostril, advancing the tube straight back toward the ear, along the floor of the nostril	1	
Advances the tube until the tape marker is at the tip of the nose	1	
Confirms tube placement by: – attaching a 20 mL syringe to the tube and aspirating stomach contents – injecting 10 to 20 mL of air into the tube while listening for gurgling sounds over the stomach with a stethoscope	2	
Secures the tube in place	1	
Verbalizes proper documentation of procedure including tube size, time of insertion, methods used to confirm tube placement and results, and any complications encountered during the procedure	1	
Total:	13	

Critical Criteria

_____ Did not take, or verbalize, body substance isolation precautions

_____ Did not insert tube to proper depth

_____ Did not ensure proper placement of the device

_____ Did not successfully place the tube

_____ Inserted tube in a manner that would be dangerous to the patient

Skill Sheet #17

••

VENTILATORY MANAGEMENT
ENDOTRACHEAL INTUBATION

Start Time: _____

Stop Time: _____ **Date:** _____

Candidate's Name: _____

Evaluator's Name: _____

*Note: If a candidate elects to initially ventilate the patient with a BVM attached to a reservoir and oxygen, full credit must be awarded for steps denoted by "**" provided the first ventilation is delivered within the initial 30 seconds*	Points Possible	Points Awarded
Takes, or verbalizes, body substance isolation precautions	1	
Opens the airway manually	1	
Elevates the patient's tongue and inserts a simple airway adjunct (oropharyngeal/nasopharyngeal airway)	1	
Note: The examiner must now inform the candidate "no gag reflux is present and the patient accepts the airway adjunct."		
**Ventilates the patient immediately using a BVM device unattached to oxygen	1	
**Hyperventilates the patient with room air	1	
Note: The examiner must now inform the candidate that ventilation is being properly performed without difficulty.		
Attaches the oxygen reservoir to the BVM	1	
Attaches the BVM to high flow oxygen (15 L/minute)	1	
Ventilates the patient at the proper volume and rate *(800 to 1200 mL/breath and 10 to 20 breaths/minute)*	1	
Note: After 30 seconds, the examiner must auscultate the patient's chest and inform the candidate that breath sounds are present and equal bilaterally and medical direction has ordered endotracheal intubation. The examiner must now take over ventilation of the patient.		
Directs assistant to hyper-oxygenate the patient	1	
Identifies/selects the proper equipment for endotracheal intubation	1	
Checks the equipment / Checks for cuff leaks	1	
Checks laryngoscope operation and bulb tightness	1	
Note: The examiner must remove the OPA and move out of the way when the candidate is prepared to intubate the patient.		
Positions the patient's head properly	1	
Inserts the laryngoscope blade into the patient's mouth while displacing the patient's tongue laterally	1	
Elevates the patient's mandible with the laryngoscope	1	
Introduces the endotracheal tube and advances the tube to the proper depth	1	
Inflates the cuff to the proper pressure	1	
Disconnects the syringe from the cuff inlet port	1	
Directs assistant to ventilate the patient	1	
Confirms proper placement of the endotracheal tube by auscultation bilaterally and over the epigastrium	1	
Note: The examiner must ask, "If you had proper placement, what would you expect to hear?"		
Secures the endotracheal tube *(may be verbalized)*	1	
Total:	21	

Critical Criteria

_____ Did not take, or verbalize, body substance isolation precautions when necessary
_____ Did not initiate ventilation within 30 seconds after applying gloves or interrupts ventilations for greater than 30 seconds at any time
_____ Did not voice or provide high oxygen concentrations *(15 L/minute or greater)*
_____ Did not ventilate the patient at a rate of at least 10 breaths per minute
_____ Did not provide adequate volume per breath (maximum of 2 errors per minute permissible)
_____ Did not hyperoxygenate the patient prior to intubation
_____ Did not successfully intubate the patient within 3 attempts
_____ Used the patient's teeth as a fulcrum
_____ Did not ensure proper tube placement by auscultation bilaterally over each lung and over the epigastrium
_____ The stylette (if used) extended beyond the end of the endotracheal tube
_____ Inserted any adjunct in a manner that was dangerous to the patient
_____ Did not immediately disconnect the syringe from the inlet port after inflating the cuff

Answer Key

....

Key Terms
1. Epigastrium
2. Preoxygenation
3. Stylet
4. Uvula
5. Sniffing
6. Arytenoid cartilage
7. Automated transport ventilator
8. Laryngoscope
9. Nasogastric
10. Nasotracheal
11. Orogastric tube
12. Compliance
13. Endotracheal tube
14. Endotracheal tube cuff

Content Review
1. Glottic opening
2. A. Sphenoidal sinus
   B. Pharyngeal tonsil
   C. Internal naris
   D. Opening of auditory tube
   E. Nasopharynx
   F. Soft palate
   G. Uvula
   H. Oropharynx
   I. Laryngopharynx
   J. Esophagus
   K. Trachea
   L. Cricoid cartilage
   M. Thyroid cartilage
   N. True vocal cord
   O. Vestibular fold
   P. Epiglottis
   Q. Lingual tonsil
   R. Tongue
   S. Oral cavity
   T. Hard palate
   U. External naris
   V. Frontal sinus
3. False
4. True
5. Vocal cords
6. A. Lip
   B. Hard palate
   C. Soft palate
   D. Uvula
   E. Tongue

7.   A. Base of tongue
     B. Epiglottis
     C. Vocal cords
     D. Trachea
8.   Vallecula
9.   Esophageal intubation
10. They are softer and more fragile in infants and children than in adults; children have a proportionally larger tongue and smaller larynx; vocal cords appear more anterior in infants and children.
11. The tongue
12. Respiratory secretions; gastric contents (food); foreign bodies; blood, and teeth.
13. Inability to adequately ventilate an apneic patient with a BVM; the patient is unresponsive to painful stimuli; the patient has no gag reflex or coughing; the patient is unable to protect the airway (e.g., unconscious, cardiac arrest).
14. ET intubation
15. Ventilate the patient with 100% oxygen
16. True
17. False
18. Esophageal intubation; inadequate oxygenation due to prolonged unsuccessful attempts; unrecognized extubation; trauma to lips, teeth, gum, tongue, and airway structures due to poor handling of the laryngoscope; stimulation of the vasus nerves causing bradycardia; and mainstem bronchi intubation
19. 30
20. 3
21. Ventilation
22. True
23. Listening to breath sounds; watching for the chest to rise; documenting end-tidal carbon dioxide; and visualizing the tube passing between the vocal cords
24. Right mainstem intubation
25. Deflate the cuff on the tube; pull back on the tube until breath sounds are heard bilaterally; then reinflate the cuff
26. Gloves; mask; and protective eye wear
27. Curved: designed to be inserted into the vallecula and pull the epiglottis anteriorly to allow vocal cord visualization
     Straight: directly lifts the epiglottis
28. False
29. 0.5
30. 7.0 to 8.0 mm
31. 8.0 to 8.5 mm
32. 5 to 10 mL
33. There are no leaks around the tube during artificial ventilation
34. Replace the tube; either the cuff has ruptured or the patient needs a larger ET tube
35. Pilot balloon
36. 20; 25
37. Take BSI precautions; manually open the airway; hyperventilate the patient; select the proper equipment; check the equipment (check the cuff for leaks and the laryngoscope for operation and bulb); position the patient in a sniffing position; insert the blade into the patient's mouth while displacing the patient's tongue laterally; elevate the patient's mandible with the laryngoscope; introduce the ET tube and advance it to the proper depth; inflate the cuff to the proper pressure; disconnect the syringe from the cuff inlet port; ventilate the patient; confirm placement; secure the ET tube in place.
38. Select the correct NG tube size; place the patient in a supine position with the patient's head turned to the left side (unless trauma is suspected); insert the lubricated tube along the floor of nose until the measured length has been inserted; confirm placement; and secure the tube in place.

39. Inject 10 to 20 mL of air into the NG tube while auscultating over the epigastrium, gurgling should be heard.
40. Measure from the tip of the nose, around the ear, to below the xiphoid process.
41. Esophageal intubation
42. R = recognition that the tube has passed through the vocal cords; I: inflation and deflation (rise and fall) of the chest during ventilations; S: sounds of air movement in both lung fields can be heard; E: epigastrium auscultation (no air sounds heard)
43. A straight blade because of better tongue displacement and vocal cord visualization
44. A curved blade because its broad base and flange provide better control and displacement of the tongue
45. 6 month to 1 year: 12 cm; 2 years: 14 cm; 4 to 6 years: 16 cm; 6 to 10 years: 18 cm; 10 to 12 years: 20 cm
46. $\dfrac{16 + \text{age of patient (in years)}}{4}$
47. 3.0 to 3.5 mm ID
48. Arrhythmias; hypoxia; bronchospasm; stimulation of cough reflex; damage of mucosa of the respiratory tissue
49. Presence of obvious secretions; development of poor compliance while ventilating with a BVM device

Chapter Quiz

1. A	6. D	11. C	16. B	21. D
2. D	7. A	12. A	17. A	22. A
3. B	8. A	13. A	18. A	23. B
4. B	9. B	14. B	19. A	24. A
5. C	10. D	15. D	20. C	25. D

Case Scenario

1. Important parts of the anatomy for intubation are the tongue and vocal cords. The tongue because it must be moved in order to facilitate visualization of the vocal cords. The vocal cords are the landmark towards which the EMT will advance the ETT and watch the cuff disappear past.

2. Ensure prior oxygenation of the patient; hyperoxygenate before intubation attempt; position the patient's head in the sniffing position; enter the blade in the patient's mouth and lift up the tongue and mandible (if using a straight blade) or begin to sweep the tongue to the left while lifting the mandible up (if using a curved blade); visualize the vocal cords; introduce the ETT from the right side of the patient's mouth and advance the tube, with stylet in place and not extending beyond the tip of the ETT, toward the vocal cords; advance the tube through the vocal cords until the tube's cuff disappears; while holding the tube, remove the laryngoscope and stylet from the cuff; fill the cuff with 10 mL of air; while continuing to hold the tube in place, have ventilation resumed using the ETT; confirm tube placement.

3. Watch for equal chest rise and fall; adequate BVM compliance; visualization of the ETT passing through the cords; verify the presence of bilateral breath sounds; auscultate the epigastrium to ensure the absence of air in the stomach; watch for an improvement in the patient's level of consciousness and skin color; use a commercially available tube placement indicator.

4. The NG tube would be indicated if noticeable distention of the patient's abdomen was present, indicating a large volume of air present in the stomach, and if there were difficulty in ventilating the patient using the BVM.

5. Determine the correct tube size; measure for the correct length (tip of the nose to the patient's stomach); lubricate the tube well; place the patient's head to the side, since trauma is not suspected, to protect from emesis; insert the tube through the nares to the desired length (if resistance is met, stop, and reattempt with the other nares; do not force the tube); confirm tube placement by observing the stomach deflate and hearing the release of air, or injecting air into the stomach, while auscultating, and hearing gurgling.

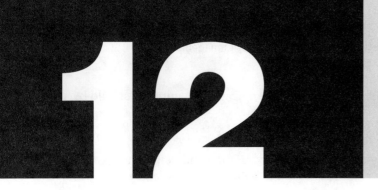

Scene Size-up and the EMS Call

Reading Assignment: Chapter 12 pages 235–252.

DOT Objectives

Upon successful completion of the EMT-Basic training program, the EMT-Basic should be able to do the following:

- Recognize hazards and potential hazards.
- Describe common hazards found at the scene of a trauma and a medical patient.
- Determine if the scene is safe for the EMT to enter.
- Discuss common mechanisms of injury and natures of illness.
- Discuss the reason for identifying the total number of patients at the scene.
- Explain the reason for identifying the need for additional help or assistance.
- Observe various scenarios and identify potential hazards.

Supplemental Objectives

- Identify the various phases of an EMS call and the different scenarios that can occur with each.
- Describe the interaction among the public, the dispatcher, EMTs, and other responding agencies.
- Describe the importance of effective communication in the processing of the EMS call.
- Describe the importance of scene evaluation, both while en route to and on arrival at the scene, and the impact on the outcome of the patient.
- Describe emergency medical dispatch and its role in helping the Emergency Medical Technician (EMT) develop strategies for delivery of the best possible patient care.
- Describe the key elements of the scene survey, gained from both the dispatcher and the survey of the scene on arrival, that can impact the outcome of patient care.
- Describe the potential threat hazardous materials present to both the EMT and the patient at the scene of a medical emergency.
- Describe the necessary safety measures to be taken for protection of both the patient and EMTs at a scene.
- Describe the importance of personal protective equipment to the EMT's safety and reduction of contamination by bloodborne pathogens or other potentially infectious materials in caring for a patient.
- Describe how bioethical considerations affect the resuscitation of patients in the prehospital setting.
- Assess the appropriateness of a do-not-resuscitate (DNR) order, a living will, advance directives, or a durable power of attorney and describe how it is used to implement or withhold resuscitation.

Key Terms

1. A legally binding document prepared and signed by an individual that clearly states personal wishes regarding the implementation of life saving techniques in the event of severe injury or terminal illness is called a(n) _____.

2. A legally binding document signed by a party that designates an individual to make health care decisions for the person executing the document is called a(n) _____.

3. Match the following abbreviations with the appropriate description of the term.

   _____ A computerized dispatch communications program
   _____ An approach to the dispatch functions that involves the dispatcher in making decisions about the type and priority of EMS response necessary
   _____ An order to withhold resuscitation efforts, issued by a physician after consultation with a patient
   _____ The medical term for a stroke
   _____ The type of dispatch based on recognition that the level of care, either basic or advanced, and the urgency of care can be identified by established criteria
   _____ Any incident involving one or more patients that cannot be handled by the first responding unit(s) to the scene
   _____ A term applied in the prehospital setting to those patients who, because of their medical condition, have no chance of survival and in which resuscitation efforts would be futile

   A. CVA
   B. CAD
   C. CBD
   D. DNR
   E. EMD
   F. MCI
   G. RNI

4. A fully integrated computerized emergency access telephone system is called _____ _____.

5. A legal document signed and witnessed outlining the types of medical interventions that may or may not be implemented is called a(n) _____.

6. The leading cause of death for children and adults under the age of 45 years and the third leading cause of deaths for all age groups is _____.

Content Review

1. List the major causes of illness and death in the geriatric population.

2. What is the leading cause of trauma related deaths and disability in the geriatric population?

3. List the information a dispatcher using EMD should provide to response personnel.

4. Why is it important that the EMT-B be notified if a call is trauma or medical in nature?

5. As the EMT-B approaches the scene, his or her first action should be to _____
   _____.

6. Whose responsibility is scene control?

7. Identify the proper procedure for the EMT-B to follow if he or she encounters an EMS DNR order.

8. If the EMT-B encounters a situation involving both a durable power of attorney and an EMS DNR order, which document prevails for EMS treatment?

9. What actions should the EMT-B take prior to leaving the Emergency Department?

Chapter Quiz

1. Lifesaving interventions should first be employed during the:
   A. Detailed physical examination
   B. Initial assessment
   C. Ongoing assessment
   D. Rapid focused history and physical examination

2. Evaluation of the mechanism of injury can assist with:
   A. Determining the number of patients that are involved
   B. Evaluating the patient(s) for possible injuries
   C. Determining the need for initiating resuscitation
   D. All of the above

3. Scene hazards may include:
   A. Downed power lines
   B. Broken gas transmission lines
   C. Toxic substances that have spilled
   D. All of the above

4. Depending on the completeness of the caller's description, dispatch information enables the EMT to determine whether the call
   A. Is a trauma or medical call
   B. Includes any life-threatening conditions
   C. Involves fire, building or other hazards
   D. All of the above

5. Scene size-up is:
   A. The best way to reduce exposure to communicable diseases
   B. A rapid assessment of the scene and scene surroundings
   C. A decision regarding priority of patient care
   D. Triage

6. When you arrive at a scene involving hazardous materials, your highest priority is:
   A. Personal safety
   B. Patient safety
   C. Public safety
   D. Triage

7. On arrival at a scene involving multiple vehicles, the EMT must consider:
   A. That additional medical personnel may be needed at the scene
   B. Whether helicopter evacuation is necessary
   C. Whether the scene requires special equipment
   D. All of the above

8. If the weather is very hot or very cold, the medical condition of the patient may be aggravated and treatment plans altered to avoid unnecessary exposure to the elements.
   A. True
   B. False

9. EMTs should never enter a scene involving reported violence until he or she confirms that the scene is secure.
   A. True
   B. False

10. Hazardous materials are transported on commercial carriers and are a regular part of EMS scene response and management. All hazardous materials should be considered a threat to the EMT until proven otherwise.
    A. True
    B. False

11. When approaching the scene, a critical clue for determining the possible injuries that a patient may have sustained at a trauma call is the mechanism of injury:
    A. True
    B. False

12. The EMT must quickly evaluate the total scene at a trauma call to help determine the probable mechanism of injury. At the scene of a motor vehicle collision this evaluation involves:
    A. Determining how the vehicle(s) collided
    B. Approximating the speed involved at the time of impact
    C. Whether safety belts were used to restrain the victims
    D. All of the above

13. At an industrial accident, evaluation might include:
    A. The height that the victim fell
    B. The amount of debris that fell on the victim
    C. The type of machinery involved in the accident
    D. All of the above

14. When considering safety concerns, the EMT should remember that any scene that involves the threat of violence should be controlled by the:
    A. Safety officer
    B. Police department
    C. Fire department
    D. EMS department

15. Personal protective equipment (PPE) is designed to protect emergency personnel from the risk of contamination by:
    A. Debris
    B. Airborne contaminants
    C. Potentially infectious materials
    D. All of the above

Case Scenario

You are dispatched to the scene of an automobile crash involving a bus. En route to the scene, the dispatcher advises you that the bus hit another car and that the bus was carrying passengers at the time. The total number of victims is unknown. The patient in the car is said to be trapped.

1. What steps should you take while traveling to the scene?

2. On arrival, what will be your initial priorities and steps of management?

On arrival at the scene, you notice a large amount of debris on the road. There is one patient trapped in the car screaming that he cannot move his legs. There are 10 patients in the bus, most complaining of minor aches, the driver of the bus is unconscious with a laceration above his left eyebrow. The windshield is cracked and the steering wheel bent.

3. What additional resources should you request for this situation?

4. Would this situation be considered a MCI?

Answer Key

Key Terms
1. Advanced directive
2. Durable power of attorney
3. B, E, D, A, C, F, G
4. E-911 (Enhanced 911)
5. Living will
6. Trauma

Content Review
1. Cardiovascular disease, cerebrovascular accident, altered mental status, pneumonia, and trauma.
2. Falls

3. Complete and accurate call information (including the type of call and any life-threats); pertinent weather information that could delay response or transport; traffic delays en route to the scene; anticipated delays from blocked railroad crossings or raised bridges; the fastest, safest route to follow; alternative routes for responding units; prearrival instructions to the caller regarding care for the patient until the EMS unit arrives; environmental hazards; and any reports of violence at the scene.
4. It helps the EMT prepare, and allows the EMT to make an informed decision as to what type of equipment to take from the unit.
5. Ensure the scene is secure and safe to enter.
6. Police, fire, and EMS personnel.
7. Perform initial assessment; verify identification of the patient; administer oxygen by mask or cannula; suction the airway; manage the airway with basic procedures (no intubation or other advanced procedures); control bleeding; make the patient comfortable; and support family members and make them comfortable.
8. The EMS DNR order
9. Ensure the vehicle is prepared for another incident; properly dispose of contaminated sharps, biohazardous waste, and linen; and disinfect non-disposable equipment.

Chapter Quiz

1. B	6. A	11. A
2. B	7. D	12. D
3. D	8. A	13. D
4. D	9. A	14. B
5. B	10. A	15. D

Case Scenario
1. Once en route to the scene, you should anticipate the potential for a large number of victims and, based on company protocol, request additional ambulance units. Ensure that fire and police have been dispatched for traffic control and law enforcement for crowd control and that the rescue unit has been dispatched to help with the entrapment.

2. Your priority on arrival at the scene is to initially ensure that the scene is secure. Ensure that law enforcement officers have removed bystanders from the scene. Don protective clothing. Once it has been determined that the scene is safe and the vehicles safe to enter, begin initial patient assessment. Determine the additional resources necessary and request their dispatch. Initiate MCI protocols and triage patients to determine those most in need of immediate attention.

3. Fire, police, law enforcement personnel, fire rescue, ALS unit additional ambulances, and fire department personnel for debris and possible gas on the roadway.

4. Yes. This is a mass casualty incident because it involves more patients than can be handled by the first responding unit.

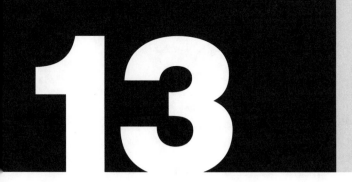

General Pharmacology

Reading Assignment: Chapter 13 pages 257–271.

DOT Objectives

Upon successful completion of the EMT-Basic training program, the EMT-Basic should be able to do the following:

- Identify which medications will be carried on the unit.
- State the medications carried on the unit by the generic names.
- Identify the medications that the EMT-Basic may assist the patient in administering.
- State the medications that the EMT-Basic may assist the patient in administering by their generic names.
- Discuss the forms in which medications may be found.
- Demonstrate general steps for assisting patients with self-administration of medications.
- Read the labels and inspect each type of medication.

Key Terms

1. Match the following abbreviations with the appropriate description.

_____ By mouth	A. BID
_____ Under the tongue	B. IM
_____ Once a day	C. PO
_____ Three times a day	D. PRN
_____ Inhaled	E. Puff
_____ Twice a day	F. QD
_____ Four times a day	G. HS
_____ As needed	H. QID
_____ Rectally	I. SQ
_____ Under the skin	J. SL
_____ At bedtime	K. Supp
_____ Intramuscular	L. TID

2. The desirable effect of a drug is called the _____.

3. _____ is the study of how chemicals work in the body.

4. The amount of drug that is absorbed from the site of administration is referred to as its _____ _____.

5. The length of time a drug is effective is called the _____.

6. The method by which a drug is put into the body is referred to as the _____
_____.

7. A drug that is applied directly to an effected area is a _____ acting medication.

8. Conditions under which a drug should be given are called _____.

9. Conditions under which a drug should not be given are called _____.

10. A simple form of a chemical name of a drug is called the _____ name.

11. A drug name created by the company that sells the drug is called the _____ name.

12. The long complex description of the structure of a drug is called the _____ name.

13. A drug that enters the blood and is carried to the whole body is a _____ acting medication.

14. Unwanted or harmful effects of a drug are referred to as _____.

Content Review

....

1. List those medications carried in the ambulance.

2. List those medications that the EMT-B can assist a patient in taking.

3. All medications have at least three names. What are they?

   1)
   2)
   3)

4. Each drug has only one generic name.
   A. True
   B. False

5. Identify each of the following as a generic name (G) or trade name (T).

   _____ Advil   _____ Nuprin
   _____ Ibuprofen   _____ Proventil
   _____ Aspirin   _____ Albuterol
   _____ Excedrine   _____ Ventolin

6. How can the EMT-B recognize a trade name versus a generic name?

7. Identify eight routes of medication administration.

    1)   5)
    2)   6)
    3)   7)
    4)   8)

8. The route of administration influences three areas. What are they?

    1)
    2)
    3)

9. The speed of absorption and availability of a drug depend on what three factors?

    1)
    2)
    3)

10. What are the two fastest routes for absorption of a drug?

11. What are the three organs through which the body removes medications?

    1)
    2)
    3)

12. What information is contained on a drug label?

13. What tasks should the EMT-B complete after administering or assisting with the administration of a medication?

Chapter Quiz

• •

1. Medications that are usually carried on the basic EMT unit include all of the following *except*:
   A. Morphine
   B. Activated charcoal
   C. Oral glucose
   D. Oxygen

2. The EMT-B, with approval from medical direction, may assist the patient in taking which of the following medications?
   A. Morphine, lasix, and atenolol
   B. Morphine, nitroglycerin, and atenolol
   C. Inhaler, ephinephrine, and nitroglycerin
   D. Inhaler, atropine, and nitroglycerin

3. The two most important medication names for the EMT-B to know are the:
   A. Chemical name and trade name
   B. Generic name and trade name
   C. Generic name and chemical name
   D. Brand name and chemical name

4. A drug can have _____ generic names.
   A. An unlimited number
   B. 2
   C. 4
   D. 1

5. The generic name is a simple form of the complex chemical name and is assigned by the government and officially listed in a book called the U.S. Pharmacopeia.
   A. True
   B. False

6. Which names are given to a drug by the company that sells the drug?
   A. Trade name or brand name
   B. Trade name and generic name
   C. Trade name and chemical name
   D. Brand name and generic name

7. Proventil and Ventolin are trade names of the same generic drug known as:
   A. Albuterol
   B. Nuprin
   C. Primatene
   D. Acetaminophen

8. Tablets are made from a:
   A. Gel
   B. Liquid
   C. Compressed powder
   D. Gas

9. Nitroglycerin spray and tablets are given to the patient:
    A. Orally
    B. Sublingually
    C. Intravenously
    D. Transdermally

10. What form of drug is oral glucose?
    A. Gel
    B. Suspension
    C. Tablet
    D. Injectable liquid

11. What form of drug is activated charcoal?
    A. Injectable liquid
    B. Gas
    C. Suspension
    D. Gel

12. How is epinephrine administered to a patient via an automatic device?
    A. SQ injection
    B. Sublingually
    C. Orally
    D. Inhalation

13. The route of medication taken by mouth is known as:
    A. PO
    B. SL
    C. IM
    D. SC

14. A drug given by subcutaneous injection in injected:
    A. Into the muscle
    B. Under the tongue
    C. Under the skin
    D. Into a vein

15. An EMT-B can assist a patient in taking medications by doing all of the following *except:*
    A. Handing the patient the medication
    B. Getting water for the patient
    C. Helping identify the medication
    D. Administering an intramuscular injection

16. Contraindications for the administration of nitroglycerin include all of the following *except:*
    A. Hypovolemia
    B. Hypotension
    C. Increased intracranial pressure
    D. Hypertension

17. Side effects of epinephrine include all of the following *except:*
    A. Tachycardia
    B. Hypotension
    C. Palpitations
    D. Dysrythmias

18. Contraindications for the administration of epinephrine include which of the following?
    A. Hypotension
    B. Pulmonary edema
    C. Severe bronchospasm
    D. All of the above

19. Indications for the use of oral glucose include all of the following *except:*
    A. Hypoglycemia
    B. Diabetes
    C. Unresponsiveness
    D. New onset seizures

20. Activated charcoal should *not* be given to patients that have ingested which of the following:
    A. Cyanide
    B. Methanol
    C. Ethanol
    D. All of the above

Case Scenario

You respond to a patient who is having difficulty breathing. On arrival, you encounter a 16-year-old patient in obvious respiratory distress. The patient states that she had been running and that she has experienced similar problems in the past. She states that she uses an inhaler but that she had not used it today.

The patient's vital signs are as follows: ventilatory rate: 38 with expiratory wheezing; blood pressure: 120/80 mm Hg; and pulse: 100 and regular. You retrieve the inhaler and note that it is albuterol that was prescribed for the patient's mother.

1. What should you do for this patient?

2. Can you assist the patient with the administration of the albuterol to relieve the respiratory distress?

3. What is the mechanism of action for albuterol?

Answer Key

Key Terms
1. C, J, F, L, E, A, H, D, K, I, G, B
2. Action
3. Pharmacology
4. Availability
5. Duration of action
6. Route of administration
7. Locally

8. Indications
9. Contraindications
10. Generic
11. Trade
12. Chemical
13. Systemically
14. Side effects

Content Review

1. Activated charcoal; oral glucose; and oxygen
2. Epinephrine; nitroglycerin; and a prescribed inhaler
3. 1) Chemical name; 2) trade name; and 3) generic name
4. True
5. T, G, G, T, T, T, G, T
6. A trade name has a ® symbol next to it.
7. 1) IV injection; 2) IM injection; 3) subcutaneous injection; 4) oral; 5) rectal; 6) sublingual; 7) inhalation; and 8) topical
8. 1) Speed of absorption; 2) availability; and 3) duration of action
9. 1) The kind of drug; 2) route of administration; and 3) form of the drug
10. IV injection and inhalation
11. 1) Lungs; 2) kidneys; and 3) liver
12. The patient's name; the name of the drug; the strength of the medication; the number of pills in the bottle; the route of administration; and directions
13. Repeat assessment of vital signs and mental status; observe for desired actions of medication (i.e., relief of symptoms); observe for unwanted side effects; document the patient's response to the interventions as it occurs; and intervene again if the patient fails to respond, has side effects, or has changing signs and symptoms.

Chapter Quiz

1. A	6. A	11. C	16. D
2. C	7. A	12. A	17. B
3. B	8. C	13. A	18. B
4. D	9. B	14. C	19. C
5. A	10. A	15. D	20. D

Case Scenario

1. Administer 100% supplemental oxygen and transport immediately to the hospital with ALS rendezvous if the transport time is prolonged.
2. Since the albuterol was not prescribed for the patient, the EMT cannot assist the patient in administering it.
3. Albuterol is a bronchodilator, which causes an opening of airways in the lungs that allows for easier breathing.

14

Respiratory Emergencies

Reading Assignment: Chapter 14 pages 272–287.

DOT Objectives

Upon successful completion of the EMT-Basic training program, the EMT-Basic should be able to do the following:

- List the indications and contraindications for inhaler medications and demonstrate the steps required to assist with inhaler administration.
- Identify the structures and function of the respiratory system.
- Establish the relationship between airway management and the patient with breathing difficulty.
- List signs of adequate air exchange.
- State the administration, action, indications and contraindications for the prescribed inhaler.
- Differentiate among the emergency medical care of the adult patient with breathing difficulty.
- List the signs and symptoms of respiratory distress and demonstrate the ability to intervene appropriately with supplemental oxygen or airway management and artificial ventilation.

Supplemental Objectives

- Define FiO_2.
- Describe the assessment and prehospital care of the patient with breathing difficulty.
- Describe the special considerations needed to care for infants and children with respiratory emergencies.
- Relate the physiology of the respiratory system to the signs and symptoms of inadequate breathing.

Key Terms

....

1. Match the following terms with their appropriate definition.

_____ Complete lack of ventilations

_____ A viral infection seen in children, characterized by a "barking" cough

_____ An infection of the lungs that may be caused by bacteria, viruses, or fungi causing fever, dyspnea and a cough

_____ Occasional, gasping breaths that occur just before death

_____ A blood clot that travels to the lung, lodging in the pulmonary arteries, causing decreased blood flow to the lungs and resulting in hypoxia

_____ A form of COPD characterized by a productive cough and obstructive airway symptoms

_____ A condition seen in patients with asthma where airways constrict tightly in response to irritants

_____ A medication that relaxes constricted airways

_____ A build up of fluid in the alveoli and small airways

_____ A bacterial infection seen most often in children causing airway obstruction and severe drooling

_____ A process in which minute ventilation is increased above normal

_____ A form of COPD characterized by destruction of alveoli, commonly seen in smokers

_____ A sign of respiratory distress often seen in children

_____ The symptom of having difficulty breathing

_____ A condition of a shortage of oxygen at the cellular level

A. Agonal ventilations
B. Apnea
C. Bronchodilator
D. Bronchospasm
E. Chronic bronchitis
F. Croup
G. Dyspnea
H. Emphysema
I. Epiglottitis
J. Hyperventilation
K. Hypoxia
L. Pneumonia
M. Pulmonary edema
N. Pulmonary embolism
O. Retractions

2. Match the following breath sounds with their appropriate description.

_____ Lower-pitched bubbling sounds produced by fluid in the lower airways

_____ Abnormal, high-pitched, musical sound caused by an obstruction in the trachea or larynx, heard on inspiration

_____ Fine breath sounds that represent opening of collapsed alveoli or fluid in small airways near alveoli, simulated by rubbing hair between fingers

_____ High-pitched sounds heard when air moves through constricted airways, commonly heard in patients with asthma

A. Crackles
B. Rales
C. Stridor
D. Wheezes

3. The percentage of inspired oxygen is referred to as _____.

4. The device designed to give a fixed dose of inhaled medications with each puff is called a(n) _____ _____.

5. The medical term for a rapid ventilatory rate is _____.

6. Widening of the nostrils that often occurs during inhalation in patients with respiratory distress is referred to as _____.

7. The term for a sensation experienced as numbness, tingling, or a "pins and needles" feeling is called _____.

8. Skin which has diffuse patches of red and white discoloration, often seen in patients with severe hypoxia, is called _____.

Content Review

1. Identify the function of the respiratory system.

2. _____ is used by the body's cells to make energy, and _____ is produced as a by-product.

3. Where do the two exchanges of oxygen and carbon dioxide take place?

   1)
   2)

4. Explain the process of the alveolar/capillary exchange in the body.

5. Explain the process of the capillary/cellular exchange in the body.

6. There are three components of COPD. List them and describe each type.

   1)
   2)
   3)

7. Patients with COPD often develop a unique shape in the thoracic cavity due to the chest becoming expanded from constant overinflation of lungs caused by the trapping of air. This unique shape is called a(n) _____.

8. Identify the signs and symptoms of asthma.

9. Explain the significance of not hearing wheezing associated with an asthma attack.

10. If hypoxia is not corrected, what may follow?

11. Hyperventilation syndrome occurs when there is _____ oxygen.
    A. Too much
    B. Too little

12. Hyperventilation and hyperventilation syndrome are two different conditions.
    A. True
    B. False

13. What are the signs and symptoms of hyperventilation?

14. List the two major causes of hyperventilation.

    1)
    2)

15. How should an EMT-B manage hyperventilation syndrome?

16. List the signs and symptoms of pulmonary edema.

17. The most common cause of pulmonary edema is _____. List the other causes.

18. How should the EMT-B care for a patient with pulmonary edema?

19. What causes a pulmonary embolism?

20. What are the signs and symptoms of pulmonary embolism?

21. What is the difference between a hemothorax and a pneumothroax?

22. List the signs and symptoms of a pneumothorax.

23. The two most common infections leading to respiratory emergencies in infants and children are
_____ and _____.

24. An infection of the lung tissue is called _____.

25. Important information for the EMT-B to obtain during assessment includes:

26. Identify the normal ventilatory rates for the following.

Adults:

Children:

Infants:

27. Why is it important to assess the depth of a patient's ventilations?

28. A patient with severe pulmonary problems assists the breathing effort by exhaling through pursed lips, which is termed _____.

29. List the interventions for management of a respiratory emergency.

30. List the indications that must be met before the EMT-B can assist with an inhaler.

31. List four contraindications for assisting with hand-held inhalers:

1)
2)
3)
4)

32. List the steps for assisting with an inhaler.

33. What is the purpose of a spacer between an inhaler and the mouth?

34. List the potential side effects of an inhaler.

Chapter Quiz
....

1. The most common respiratory or breathing disorders the EMT-B will encounter in the field are:
   A. COPD and hyperventilation
   B. Pulmonary embolism and hemothorax
   C. COPD and asthma
   D. Pulmonary edema and pneumothorax

2. Signs and symptoms of respiratory distress related to COPD may include:
   A. Dyspnea
   B. Productive cough
   C. Agitation
   D. All of the above

3. Signs and symptoms of a severe asthma attack may include all of the following *except:*
   A. No lung sounds and cardiac arrest
   B. Respiratory arrest and irritability
   C. Confusion and lethargy
   D. Crepitus and abdominal distention

4. Chronic obstructive pulmonary disease is most often seen in:
   A. Infants that cannot drink milk
   B. Children that eat smoked meat
   C. Older people with a history of smoking
   D. Young adults that drink

5. Signs and symptoms of hyperventilation may include:
    A. An increased ventilatory rate
    B. Paresthesia
    C. Agitation
    D. All of the above

6. A patient who appears to be hyperventilating, with signs of another respiratory condition, should be:
    A. Instructed to increase the rate of breathing
    B. Instructed to relax and slow their breathing
    C. Be fitted with an oxygen mask without oxygen
    D. All of the above

7. Hyperventilation is always caused by anxiety.
    A. True
    B. False

8. The most common cause of pulmonary edema is:
    A. Pulmonary embolism
    B. Bee stings
    C. Congestive heart failure
    D. Fluid overload

9. The signs and symptoms of pulmonary edema may include:
    A. Pink frothy sputum and distended neck veins
    B. Dyspnea and hypoxia
    C. Breath sounds with coarse crackles
    D. All of the above

10. Patients with pulmonary edema should be given high-flow oxygen and transported immediately.
    A. True
    B. False

11. Croup is caused by:
    A. A virus
    B. Bacteria
    C. Parasites
    D. Drugs

12. Croup is usually seen in what age group?
    A. 1 month to 3 months
    B. 6 months to 3 years
    C. 3 years to 6 years
    D. 5 years to 8 years

13. Signs and symptoms of croup include all of the following *except:*
    A. Agitation
    B. "Barking" cough
    C. Low-grade fever
    D. Drooling

14. Epiglottitis is caused by:
    A. Parasite
    B. Bacteria
    C. A virus
    D. Poisoning

15. Signs and symptoms of epiglottitis include:
    A. A quiet child that sits still
    B. An excessive amount of saliva
    C. A high fever
    D. All of the above

16. Chronic bronchitis is a form of obstructive lung disease characterized by excess mucus production in the airways, causing cough and airway obstruction.
    A. True
    B. False

17. Signs and symptoms of asthma include all of the following *except:*
    A. Dyspnea and difficulty exhaling
    B. Wheezing and a dry cough
    C. An overexpanded chest
    D. Bradycardia and jaundice

18. A pulmonary embolism causes hypoxia by:
    A. Blocking the aorta
    B. Blocking the inferior vena cava
    C. Blocking the carotid artery
    D. Blocking a pulmonary artery

19. A pneumothorax is caused by:
    A. Air in the pleural space
    B. Blood in the pleural space
    C. Blood and air in the pleural space
    D. Plasma in the pleural space

20. A hemothorax is caused by:
    A. Air in the pleural space
    B. Blood in the pleural space
    C. Blood and air in the pleural space
    D. Plasma in the pleural space

21. Pneumonia is caused by:
    A. Bacteria
    B. Viruses
    C. Fungi
    D. All of the above

22. Signs and symptoms of pneumonia include:
    A. Fever and chills
    B. Productive cough
    C. Dyspnea and hypoxia
    D. All of the above

23. Which of the following indications must be present before the EMT-B can assist with an inhaler?
    A. The patient exhibits signs and symptoms of respiratory distress.
    B. The patient has a currently prescribed hand-held inhaler.
    C. The EMT-B has specific authorization by medical control to assist with inhalers.
    D. All of the above

24. Which of the following is important information about the patient with respiratory difficulties?
    A. Onset and duration of symptoms
    B. The presence of associated symptoms
    C. The patient's previous medical history
    D. All of the above

25. Patients who are in acute respiratory distress are often unable to talk or may talk in one- to two-word sentences.
    A. True
    B. False

26. A patient with COPD and signs of hypoxia needs high-flow oxygen.
    A. True
    B. False

27. The EMT-B should let the non-trauma patient stay in whatever position is most comfortable.
    A. True
    B. False

28. Side effects of bronchodilators include:
    A. Increased pulse rate
    B. Tremors
    C. Nervousness and agitation
    D. All of the above

29. An alternative to oxygen administration by mask for children is the blow-by method.
    A. True
    B. False

Case Scenario

You are called to the scene of a 58-year-old male patient who is complaining of shortness of breath. On your arrival, you find a patient who appears anxious and cyanotic, especially around the lips. He is sitting upright, leaning forward to try and catch his breath. His breathing is rapid and labored. He is conscious, alert, and oriented. When you ask him questions, he responds with one and two word sentences and appears very agitated. On ausculation of his lung sounds, you notice coarse crackles in the base of both lungs. His skin is cool and clammy.

The patient's wife states that he is a very heavy smoker and has been coughing more lately, producing thick mucus. He has been getting worse all week and today he could hardly take two steps without gasping for air. He has no significant past medical history and is not currently taking any medication.

1. What are the two first actions the EMT should take on arrival at the scene?

2. What signs and symptoms of respiratory distress are present in this patient?

3. What is most likely wrong with this patient?

4. What steps should you take to manage this patient?

Skill Sheet #18

••

PRESCRIBED INHALER
Assisting with Administration

Start Time: _____

Stop Time: _____   Date: _____

Candidate's Name: _____

Evaluator's Name: _____

	Points Possible	Points Awarded
Takes, or verbalizes, body substance isolation precautions	1	
Obtains an order from medical direction (either on-line or off-line)	1	
Assures right medication, right patient, right route, and patient alert enough to use inhaler	1	
Checks the expiration date of the inhaler	1	
Checks to see if the patient has already taken any doses	1	
Assures the inhaler is at room temperature or warmer	1	
Attaches a spacer device, if available	1	
Shakes the inhaler vigorously several times	1	
Removes oxygen adjunct from the patient	1	
Has the patient exhale deeply	1	
Has the patient put his or her lips around the opening of the inhaler	1	
Has the patient depress the hand-held inhaler as he or she begins to inhale deeply	1	
Instructs the patient to hold his or her breath for as long as he or she comfortably can (so the medication can be absorbed)	1	
Replaces oxygen on the patient	1	
Allows the patient to breathe a few times and repeats the second dose per medical direction	1	
Records the name, dose, route, time, and results of administration of the medication	1	
Total:	16	

Critical Criteria

_____ Did not take, or verbalize, body substance isolation precautions

_____ Did not check the medication for correct prescription and for the expiration date

_____ Did not check to see if the patient has already taken any doses

_____ Did not instruct the patient correctly on how to use the inhaler

_____ Did not replace the oxygen on the patient

_____ Did not properly record medication administration

Answer Key

....

Key Terms
1. B, F, L, A, N, E, D, C, M, I, J, H, O, G, K
2. A, C, B, D
3. FiO_2
4. Metered dose inhaler
5. Tachypnea
6. Nasal flaring
7. Paresthesia
8. Mottling

Content Review
1. It supplies oxygen to and removes carbon dioxide from the tissue cells.
2. Oxygen; carbon dioxide
3. 1) Alveolar/capillary exchange; and 2) Capillary/cellular exchange
4. It is the exchange of oxygen from the alveoli into the blood, where it is taken up by RBCs and where carbon dioxide moves from the plasma into the alveoli to be exhaled.
5. It is the exchange of oxygen involving the transfer of oxygen to body cells and removal of carbon dioxide throughout the body tissues.
6. 1) Emphysema—alveoli in the lung are destroyed, reducing the alveolar/capillary surface area for gas exchange; 2) Chronic bronchitis—characterized by excess mucus production in the airways causing cough and airway obstruction; 3) Infection—which occurs when alveoli cannot completely empty due to obstruction by the mucus, causing bacteria to grow and produce infections
7. Barrel chest deformity
8. Dyspnea, wheezing, dry cough, overexpanded chest, and altered LOC (confusion, irritability, lethargy)
9. The patient may not move enough air to cause wheezing, indicating severe respiratory distress.
10. Respiratory arrest and then cardiac arrest
11. A. Too much
12. False
13. Tingling and spasm of the forearm, muscles drawing hands into a claw, tingling in the fingertips and around the mouth, hunger for air, and an increased ventilatory rate
14. 1) Anaerobic metabolism secondary to hypoxia and decreased oxygen delivery to tissue cells; and 2) hyperventilation syndrome resulting from pain and anxiety
15. Provide calm reassurance; "talk down" the patient to calm him or her
16. Severe dyspnea, hypoxia, coarse crackles in the lower part of the lungs, pink frothy sputum, and distended neck veins
17. Congestive heart failure; severe infection, smoke or toxin inhalation, high altitudes, narcotic overdose, and fluid overload
18. High-flow oxygen and rapid transport; be prepared with BVM in case assisted ventilations are necessary
19. A blood clot breaks off and travels to the lung, lodges in a branch of the pulmonary arteries, and causes a decrease in blood flow to the lungs.
20. Sudden dyspnea and tachypnea
21. Pneumothorax is an accumulation of air in the pleural space, and a hemothorax is the accumulation of blood in the pleural space.
22. Severe dyspnea, chest pain, tachypnea, diminished breath sounds on the affected side, and signs and symptoms of hypoxia (agitation, disorientation, cyanosis)

23. Croup; epiglottitis
24. Pneumonia
25. The onset and duration of symptoms; the presence of associated symptoms; past medical history; medications; and any allergies
26. Adults: 12 to 20; children: 15 to 30; infants: 25 to 50 breaths per minute
27. Insufficient tidal volume can lead to hypoxia, if not corrected.
28. Huffing
29. Establish and maintain an adequate airway; administer supplemental oxygen; provide assisted ventilations when needed; monitor vital signs; maintain patient comfort; and assist with inhaler medications as needed
30. The patient exhibits signs and symptoms of respiratory distress; the patient has a currently prescribed hand-held inhaler; and the EMT-B has specific authorization from the medical director to assist with the inhaler.
31. 1) The patient is unable to use the device (due to severe symptoms); 2) the inhaler is not prescribed for the patient (e.g., it is a family member's); 3) the patient has already taken the maximum number of doses; or 4) the EMT-B does not have authority to assist with the inhaler.
32. Ensure the prescription is for the patient, that the medication has not expired, and that the patient is alert enough to use the inhaler; ask the patient how many doses he or she has taken and verify that the maximum dose has not been reached; shake the inhaler vigorously several times; remove any oxygen adjunct from the patient; have the patient exhale deeply and place his or her lips around the opening; have the patient inhale causing the device to be triggered; have the patient hold his or her breath as long as possible to improve absorption of the medication; reapply the oxygen adjunct; and repeat a second dose, if indicated and allowed.
33. It helps to increase the amount of medication that becomes airborne and reaches the lungs. Without a spacer, most of the medication sticks to the walls of the mouth before it becomes completely airborne.
34. Nervousness, tremors, headache, hypertension, dysrhythmia, chest pain, palpitations, nausea, and vomiting

Chapter Quiz

1. C	6. B	11. A	16. A	21. D	26. A
2. D	7. B	12. B	17. D	22. D	27. A
3. D	8. C	13. D	18. D	23. D	28. D
4. C	9. D	14. B	19. A	24. D	29. A
5. D	10. A	15. D	20. B	25. A	

Case Scenario

1. Establish scene safety and take BSI precautions.
2. Dyspnea; anxiety; skin (cool, clammy, and cyanotic); inability to speak in more than one- and two-word sentences; position of patient (sitting upright, leaning forward); labored breathing; increased ventilatory rate; agitation; and noisy ventilations (coarse crackles)
3. Respiratory distress from COPD—most likely emphysema
4. Administer high-flow oxygen, monitor vital signs, rapid transport allowing the patient to sit in the position of comfort, and complete a detailed history and physical en route to the hosptial.

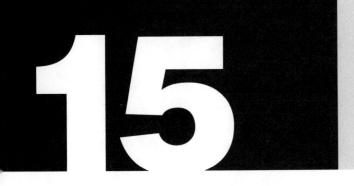

Cardiovascular Emergencies

Reading Assignment: Chapter 15 pages 288–305.

DOT Objectives

Upon successful completion of the EMT-Basic training program, the EMT-Basic should be able to do the following:

- Describe the anatomy and function of the cardiovascular system.
- Identify signs and symptoms of patients experiencing a cardiovascular problem and perform the necessary interventions for standard cardiac care.
- Describe the emergency cardiac care system, including the rationale, indications, and contraindications for early defibrillation; the importance of early advanced cardiac life support (ACLS); the relationship between basic life support and ACLS providers; and the role of the emergency medical technician (EMT) within this system.
- Explain the rationale for facilitating the use of nitroglycerin for patients with chest pain, including the indications, contraindications, and side effects of the drug.
- Discuss the position of comfort for patients with various cardiac emergencies.
- Establish the relationship between airway management and the patient with cardiovascular compromise.
- Predict the relationship between the patient experiencing cardiovascular compromise and basic life support.
- Explain that not all chest pain patients result in cardiac arrest and not all need to be attached to an automated external defibrillator.
- Explain the importance of urgent transport to a facility with Advanced Cardiac Life Support if it is not available in the prehospital setting.
- Discuss the components that should be included in a case review.
- Recognize the need for medical direction of protocols to assist in the emergency medical care of the patient with chest pain.

Key Terms

••

1. Match the following terms with their description.

_____ Fluid build up in the alveoli causing hypoxia and dyspnea
_____ Chest pain brought on by exercise and relieved by rest
_____ Plaque build up on the inside of arteries
_____ Irreversible death of part of the heart muscle
_____ Abnormally high blood pressure
_____ Hypoperfusion from inadequate pumping of the heart
_____ An irregular heart beat
_____ Heart in state of disorganized electrical and mechanical activity
_____ Abnormally low blood pressure
_____ Dysrhythmia where electrical impulses are separated from normal conduction system
_____ Heartbeat greater than 100 beats per minute
_____ Inadequate pumping of the heart caused by fluid in the lungs
_____ Delivery of an electrical shock to restore a normal heart rhythm
_____ An electrical flat line

A. CHF
B. Cardiogenic shock
C. Hypotension
D. Atherosclerosis
E. Asystole
F. Dysrhythmia
G. Ventricular fibrillation
H. Tachycardia
I. Angina pectoris
J. Hypertension
K. Ventricular tachycardia
L. Myocardial infarction
M. Pulmonary edema
N. Defibrillation

2. Match the following terms with their description.

_____ The upper chamber of the heart
_____ The vein that returns blood from the lower extremities, pelvis, and abdomen to the right atrium
_____ The smallest blood vessels in the body
_____ Vessels that carry blood from the heart to the lungs
_____ Vessels that carry blood back to the heart
_____ Vessels that supply capillaries with oxygenated blood
_____ Vessels that carry blood from capillaries to veins
_____ The largest artery in the body
_____ The lower chambers of the heart
_____ The large vein that returns blood from the thorax, arms, head, and neck to the right atrium
_____ Vessels that carry blood away from the heart
_____ Vessels that carry blood from the lungs to the left side of the heart

A. Aorta
B. Artery
C. Arteriole
D. Atria
E. Capillary
F. Inferior vena cava
G. Pulmonary artery
H. Pulmonary vein
I. Superior vena cava
J. Ventricles
K. Vein
L. Venule

Content Review

1. Identify each of the following ECG tracings.

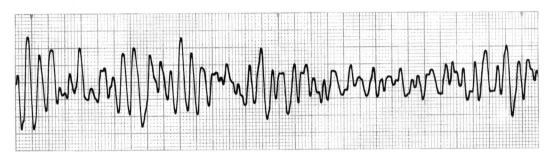

A. _____

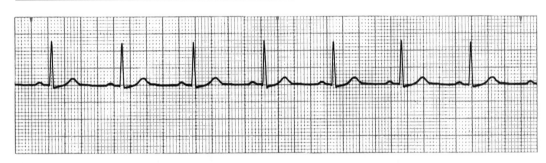

B. _____

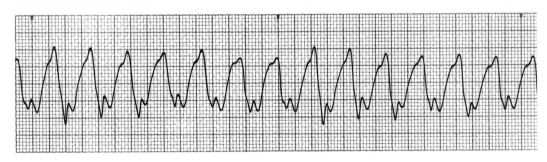

C. _____

2. Inadequate blood flow to tissue is called _____.

3. Many patients with a history of angina take a medication called _____.

4. Identify each of the arteries and veins identified in the diagram below.

Anterior tibial artery   Femoral artery   Posterior tibial artery
Aorta   Femoral vein   Pulmonary arteries and veins
Axillary vein   Great saphenous vein   Radial artery
Brachial artery   Inferior vena cava   Right common iliac artery
Dorsalis pedis artery   Left common iliac vein Superior vena cava

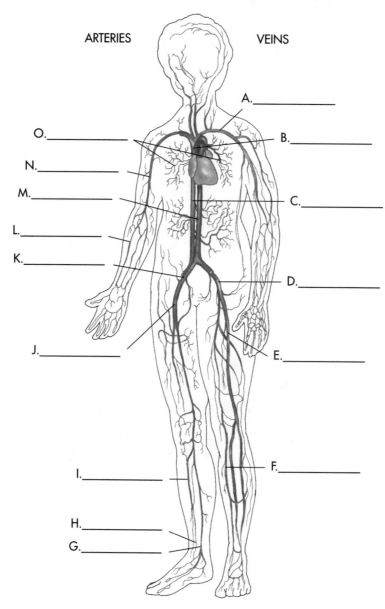

5. Identify the order of the flow of blood to and from tissues.

_____ A. Arterioles
_____ B. Artery
_____ C. Capillaries
_____ D. Heart
_____ E. Veins
_____ F. Venules

6. The right half of the heart pumps blood to the _____ and the left half pumps blood to the _____.

7. What anatomical structure prevents the backflow of blood within the heart? _____

8. Identify each of the following components of the heart.

Aorta
Aortic valve
Bicuspid or mitral valve
Endocardium
Inferior vena cava
Left atrium

Left ventricle
Myocardium
Pericardium
Pulmonary artery
Pulmonary valve
Right atrium

Right ventricle
Septum
Space for pericardial fluid
Superior vena cava
Tricuspid valve

Q._____

P._____

O._____

N._____

M._____

A._____

B._____

C._____

D._____

E._____

F._____

G._____

H._____

I._____

J._____

K._____

L._____

9. There are four valves in the heart. Where are they located?

1)
2)
3)
4)

10. All arteries carry oxygen-rich blood except for the _____ which carry deoxygenated blood from the right ventricle to the lungs.

11. The largest artery in the body is the _____, which extends to the navel, where it divides into the _____.

12. The _____ supplies blood to all other arteries.

13. The _____ arteries supply the myocardium with blood.

14. If coronary arteries become occluded, preventing adequate blood flow, _____ may result.

15. Identify which arteries supply the following parts of the body.

    Head:
    Upper arm:
    Lower forearm and hand:
    Lower extremities and groin:
    Ankle:
    Upper foot:

16. _____ carry blood toward the heart, except for the _____, which carry oxygenated blood from the lungs to the left atria.

17. The smallest veins in the body are called _____.

18. The largest veins in the body are the _____.

19. Electrical impulses of the heart are observed on a(n) _____.

20. Two dysrhythmias that require defibrillation are _____ and _____.

21. The measurement of the force applied to the arterial walls by blood is a(n) _____
    _____.

22. The _____ pressure is the pressure exerted against walls of the arteries when the left ventricle contracts and forces blood out of the heart.

23. The _____ pressure is the pressure that remains in the blood vessels when the left ventricle is refilling from the left atria.

24. The _____ is the difference between the systolic and diastolic pressures.

25. A patient with a blood pressure of 150/90 mm Hg has a pulse pressure of _____.

26. The medical condition that involves periods of intermittent ischemia is called _____
    _____.

27. The medical condition that involves irreversible death of part of the heart muscle is _____
    _____.

28. A myocardial infarction and heart attack are the same thing.
    A. True
    B. False

29. A heart attack is the same as a cardiac arrest.
    A. True
    B. False

30. What are the two most common signs of right-sided heart failure?

    1)
    2)

31. Coarse rales heard when auscultating breath sounds are a sign of _____.

32. Why is accumulation of fluid in the lungs so dangerous?

33. The most common cause of acute cardiogenic shock is _____.

34. List six signs or symptoms of cardiogenic shock.

    1)
    2)
    3)
    4)
    5)
    6)

35. Cardiogenic shock can quickly lead to death.
    A. True
    B. False

36. What are the two most common symptoms associated with cardiovascular system problems?

    1)
    2)

37. Chest pain should be assessed by determining six primary factors. What are they?

    1)
    2)
    3)
    4)
    5)
    6)

38. Identify symptoms commonly associated with cardiac compromise.

39. What does the following mnemonic stand for and when is it used?

    O:
    P:
    Q:
    R:
    S:
    T:

40. What steps should the EMT-B take when caring for a patient with cardiac symptoms?

41. Distended neck veins and swollen extremities are signs of what condition?

42. Most patients with chest pain and shortness of breath prefer to be transported in what position?

43. What is the mechanism of action for nitroglycerin?

44. Identify three side effects of nitroglycerin.

    1)
    2)
    3)

45. Identify three criteria that must be met in order for the EMT-B to administer nitroglycerin.

    1)
    2)
    3)

46. Identify four contraindications for the administration of nitroglycerin.

    1)
    2)
    3)
    4)

47. What is the correct dosage of nitroglycerin?

48. The maximum number of nitroglycerin tablets that can be given in the prehospital environment is _____.

49. The systolic blood pressure must be _____ before the EMT-B can administer nitroglycerin.

Chapter Quiz

· ·

1. How many chambers are in the heart?
   A. 5
   B. 3
   C. 4
   D. 6

2. The two upper chambers of the heart are the:
   A. Ventricles
   B. Atria
   C. Aorta
   D. Vena cava

3. The right half of the heart receives blood from the veins of the body, which empty into the right atrium through the superior and inferior vena cava.
   A. True
   B. False

4. The right ventricle pumps oxygen-poor blood to the lungs through the:
   A. Pulmonary veins
   B. Aorta
   C. Vena cava
   D. Pulmonary arteries

5. What happens to the blood as it passes through the pulmonary capillaries?
   A. Oxygen is added and carbon dioxide is removed.
   B. Carbon dioxide is added and oxygen is removed.
   C. Oxygen is added and carbon dioxide is added.
   D. Oxygen is removed and carbon dioxide is removed.

6. After receiving oxygen and eliminating carbon dioxide in the lungs, the blood enters the left atrium via the:
   A. Pulmonary veins
   B. Aorta
   C. Pulmonary arteries
   D. Vena cava

7. How many valves are in the heart?
   A. 5
   B. 6
   C. 4
   D. 8

8. Where are the valves located in the heart?
   A. Between the atria and ventricles
   B. Between the right ventricle and pulmonary artery
   C. Between the left ventricle and the aorta
   D. All of the above

9. Bradycardia usually refers to a heart rate of:
   A. Less than 70 bpm
   B. Less than 60 bpm
   C. Greater than 60 bpm
   D. Less than 100 bpm

10. Tachycardia usually refers to a heart rate of:
    A. Greater than 100 bpm
    B. Greater than 80 bpm
    C. Less than 100 bpm
    D. Less than 60 bpm

11. Ventricular fibrillation is an arrhythmia in which the entire heart is receiving random, disorganized, electrical impulses, and a coordinated contraction cannot take place.
    A. True
    B. False

12. Defibrillation is designed to temporarily halt the electrical activity of the heart, to allow the normal conduction system to regain control in the heart, enabling effective contraction.
    A. True
    B. False

13. Which of the following is an arrhythmia that may require defibrillation?
    A. Normal sinus rhythm
    B. Pulseless ventricular tachycardia
    C. An agonal rhythm
    D. Atrial fibrillation

14. Arteries are blood vessels that carry blood to the heart.
    A. True
    B. False

15. The pulmonary arteries carry:
    A. Deoxygenated blood
    B. Plasma only
    C. Oxygen-rich blood
    D. Oxygenated blood

16. The largest artery in the body is the:
    A. Femoral
    B. Aorta
    C. Carotid
    D. Pulmonary

17. The heart is supplied with blood from the:
    A. Coronary arteries
    B. Carotid arteries
    C. Radial arteries
    D. Pulmonary arteries

18. The smallest branches of the arteries are the:
    A. Venules
    B. Veins
    C. Vena cava
    D. Arterioles

19. Capillaries surround the body's cells and supply them with oxygen and nutrients.
    A. True
    B. False

20. The largest veins in the body are the:
    A. Ascending and descending aorta
    B. Jugular veins
    C. Superior and inferior vena cavae
    D. Saphenous veins

21. If the EMT-B is able to palpate a carotid pulse, the patient's systolic blood pressure is estimated to be at least _____ mm Hg.
    A. 60
    B. 70
    C. 80
    D. 100

22. Inadequate blood flow to a tissue is called:
    A. Perfusion
    B. Ischemia
    C. Anemia
    D. Hypertension

23. The most common signs of right-sided heart failure are:
    A. Distended neck veins and swelling of the upper extremities
    B. Flat neck veins and swelling of the upper extremities
    C. Flat neck veins and swelling of the lower extremities
    D. Distended neck veins and swelling of the lower extremities

24. If a patient complains of severe substernal chest pain and shortness of breath, the EMT-B should immediately:
    A. Check the patient's blood pressure
    B. Administer a high concentration of oxygen
    C. Call medical direction
    D. Place the patient in a prone position

25. Typical findings with cardiac related chest pain include all of the following *except:*
    A. Originates in the center of the chest
    B. Is dull or squeezing in nature
    C. Radiates down the left arm
    D. Radiates down the right leg

26. Standard cardiac care for the EMT-B includes all of the following *except:*
    A. Placing the patient in a position of comfort
    B. Providing supplemental oxygen
    C. Assisting with administration of NTG when indicated
    D. Administration of lidocaine when indicated

27. Nitroglycerin:
    A. Relaxes and dilates blood vessels
    B. Dilates the coronary arteries
    C. Can cause hypotension
    D. All of the above

28. Indications for NTG include:
    A. Chest pain
    B. Hypotension
    C. An allergic reaction
    D. All of the above

29. The maximum number of doses for NTG is:
    A. 2
    B. 3
    C. 4
    D. 5

30. The four links in the chain of survival are:
    A. Early access, early CPR, early defibrillation, early ACLS
    B. Early access, early CPR, early defibrillation, early definitive treatment
    C. Early access, early CPR, early reporting, early ACLS
    D. Early access, early CPR, early dispatch, early ACLS

Case Scenario

You are dispatched to the Denton Corporate Center for a patient with chest pain. On your arrival, you are directed to the President's office where you find a 58-year-old male patient sitting in a chair with his head down on the table in obvious pain. When asked to describe the pain, he states it is the worst pain he has ever felt, like someone was standing on his chest, and that it radiates down his left arm. He is extremely anxious and short of breath. His skin is pale, cool, and clammy. His pulse rate is 132 and weak and respiratory rate is 28 per minute.

1. What is most likely wrong with this patient?

2. What symptoms does the patient have that would indicate a cardiac problem?

While interviewing the patient, you learn that he has been under extreme stress recently. He has had episodes like this before, but they have never been this bad. He said that he had some pills but couldn't find them. As you are assessing the patient, his secretary enters with a bottle of pills. You observe the label and note that they are nitroglycerin tablets.

3. What is the mechanism of action for NTG?

4. What is the procedure for assisting a patient take NTG?

5. What are the contraindications for NTG?

6. After assisting the patient in taking the NTG, what should you do?

Skill Sheet #19

••

NITROGLYCERIN
Assisting with Administration

Start Time: _____

Stop Time: _____   **Date:** _____

Candidate's Name: _____

Evaluator's Name: _____

	Points Possible	Points Awarded
Takes, or verbalizes, body substance isolation precautions	1	
Obtains an order from medical direction (either on-line or off-line)	1	
Verifies indications for administration of this medication are met	1	
Assesses for evidence of or suspected head injury or other contraindications for medication administration	1	
Takes the patient's blood pressure and assures that it is above 100 mm Hg systolic	1	
Assures the right medication, right patient, right route, and patient alert enough to use inhaler	1	
Checks the expiration date of the nitroglycerin	1	
Questions the patient on the last does administration, effects, and assures the understanding of the route of administration	1	
Asks the patient to lift tongue and places a tablet or spray dose under the tongue (while wearing gloves) or has the patient place the tablet or spray under tongue	1	
Has the patient keep mouth closed with tablet under tongue (without swallowing) until dissolved and absorbed	1	
Rechecks blood pressure within 2 minutes	1	
Records name, dose, route, time, and results of administration time	1	
Performs reassessment	1	
Repeats administration every 3 to 5 minutes until pain is relieved, up to a maximum of three doses, reassessing vital signs and chest pain after each dose, and assuring that the systolic blood pressure is greater than 100 mm Hg before each dose	1	
Total:	14	

Critical Criteria

_____ Did not take, or verbalize, body substance isolation precautions

_____ Did not obtain authorization from medical director (on-line or off-line)

_____ Did not check the medication for correct prescription and for the expiration date

_____ Did not check to see if the patient has already taken any doses

_____ Did not assess the patient's blood pressure to assure systolic of at least 100 mm Hg

_____ Did not reassess blood pressure within 2 minutes

_____ Did not provide additional doses as indicated

_____ Did not appropriately record administration

Skill Sheet #20

● ●

CARDIOPULMONARY RESUSCITATION
Adult—One-Rescuer—EMS Responder

Start Time: _____

Stop Time: _____   **Date:** _____

Candidate's Name: _____

Evaluator's Name: _____

	Points Possible	Points Awarded
Takes, or verbalizes, body substance isolation precautions	1	
Establishes unresponsiveness	1	
Opens the airway (head tile – chin lift or jaw thrust maneuver)	1	
Assesses breathing (look, listen and feel) to identify absent or inadequate breathing—taking no more than 10 seconds	1	
If victim is breathing or resumes effective breathing, place victim in recovery position	1	
If victim is not breathing, gives 2 slow breaths (without O_2 supplement over 2 seconds each; with O_2 supplement over 1 to 2 seconds)	1	
If unable to give initial breaths, repositions the head and reattempts ventilation. If still unsuccessful, follows unresponsive FBAO sequence	1	
Assess for signs of circulation by feeling for a carotid pulse—taking no more than 10 seconds	1	
If there are no signs of circulation, begins chest compressions by locating proper hand position; considers AED use if available and appropriate	1	
Performs 15 chest compressions at a rate of approximately 100 per minute, depressing the chest 1-1/2 to 2 inches with each compression	1	
Opens the airway and delivers 2 slow rescue breaths (2 seconds each)	1	
Finds the proper hand position and begins 15 more compressions at a rate of 100 per minute	1	
Performs 4 complete cycles of 15 compressions and 2 ventilations	1	
Re-assesses for signs of circulation (10 seconds)	1	
If there are still no signs of circulation, resumes CPR, beginning with chest compressions, checking for signs of circulation and spontaneous breathing every few minutes	1	
If signs of circulation are present, checks for breathing	1	
If breathing is present, places the victim in a recovery position and monitors breathing and circulation	1	
If breathing is absent but signs of circulation are present, provides rescue breathing at 10 to 12 times per minute (1 breath every 4 to 5 seconds) and monitors for signs of circulation every few minutes	1	
Total:	18	

Critical Criteria

_____ Did not take, or verbalize, body substance isolation precautions
_____ Did not establish unresponsiveness
_____ Did not open the victim's airway
_____ Did not establish that the victim was not breathing
_____ Did not deliver two adequate rescue breaths
_____ Took longer than 10 seconds to establish the patient was not breathing
_____ Did not assess for a pulse
_____ Took longer than 10 seconds to establish the patient had no pulse
_____ Did not consider AED use
_____ Did not deliver compressions at an appropriate depth, location, or rate
_____ Did not reassess the patient's circulatory or respiratory status
_____ Did not assess breathing status after the return of a pulse
_____ Did not provide rescue breathing as necessary after the return of a pulse

Skill Sheet #21

CARDIOPULMONARY RESUSCITATION
Adult—Two-Rescuers—EMS Responder

Start Time: _____

Stop Time: _____ **Date:** _____

Candidate's Name: _____

Evaluator's Name: _____

	Points Possible	Points Awarded
Takes, or verbalizes, body substance isolation precautions	1	
Establishes unresponsiveness	1	
RESCUER #1 Remains at the victim's head		
Opens the airway (head tilt – chin lift or jaw thrust maneuver)	1	
Assesses breathing (look, listen and feel) to identify absent or inadequate breathing—taking no more than 10 seconds	1	
If victim is breathing or resumes effective breathing, places victim in recovery position	1	
If victim is not breathing, gives 2 slow breaths (without O_2 supplement over 2 seconds each; with O_2 supplement over 1 to 2 seconds)	1	
If unable to give initial breaths, repositions the head and re-attempts ventilation. If still unsuccessful, follows unresponsive FBAO sequence	1	
Assesses for signs of circulation by feeling for a carotid pulse—taking no more than 10 seconds	1	
RESCUER #2 Positioned at the victim's side		
If there are no signs of circulation, begins chest compressions by locating proper hand position; considers AED use if available and appropriate	1	
Performs 15 chest compressions at a rate of approximately 100 per minute. depressing the chest 1-1/2 to 2 inches with each compression	1	
RESCUERS #1 and #2		
Continues CPR with a compression to ventilation ratio of 15:2, with a pause for ventilation of 2 seconds each until the airway is secured by a cuffed endotracheal tube	1	
When the person performing chest compressions becomes fatigued, the rescuers should change positions with minimal interruption of chest compressions	1	
RESCUER #1		
Assesses the effectiveness of the partner's chest compressions by checking the pulse during compressions	1	
Determines whether the victim has resumed spontaneous breathing and circulation by stopping compressions for 10 seconds at approximately the end of the first minute of CPR and every few minutes thereafter	1	
If signs of circulation are present, checks for breathing	1	
If breathing is present, places the victim in a recovery position and monitors breathing and circulation	1	
If breathing is absent but signs of circulation are presend, provides rescue breathing at 10 to 12 times per minute (1 breath every 4 to 5 seconds) and monitors for signs of circulation every few minutes	1	
Total:	17	

Critical Criteria

_____ Did not take, or verbalize, body substance isolation precautions
_____ Did not establish unresponsiveness
_____ Did not open the victim's airway
_____ Did not establish that the victim was not breathing
_____ Took longer than 10 seconds to establish the patient was not breathing
_____ Did not assess for a pulse
_____ Took longer than 10 seconds to establish the patient had no pulse
_____ Did not consider AED use
_____ Did not deliver two adequate rescue breaths
_____ Did not deliver compressions at an appropriate depth, location, or rate
_____ Did not reassess the patient's circulatory or respiratory status
_____ Did not assess breathing status after the return of a pulse
_____ Did not provide rescue breathing as necessary after the return of a pulse

skill sheet #22

••

CARDIOPULMONARY RESUSCITATION
Child Victim—EMS Responder

Start Time: _____

Stop Time: _____   **Date:** _____

Candidate's Name: _____

Evaluator's Name: _____

	Points Possible	Points Awarded
Takes, or verbalizes, body substance isolation precautions	1	
Establishes unresponsiveness	1	
Opens the airway (head tilt – chin lift or jaw thrust maneuver)	1	
Assesses breathing (look, listen and feel) to identify absent or inadequate breathing—taking no more than 10 seconds	1	
If victim is breathing or resumes effective breathing, place victim in recovery position	1	
If victim is not breathing, gives 2 slow breaths (mouth-to-mouth, with enough volume to make the chest rise, taking 1 – 1-1/2 seconds per breath)	1	
If unable to give initial breaths, repositions the head and reattempts ventilation. If still unsuccessful, follows unresponsive FBAO sequence	1	
Assesses for signs of circulation by feeling for a carotid pulse—taking no more than 10 seconds	1	
If there are no signs of circulation, begins chest compressions by locating proper hand position	1	
Performs 5 chest compressions at a rate of approximately 100 per minute	1	
Opens the airway and delivers 1 ventilation (1 – 1-1/2 seconds per breath; use bagmask ventilation if readily available)	1	
Performs 10 complete cycles of 5 compressions and 1 ventilation (5:1 ratio)	1	
Re-assesses for signs of circulation (10 seconds)	1	
If there are still no signs of circulation, resumes CPR, beginning with chest compressions, checking for signs of circulation and spontaneous breathing every few minutes	1	
If signs of circulation are present, checks for breathing	1	
If breathing is present, places the victim in a recovery position and monitors breathing and circulation	1	
If breathing is absent but signs of circulation are present, provides rescue breathing at 20 breaths per minute (1 breath every 3 seconds) and monitors for signs of circulation every few minutes	1	
Total:	17	

Critical Criteria
_____ Did not take, or verbalize, body substance isolation precautions
_____ Did not establish unresponsiveness
_____ Did not open the victim's airway
_____ Did not establish that the victim was not breathing
_____ Took longer than 10 seconds to establish the patient was not breathing
_____ Did not assess for a pulse
_____ Took longer than 10 seconds to establish the patient had no pulse
_____ Did not deliver two adequate rescue breaths
_____ Did not deliver compressions at an appropriate depth, location, or rate
_____ Did not reassess the patient's circulatory or respiratory status
_____ Did not assess breathing status after the return of a pulse
_____ Did not provide rescue breathing as necessary after the return of a pulse

Skill Sheet #23

••

CARDIOPULMONARY RESUSCITATION
Infant Victim—EMS Responder

Start Time: _____

Stop Time: _____   **Date:** _____

Candidate's Name: _____

Evaluator's Name: _____

	Points Possible	Points Awarded
Takes, or verbalizes, body substance isolation precautions	1	
Establishes unresponsiveness—attempts to stimulate	1	
Opens the airway (head tilt – chin lift or jaw thrust maneuver)	1	
Assesses breathing (look, listen and feel) to identify absent or inadequate breathing—taking no more than 10 seconds	1	
If victim is breathing or resumes effective breathing, place victim in recovery position	1	
If victim is not breathing, gives 2 slow breaths (mouth-to-mouth-and nose, with enough volume to make the chest rise, taking 1 – 1-1/2 seconds per breath)	1	
If unable to give initial breaths, repositions the head and reattempts ventilation. If still unsuccessful, follows unresponsive FBAO sequence	1	
Assesses for signs of circulation by feeling for a brachial pulse—taking no more than 10 seconds	1	
If there are no signs of circulation or if the pulse rate is <60 bpm with signs of poor perfusion, begins chest compressions by locating proper hand position	1	
Performs 5 chest compressions at a rate of approximately 100 per minute at a depth of 1/2 to 1 inch, using the 2 finger technique for 1 rescuer and 2 thumb technique for 2 rescuers	1	
Opens the airway and delivers 1 slow rescue breath (1 – 1-1/2 seconds, using a bagmask ventilation for 2 rescuers, if readily available)	1	
Finds the proper hand position and continues with a series of 5 compressions and 1 breath at a rate of 100 per minute	1	
Performs 10 complete cycles of 5 compressions and 1 ventilation each	1	
Re-assesses for signs of circulation (taking no more than 10 seconds)	1	
If there are still no signs of adequate circulation, resumes CPR, beginning with chest compressions at a ratio of 5 compressions to 1 ventilation, checking for signs of circulation and spontaneous breathing every few minutes	1	
If signs of adequate circulation are present, checks for breathing	1	
If breathing is present, places the victim in a recovery position and monitors breathing and circulation	1	
If breathing is absent but signs of adequate circulation are present, provides rescue breathing at a rate of 20 per minute (1 breath every 3 seconds) until breathing resumes, and monitors for signs of circulation every few minutes	1	
Total:	18	

Critical Criteria

_____ Did not take, or verbalize, body substance isolation precautions
_____ Did not open the victim's airway
_____ Did not establish that the victim was not breathing
_____ Took longer than 10 seconds to establish the patient was not breathing
_____ Did not assess for a pulse
_____ Took longer than 10 seconds to establish the patient had no pulse
_____ Did not begin chest compressions with heart rate of 60 bpm or less with signs of poor perfusion
_____ Did not deliver two adequate rescue breaths
_____ Did not deliver compressions at an appropriate depth, location, or rate
_____ Did not reassess the patient's circulatory or respiratory status
_____ Did not assess breathing status after the return of a pulse
_____ Did not provide rescue breathing as necessary after the return of a pulse

Skill Sheet #24

• •

CARDIOPULMONARY RESUSCITATION
Newborn Infant Victim—EMS Responder

Start Time: _____

Stop Time: _____   **Date:** _____

Candidate's Name: _____

Evaluator's Name: _____

	Points Possible	Points Awarded
Takes, or verbalizes, body substance isolation precautions	1	
Establishes unresponsiveness—attempts to stimulate	1	
Prevents heat loss—keeps newborn as warm as possible	1	
Opens the airway (head tilt – chin lift or jaw thrust maneuver to a neutral position)	1	
Assesses breathing (look, listen, and feel) to identify absent or inadequate breathing—taking no more than 10 seconds	1	
If victim is not breathing, gives 2 slow breaths (mouth-to-mouth-and-nose with enough volume to make the chest rise, taking 1/2 to 1 second per breath)	1	
Assesses for signs of circulation by feeling for a brachial pulse—taking no more than 10 seconds	1	
If heart rate is 60 to 80 bpm and not rising, ventilation should be the priority in resuscitation. If there are no signs of circulation or if heart rate is <60 bpm, begins chest compressions by locating proper hand position.	1	
Performs 3 chest compressions at a rate of approximately 120 per minute at a depth of 1/2 to 1 inch, using the 2 finger technique for 1 rescuer and 2 thumb technique for 2 rescuers [unless local protocols require a 5:1 ratio]	1	
Opens the airway and delivers 1 slow rescue breath (1/2 second, using a bag-mask ventilation for 2 rescuers, if readily available)	1	
Finds the proper hand position and continues with a series of 3 compressions and 1 breath at a rate of 120 per minute (unless local protocols require a 5:1 ratio)	1	
After approximately 1 minute, reassesses for signs of circulation—taking no more than 10 seconds	1	
If there are still no signs of circulation, resumes CPR, beginning with chest compressions, checking for signs of circulation and spontaneous breathing every few minutes	1	
If signs of circulation are present, checks for breathing	1	
If breathing is present, places the victim in a recovery position and monitors breathing and circulation	1	
If breathing is absent but signs of adequate circulation are present or if heart rate continues at a rate <100 bpm, provides rescue breathing at 40 to 60 per minute using a neonatal BVM and monitors for signs of circulation every few minutes	1	
Total:	16	

Critical Criteria
_____ Did not take, or verbalize, body substance isolation precautions
_____ Did not take steps to prevent heat loss
_____ Did not open the victim's airway
_____ Did not establish that the victim was not breathing or that breathing was inadequate
_____ Took longer than 10 seconds to establish the patient was not breathing
_____ Did not assess for a pulse
_____ Took longer than 10 seconds to establish the patient had no pulse
_____ Did not begin assisted ventilations with heart rate of 100 bpm or less
_____ Did not begin chest compressions with heart rate of 60 bpm or less
_____ Did not deliver adequate rescue breaths
_____ Did not deliver compressions at an appropriate depth, location, or rate
_____ Did not reassess the patient's circulatory or respiratory status
_____ Did not assess breathing status after the return of a pulse
_____ Did not provide appropriate rescue breaths as necessary after the return of a pulse

Answer Key

● ●

Key Terms
1. M, I, D, L, J, B, F, G, C, K, H, A, N, E
2. D, F, E, G, K, C, L, A, J, I, B, H

Content Review
1. Ventricular fibrillation
   Normal sinus rhythm
   Ventricular tachycardia
2. Ischemia
3. Nitroglycerin
4. A. Axillary vein
   B. Superior vena cava
   C. Inferior vena cava
   D. Left common iliac vein
   E. Femoral vein
   F. Great saphenous vein
   G. Posterior tibial artery
   H. Dorsalis pedis artery
   I. Anterior tibial artery
   J. Femoral artery
   K. Right common iliac artery
   L. Radial artery
   M. Aorta
   N. Brachial artery
   O. Pulmonary arteries and veins
5. A, C, E, B, F, D, A
6. Lungs; body
7. Valves
8. A. Aorta
   B. Pulmonary artery
   C. Left atrium
   D. Bicuspid or mitral valve
   E. Aortic valve
   F. Endocardium
   G. Myocardium
   H. Pericardium
   I. Space for pericardial fluid
   J. Left ventricle
   K. Septum
   L. Right ventricle
   M. Inferior vena cava
   N. Tricuspid valve
   O. Pulmonary valve
   P. Right atrium
   Q. Superior vena cava
9. 1) Between the right ventricle and right atrium; 2) between the left ventricle and left atrium; 3) between the right ventricle and pulmonary artery; and 4) between the left ventricle and aorta
10. Pulmonary arteries
11. Aorta; iliac arteries

12. Aorta
13. Coronary
14. Myocardial infarction
15. Head: carotid; upper arm: brachial; lower forearm and hand: radial; lower extremities and groin: femoral; ankle: posterior tibial; upper foot: dorsalis pedis
16. Veins; pulmonary veins
17. Venules
18. Superior and inferior vena cava
19. Electrocardiogram (ECG)
20. Ventricular fibrillation; pulseless ventricular tachycardia
21. Blood pressure
22. Systolic
23. Diastolic
24. Pulse pressure
25. 60 mm Hg
26. Angina pectoris
27. Myocardial infarction
28. True
29. False
30. 1) Distended neck veins; and 2) edema in the lower extremities
31. Pulmonary edema
32. It prevents oxygen and carbon dioxide exchange within the blood.
33. Myocardial infarction
34. 1) Pale or cyanotic skin; 2) diaphoresis; 3) restlessness; 4) rapid and weak pulse; 5) rapid and shallow respirations; and 6) decreased blood pressure
35. True
36. Chest pain and dyspnea
37. 1) Location; 2) quality; 3) severity; 4) presence of radiation; 5) aggravating and relieving features; and 6) associated symptoms
38. Shortness of breath, nausea, anxiety, feeling of impending doom, cool and diaphoretic skin, abnormal and/or irregular pulse rate, and an abnormal blood pressure (high or low)
39. O: onset of pain; P: provocation; Q: quality of pain; R: radiation of pain; S: severity of pain; T: time when pain started. OPQRST is used to assess the severity of a patient complaining of pain.
40. Place the patient in a position of comfort; provide supplemental oxygen; assist with administration of nitroglycerin when indicated; rapid transport; and monitor vital signs frequently
41. Congestive heart failure
42. Sitting
43. Nitroglycerin relaxes and dilates blood vessels, decreases workload of the heart, decreases the heart's demand for oxygen, and dilates coronary arteries improving blood supply to the heart.
44. 1) Decreased blood pressure; 2) headache; and 3) changes in pulse rate
45. 1) The patient has signs and symptoms of chest pain; 2) the patient has a current prescription for nitroglycerin, and 3) the EMT-B has authorization by the medical director to administer the drug
46. 1) A systolic blood pressure less than 100 mm Hg; 2) a head injury; 3) the patient is an infant or child; or 4) the patient has taken 3 NTG tablets prior to the EMT-B's arrival.
47. 1 tablet (or 1 to 2 puffs of spray) every 3 to 5 minutes until the pain is relieved; up to 3 doses
48. 3
49. Greater than 100 mm Hg

Chapter Quiz

1. C	6. A	11. A	16. B	21. A	26. D
2. B	7. C	12. A	17. A	22. B	27. D
3. A	8. D	13. B	18. D	23. D	28. A
4. D	9. B	14. B	19. A	24. B	29. B
5. A	10. A	15. A	20. C	25. D	30. A

Case Scenario

1. Cardiac compromise from angina pectoris or an acute myocardial infarction.

2. Substernal chest pain radiating to the arm; chest pain, shortness of breath; pale, cool, and clammy skin; anxiety; increased ventilations; and increased pulse

3. NTG dilates large veins and decreases workload on the heart; it dilates large coronary arteries; and helps relieves the pain of angina.

4. Check the prescription to make certain it is for the patient and that it is current (has not expired); document that the blood pressure is greater than 100 mm Hg; place one tablet under the patient's tongue and have him close his mouth; instruct the patient not to swallow or chew the tablet; take the patient's blood pressure two minutes after administration; record vital signs, symptoms, and time of administration for each dose.

5. Head injury; systolic BP less than 100 mm Hg; infant or child patient; or the patient has already taken three tablets prior to the EMT's arrival

6. Administer high-flow oxygen (if not already in place); watch for the effects of the medication (i.e., relief of symptoms) reassess vital signs; assist with additional NTG tablets every 3 to 5 minutes as needed to a maximum of 3 doses; watch for side effects (hypotension, increased heart rate, or headache); make the patient comfortable; and transport immediately, considering ALS rendezvous en route.

Reading Assignment: Chapter 16 pages 306–322.

DOT Objectives

Upon successful completion of the EMT-Basic training program, the EMT-Basic should be able to do the following:

- List the indications for use of the automated external defibrillator.
- List the contraindications for use of the automated external defibrillator.
- Explain the role of age and weight in use of the automated external defibrillator.
- Discuss the fundamentals of and explain the rationale for early defibrillation.
- Explain the importance of early ALS interventions to the cardiac arrest patient, if available.
- Discuss the types of automated external defibrillators.
- Differentiate between a fully automatic and a semi-automatic automated external defibrillator.
- Discuss procedures that must be taken into account for use of the automated external defibrillator.
- Discuss circumstances in which inappropriate shocks could occur while using the automated external defibrillator.
- Discuss advantages and summarize speed of operation in the use of the automated external defibrillator.
- List the steps in use of the automated external defibrillator.
- Discuss procedures for management of a patient who remains in cardiac arrest after use of the automated external defibrillator.
- Discuss the importance of post-resuscitation patient care.
- List the importance of regular skills practice in using the automated external defibrillator.
- Explain the role medical direction plays in the use of the automated external defibrillator.
- Discuss the components of and why case reviews are important in the use of automated external defibrillation.
- Define the function of all controls found on an automated external defibrillator.
- Demonstrate the application and use of the automated external defibrillator
- Demonstrate the maintenance procedures for the automated external defibrillator.
- Demonstrate patient assessment while using and following use of the automated external defibrillator.
- Demonstrate skills to complete the operator's skills checklist for the automated external defibrillator.

Key Terms

1. The condition in which a human body no longer exists in a conscious state, caused by extended periods of anoxia to brain tissue resulting in no conscious activity within the nervous system is called a(n) _____.

2. A device that uses computer technology to interpret a patient's electrical heart rhythm and deliver an electrical current on its own when indicated is called a(n) _____ _____.

3. The use of electroshock to terminate ventricular fibrillation is called _____.

4. A dysrhythmia in which the heart is in a state of disorganized electrical and mechanical activity, resulting in a lack of blood flow, is called _____.

5. Death to a portion of the heart muscle caused by interruption of normal blood supply and oxygen is called _____.

6. A form of arteriosclerosis in which deposits of yellowish plaque containing cholesterol and lipid material become deposited in the walls of the arteries, generally resulting in decreased blood supply is called _____.

7. Another frequently used term for cardiac arrest is _____.

Content Review

1. List the four components of the "chain of survival."

   1)

   2)

   3)

   4)

2. The highest priority for care of a patient in ventricular fibrillation is _____.

3. A brain deprived of oxygen for _____ minutes generally will not recover.

4. The most common dysrhythmia that occurs in the initial minutes of a cardiac arrest is _____ _____.

5. When the heart is in ventricular fibrillation, it produces no cardiac output.
   A. True
   B. False

6. The only definitive treatment for a patient in ventricular fibrillation is _____.

7. The delivery of high-voltage current through the patient's skin, causing it to traverse the myocardium and terminate ventricular fibrillation is called _____.

8. What is the purpose of CPR?

9. The energy levels transmitted through an AED are measured in _____.

10. What is the difference between a fully automatic or semi-automatic AED?

11. On whom should the AED unit be applied?

12. CPR should be continued until the AED is attached.
    A. True
    B. False

13. List the voice prompts that are normally heard from an AED.

14. When will an AED unit instruct the EMT to check breathing and pulse?

15. All AEDs are programmed to deliver shocks in stacked sets of _____.

16. Treatment protocol for AED indicate a patient in cardiac arrest should receive the following in what order.

    _____ 1 minute of CPR
    _____ 3 stacked defibrillation shocks

17. Why is CPR provided between sets of shock?

18. When faced with a patient in cardiac arrest, the EMT should not take time to call for additional help or contact medical direction until:

19. The use of an AED requires the presence of ALS personnel on the scene.
    A. True
    B. False

20. Currently available AEDs should not be used on anyone under age _____ years or weighing less than _____ pounds

21. AED is not a method of management for cardiac arrest secondary to major trauma.
    A. True
    B. False

22. Identify three safety issues regarding the use of the AED.

    1)
    2)
    3)

23. If there is a return of spontaneous pulse after delivery of an electrical shock, what should the EMT do?

24. What information should be recorded on a prehospital care report?

25. One of the most important maintenance items for the AED is _____ _____.

26. Current guidelines recommend that review and practice of AED skills be conducted every _____ days.

Chapter Quiz

1. What is the normal order of the electrical conduction system of the heart?
   A. AV node, SA node, ventricles
   B. Ventricles, AV node, SA node
   C. SA node, ventricles, AV node
   D. SA node, AV node, ventricles

2. An abnormal rhythm of the heart is called a(n):
   A. Dysrhythmia
   B. Paranormal rhythm
   C. Rhythmia
   D. Pararhythm

3. The most common initial rhythm in cardiac arrest is VF and:
   A. The definitive treatment for VF is defibrillation
   B. The likelihood of successful defibrillation diminishes rapidly after onset of VF
   C. Normal sinus rhythm
   D. A and B

4. Proper AED operation depends on:
   A. Thorough knowledge of established protocols
   B. Frequent practice with the device
   C. Routine defibrillator and battery maintenance
   D. All of the above

5. A fully automated defibrillator delivers shocks to the patient without any action by the EMT except turning the power on and applying the electrodes.
   A. True
   B. False

6. A semi-automated defibrillator delivers shocks to the patient without any action by the EMT except turning the power on and applying the electrodes.
   A. True
   B. False

7. Unless ALS personnel are on the scene or a variance is permitted by local medical control, the patient should be transported when which of the following occurs?
   A. The patient regains a pulse
   B. Six shocks are delivered
   C. Three consecutive no shock messages are given separated by 1 minute of CPR
   D. All of the above

8. The most common cause of cardiac arrest in children is:
   A. Cardiac failure
   B. Brain abnormalities
   C. Respiratory compromise
   D. Congenital abnormalities

9. An AED cannot accurately analyze a patient in a moving vehicle.
   A. True
   B. False

10. Defibrillation is more important than CPR when VF or pulseless VT is present.
    A. True
    B. False

11. Postresuscitation care components include:
    A. Breathing assessment
    B. Pulse assessment
    C. Oxygen administration
    D. All of the above

12. Automated external defibrillator operation by EMTs can only take place under the authority of local medical control and each case in which an AED is used should be reviewed by the local medical director.
    A. True
    B. False

13. Documented use of the AED for case reviews should include written reports, voice-electrocardiogram tape recordings, and digitized ECG.
    A. True
    B. False

Case Scenario

You and your partner have been dispatched to the airport in reference to a call from airport police that an inbound commercial airliner has a passenger who is experiencing chest pain. The pilot reported that the patient, a male, developed severe chest pain approximately 5 minutes ago, and is sweating and complaining of difficulty getting his breath. No other information is available.

The plane touches down approximately 5 minutes after your arrival. You and your partner enter the plane where you are directed to the patient. You observe a middle age male sitting in the rear seat with oxygen being administered. Your initial assessment reveals a conscious, alert, and oriented 48-year-old patient who is breathing at a rate of 26 breaths per minute with some distress, with a radial pulse of 112 and irregular, and who is pale and diaphoretic.

As you finish your initial assessment, the patient suddenly gasps, grabs his chest, and becomes unresponsive in the seat. A quick evaluation reveals that he is pulseless and apneic. You quickly move him from the seat to the floor, open your AED and place the pads on his exposed chest. After turning the AED on, you are advised to stop CPR and the machine assesses the patient's cardiac rhythm. You are advised to stand back as the machine charges and delivers the first shock. Reassessment by the AED reveals the need for a second shock that is then delivered to the patient. The machine then advises, after again reassessing the patient, to check for breathing and pulse.

Assessment then reveals the patient's pulse has returned and he is breathing shallow and irregular at 12 breaths per minute. You advise your partner to assist his ventilations while you prepare to move the patient to the ambulance for transport.

1. Why was your first action on this patient to apply the AED? Are their any limitations to its use?

2. What would you have done for this patient if the AED had advised that no shock was indicated?

3. What are the basic voice commands of the AED?

4. What steps should you take in the postresuscitation care of this patient?

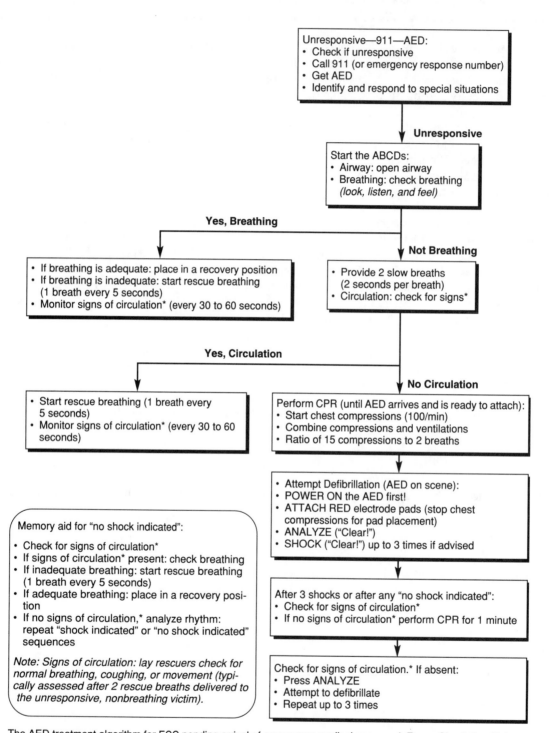

Unresponsive—911—AED:
- Check if unresponsive
- Call 911 (or emergency response number)
- Get AED
- Identify and respond to special situations

Unresponsive

Start the ABCDs:
- Airway: open airway
- Breathing: check breathing *(look, listen, and feel)*

Yes, Breathing

Not Breathing

- If breathing is adequate: place in a recovery position
- If breathing is inadequate: start rescue breathing (1 breath every 5 seconds)
- Monitor signs of circulation* (every 30 to 60 seconds)

- Provide 2 slow breaths (2 seconds per breath)
- Circulation: check for signs*

Yes, Circulation

No Circulation

- Start rescue breathing (1 breath every 5 seconds)
- Monitor signs of circulation* (every 30 to 60 seconds)

Perform CPR (until AED arrives and is ready to attach):
- Start chest compressions (100/min)
- Combine compressions and ventilations
- Ratio of 15 compressions to 2 breaths

Memory aid for "no shock indicated":

- Check for signs of circulation*
- If signs of circulation* present: check breathing
- If inadequate breathing: start rescue breathing (1 breath every 5 seconds)
- If adequate breathing: place in a recovery position
- If no signs of circulation,* analyze rhythm: repeat "shock indicated" or "no shock indicated" sequences

Note: Signs of circulation: lay rescuers check for normal breathing, coughing, or movement (typically assessed after 2 rescue breaths delivered to the unresponsive, nonbreathing victim).

- Attempt Defibrillation (AED on scene):
- POWER ON the AED first!
- ATTACH RED electrode pads (stop chest compressions for pad placement)
- ANALYZE ("Clear!")
- SHOCK ("Clear!") up to 3 times if advised

After 3 shocks or after any "no shock indicated":
- Check for signs of circulation*
- If no signs of circulation* perform CPR for 1 minute

Check for signs of circulation.* If absent:
- Press ANALYZE
- Attempt to defibrillate
- Repeat up to 3 times

The AED treatment algorithm for ECC pending arrival of emergency medical personnel. From: *Circulation*, Vol. 102, No. 8, Aug. 22, 2000, ISSN 009-7322.

Skill Sheet #25

CARDIAC ARREST MANAGEMENT/AED

Start Time: _____

Stop Time: _____   Date: _____

Candidate's Name: _____

Evaluator's Name: _____

	Points Possible	Points Awarded
ASSESSMENT		
Takes, or verbalizes, body substance isolation precautions	1	
Briefly questions the rescuer about arrest events	1	
Directs rescuer to stop CPR	1	
Verifies absence of spontaneous pulse (skill station examiner states "no pulse")	1	
Directs resumption of CPR	1	
Turns on defibrillator power	1	
Attaches automated defibrillator to the patient	1	
Directs rescuer to stop CPR and ensures all individuals are clear of the patient	1	
Initiates analysis of the rhythm	1	
Delivers shock (up to three successive shocks)	1	
Verifies absence of spontaneous pulse (skill station examiner states "no pulse")	1	
TRANSITION		
Directs resumption of CPR	1	
Gathers additional information about arrest event	1	
Confirms effectiveness of CPR (ventilation and compressions)	1	
INTEGRATION		
Verbalizes or directs insertion of a simple airway adjunct (oral/nasal airway)	1	
Ventilates, or directs ventilation of, the patient	1	
Assures high concentration of oxygen is delivered to the patient	1	
Assures CPR continues without unnecessary/prolonged interruption	1	
Re-evaluates patient/CPR in approximately 1 minute	1	
TRANSPORTATION		
Verbalizes transportation of patient	1	
Total:	21	

Critical Criteria

_____ Did not take, or verbalize, body substance isolation precautions

_____ Did not evaluate the need for immediate use of the AED

_____ Did not direct initiation/resumption of ventilation/compressions at appropriate times.

_____ Did not assure all individuals were clear of patient before delivering each shock

_____ Did not operate the AED properly (inability to deliver shock)

_____ Prevented the defibrillator from delivering indicated stacked shocks

Answer Key

· ·

Key Terms
1. Permanent vegetative state
2. Automated external defibrillator
3. Defibrillation
4. Ventricular fibrillation
5. Myocardial infarction
6. Atherosclerosis
7. Sudden cardiac death

Content Review
1. 1) Early access; 2) early CPR; 3) early defibrillation; and 4) early advanced care
2. Defibrillation
3. 10
4. Ventricular fibrillation
5. True
6. Defibrillation
7. Defibrillation
8. CPR artificially circulates blood and oxygen to the central circulation of the body, thereby extending the window of opportunity for resuscitation.
9. Joules
10. Whether or not the operator has to manually push the shock button or the device will perform the delivery automatically
11. A patient who is unconscious, unresponsive, and pulseless
12. True
13. Attach electrode pads; Assessing—do not touch patient; Charging—stand back; Push to shock; check patient (or check breathing and pulse)
14. After every third shock (3, 6, 9) during the initial defibrillation and if the initial analysis of the patient's heart rhythm reveals a non-ventricular fibrillation pattern or if the patient's ECG rhythm is changed from v-fib to a non-ventricular fibrillation pattern by any single defibrillation shock
15. 3
16. 2, 1
17. After the third shock, a patient still in VF needs the myocardium to be oxygenated with CPR before any further attempts at defibrillation are made.
18. After the first three shocks have been given or the voice prompts you to check breathing and pulse.
19. False
20. 8; 55
21. True
22. 1) Do not use on patients weighing less than 55 pounds; 2) do not use in wet environments as this could result in energy being transferred to the rescuers; and 3) make sure no one is touching the patient at the time of shock
23. Ensure the patient has a patent airway and that ventilations are adequate. If not, immediately deliver rescue breaths with supplemental oxygen; if ventilations are adequate, apply supplemental oxygen as soon as possible; continually monitor the patient's ABCs; and leave the AED unit applied.
24. Times; number of shocks given; any treatment given prior to, during, or in the postresuscitation periods; attachment of any ECG tracings from AED unit; and any interactions with family, bystanders, or other rescuers.
25. Ensuring batteries are current and fully charged
26. 90

Chapter Quiz

1. D	5. A	8. C	11. D
2. A	6. B	9. A	12. A
3. D	7. D	10. A	13. A
4. D			

Case Scenario

1. The majority of cardiac arrest patients will present with ventricular fibrillation as their primary dysrythmia. The only definitive treatment for VF is defibrillation. Also, for every 1 minute a patient is in cardiac arrest, they lose 7% chance for resuscitation. Limitations for use include age greater than 8 or a minimum weight of less than 55 lbs. and a wet environment.

2. Ensure that the patient was not being moved while the AED unit was assessing the patient. Check for a pulse. If there is a pulse and the patient is breathing, apply supplemental oxygen and transport immediately. If there is no pulse, administer CPR per local protocols.

3. "Attach electrode pads"; "Assessing - do not touch patient": "Charging—stand back"; "Push to shock"; "Check breathing and pulse."

4. Immediate postresuscitative care should be directed at ensuring a patent airway, adequate ventilations, and the administration of supplemental oxygen. Assess the location, rate, and quality of the pulse. Initiate immediate transport to the hospital with an ALS rendevous, if possible.

17

Altered Mental Status

Reading Assignment: Chapter 17 pages 323–334.

DOT Objectives

- Identify the patient taking diabetic medications with altered mental status and the implications of a diabetes history.
- State the steps in the emergency medical care of the patient taking diabetic medicine with an altered mental status and a history of diabetes.
- Establish the relationship between airway management and the history of diabetes.
- State the trade names, administration, action, and contraindications of oral glucose.
- Evaluate the need for medical direction in the emergency care of a diabetic patient.

Supplemental Objectives

- Describe the different levels of altered mental states.
- Describe and differentiate the following possible causes for altered mental states:
  - Neurologic (i.e., stroke, seizure, organic brain syndrome, or Alzheimer's disease)
  - Toxicologic (drug or alcohol induced)
  - Traumatic (injury)
  - Hypoxia (impaired respirations or circulation)
  - Metabolic or organic (diabetes)
- Demonstrate the assessment and documentation process of patients with altered mental status.
- Identify the appropriate management of patients with altered mental states.
- Identify specific prehospital management appropriate for diabetic patients.
- Identify medications that reveal important history in regard to patients with altered mental states.
- Identify special safety concerns for both the patient and the rescuer when working with patients with altered mental states.

Key Terms

••

1. A phenomenon of increasing intracranial pressure, distinguished by an increase in blood pressure, bizarre respirations, and decrease in pulse is called _____.

2. The hormone produced in the pancreas that is necessary for the proper metabolism of blood sugar is _____.

3. The period of time immediately following a seizure is called the _____.

4. A starch that is the major storage form of glucose is called _____.

5. The medical term for a low blood glucose level is _____.

6. The standardized rating system used to evaluate the degree of LOC impairment based on three categories is called the _____.

7. The medical term for an elevated blood glucose level is _____.

8. The cluster of cells in the pancreas that produce insulin are the _____.

9. A partial paralysis affecting only one side of the body is called _____.

10. A total paralysis that affects only one side of the body is termed _____.

11. A metabolic disorder that is the result of inadequate insulin secretion is called _____.

12. The hormone secreted by the pancreas that stimulates the breakdown of glycogen and the release of glucose by the liver is _____.

13. A temporary disruption in blood flow to the brain that results in dizziness, imbalance, and generalized weakness is called a(n) _____.

14. A continuous seizure that lasts more than 30 minutes is called _____.

15. A subjective sensation experienced as numbness or tingling or a "pins and needles" feeling is called _____.

16. A simple sugar used by cells for energy is called _____.

17. The term for a group of neurologic disorders that is characterized by recurrent episodes of convulsive seizures or sensory disturbances is _____.

18. A generalized full tonic/clonic seizure is called a _____ seizure.

19. A partial seizure, often seen in children, is called a _____ seizure.

20. The rhythmic motion of the body and extremities that occurs with a seizure is called _____.

Content Review

1. The Glasgow coma scale evaluates LOC based on what three categories?

   1)
   2)
   3)

2. The type of diabetes that can usually be controlled by diet and oral hypoglycemics is _____ _____.

3. The gland that produces insulin is the _____.

4. The most common cause of altered mental states is _____.

5. If too much insulin is given or not enough food is eaten, the blood glucose level will fall, a condition called _____.

6. Brain cells can only use glucose for fuel. Therefore a patient with low blood sugar may have dysfunctioning brain cells resulting in an altered mental status.
   A. True
   B. False

7. The normal blood glucose level is _____

8. Treatment of hyperglycemia can begin in the field.
   A. True
   B. False

9. The cells in the pancreas which produce insulin are called _____.

10. Type 1 diabetes is also known as _____.

11. Type 2 diabetes is also known as _____.

12. Patients with Type _____ diabetes usually require insulin injections.

13. Type _____ diabetes usually occurs in adolescence or early adulthood.

14. Type _____ diabetes is more common in older patients and frequently associated with obesity.

15. What is the classic triad of symptoms of diabetes?

16. The medical term for frequent urination is _____.

17. What are the three types of emergencies specific to patients with diabetes?

    1)
    2)
    3)

18. List the steps for proper management of a patient with a diabetic problem.

19. If a diabetic patient has an altered mental state, the EMT-B should administer sugar, even if he or she is uncertain whether the problem is hyperglycemia or hypoglycemia.
    A. True
    B. False

20. The left side of the brain controls the _____ side of the body and the right side of the brain controls the _____ side of the body.

21. Identify two causes of stroke.

    1)
    2)

22. What is the most common cause of seizures in children?

23. The postictal state of a seizure usually lasts _____ minutes.

24. How should the EMT care for a seizure patient?

25. The EMT should use a "bite stick" in the mouth of a seizure patient to prevent the patient from biting the tongue.
    A. True
    B. False

26. A slow, progressive loss of awareness for time and place, usually with the inability to learn new things or remember recent events, is a condition called _____.

27. An abrupt disorientation for time and place, usually with illusions and hallucinations, where the mind wanders, speech may be incoherent, and the patient is in a state of mental confusion and excitement is a condition called _____.

28. What is organic brain syndrome?

29. A chronic, organic mental disorder that results from atrophy of the frontal and occipital lobes of the brain and involves progressive and irreversible loss of memory, disturbance of intellectual functions, apathy, speech and gait disturbances, and disorientation is a condition known as _____ _____.

30. Narcotics cause what symptoms?

31. Cocaine and amphetamines are classified as which type of drugs?

32. What are the signs and symptoms of cocaine use?

33. A patient taking LSD or PCP may exhibit what signs and symptoms?

34. Why might a patient with kidney disease appear with an altered mental status?

35. What does the acronym AVPU stand for?

   A:
   V:
   P:
   U:

Chapter Quiz

1. What substances are used by all cells of the body to produce energy?
   A. Oxygen and carbon dioxide
   B. Sugar and oxygen
   C. Hemoglobin and nitrogen
   D. Sugar and carbon monoxide

2. The hormone insulin facilitates the:
   A. Transmission of glucose from the blood into the cell
   B. Transmission of glucose from the cell into the blood
   C. Excretion of glucose from the cell
   D. Metabolization of ketones for energy

3. Insulin is made in special cells found in the:
   A. Stomach
   B. Liver
   C. Pancreas
   D. Spleen

4. Type 1 diabetics:
   A. Usually require insulin treatment and have adolescent onset
   B. Do not require insulin treatment and start in late adulthood
   C. Do not have the normal signs and symptoms of diabetes
   D. Produce too much insulin and therefore must eat often

5. Type 2 diabetics are:
    A. Very rare
    B. Common in early adulthood and often associated with smoking
    C. Common in slim adolescents
    D. More common in older patients and often associated with obesity

6. Polyuria is a classic symptom of diabetes.
    A. True
    B. False

7. Which of the following signs of diabetes can be attributed to the effects of low insulin levels?
    A. Increased blood glucose levels
    B. Decreased fat use
    C. Decreased protein use
    D. Increased protein in the urine

8. Oral hypoglycemics are drugs that act to:
    A. Reduce glucose levels by increasing caloric intake
    B. Decrease insulin production and increase glucose levels
    C. Stimulate insulin release from the pancreas
    D. Stimulate the use of fats and increase ketones

9. Diabetic ketoacidosis may be caused by:
    A. Lack of adequate insulin
    B. An infection
    C. Significant stress
    D. All of the above

10. In DKA, the cells are not able to metabolize glucose, therefore the body begins to metabolize fats and proteins to provide an energy source for cells.
    A. True
    B. False

11. The DKA patient may present with which of the following signs and symptoms?
    A. A fruity odor on the breath
    B. Diuresis and dehydration
    C. A change in level of consciousness
    D. All of the above

12. Which of the following are true concerning non-ketotic, hyperosmolar states (NKHS)?
    A. Fat and protein breakdown does not occur to the extent of DKA
    B. The patient will present with altered mental status
    C. The patient has extreme hyperglycemia
    D. All of the above

13. Hypoglycemia is:
    A. High blood sugar
    B. Low blood sugar
    C. High calorie intake
    D. Low calorie intake

14. Low blood sugar can cause:
    A. Altered levels of consciousness
    B. Seizures
    C. Brain damage
    D. All of the above

15. Diabetic patients with altered mental status may have problems maintaining their airway.
    A. True
    B. False

16. Characteristics of Kussmaul's respirations are:
    A. Slow, deep breathing
    B. Rapid, deep breathing
    C. Shallow, agonal breathing
    D. Rapid, shallow breathing

17. Which of the following is not a finding of the severely ill diabetic?
    A. Consciousness and alertness
    B. Restlessness and confusion
    C. Combativeness
    D. Seizures or coma

18. Diabetic patients who are drooling should not be given oral glucose.
    A. True
    B. False

Case Scenario

You are called to a residence where you find a 32-year-old female patient lying on the couch. The patient's husband informs you that the patient has a history of diabetes for which she takes insulin. He states that she has not been feeling well for the past few days.

The husband said that this morning while she was making coffee, she started to "feel shaky" and went to lie down on the couch. A few minutes later he found her "not looking well," so he called 911.

On initial assessment, you find that the patient responds to verbal stimuli. Her skin is pale, cool, and clammy.

1. List the pertinent questions that you should ask the patient, her husband, or both to help you better understand the situation at hand.

2. What is most likely wrong with this patient?

3. What assessment and management steps should you take for this patient?

Skill Sheet #26

. . . .

ORAL GLUCOSE ADMINISTRATION

Start Time: _____

Stop Time: _____   **Date:** _____

Candidate's Name: _____

Evaluator's Name: _____

	Points Possible	Points Awarded
Takes, or verbalizes, body substance isolation precautions	1	
Performs initial assessment, establishes and maintains an open airway	2	
Assures signs and symptoms of altered mental status with known history of diabetes (looks for medical identification tag)	2	
Determines last meal/oral intake, medication dose, any related illness	3	
Obtains baseline vital signs	1	
Determines if patient is awake enough to swallow	1	
Obtains order from medical direction to administer medication (either on-line or off-line)	1	
Connects rigid suction catheter to suction and ensures equipment is readily available	1	
Confirms medication name and expiration date	2	
Places glucose gel onto a tongue depressor	1	
Places tongue depressor between patient's cheek and gum	1	
Performs ongoing assessment reassessing and recording vital signs and patient's response to treatment	3	
Total:	19	

Critical Criteria

_____ Did not take, or verbalize, body substance isolation precautions

_____ Did not perform initial assessment before medication administration

_____ Did not confirm diabetic history

_____ Did not obtain on-line or off-line medical direction

_____ Did not confirm patient is awake enough to swallow

_____ Did not confirm drug and expiration date before administration

_____ Did not reassess patient after medication administration

Answer Key

Key Terms
1. Cushing's triad
2. Insulin
3. Postictal state
4. Glycogen
5. Hypoglycemia
6. Glasgow coma scale
7. Hyperglycemia
8. Islets of Langerhans
9. Hemiparesis
10. Hemiplegia
11. Diabetes
12. Glucagon
13. Transient ischemic attacks (TIA)
14. Status epilepticus
15. Paresthesia
16. Glucose
17. Epilepsy
18. Grand mal
19. Petit mal
20. Tonic-clonic

Content Review
1. 1) Eye opening; 2) motor response; and 3) verbal response
2. Non-insulin-dependant diabetes
3. Pancreas
4. Diabetes
5. Hypoglycemia
6. True
7. 80 to 120 mg/dL (milligrams per deciliter)
8. False
9. Beta cells
10. Insulin-dependent diabetes mellitis (IDDM)
11. Non-insulin-dependent diabetes mellitis (NIDDM)
12. 1
13. 1
14. 2
15. Increased urination, increased thirst, and increased hunger
16. Polyuria
17. 1) Diabetic ketoacidosis (DKA); 2) nonketonic hyperosmolar syndrome (NKHS); and 3) hypoglycemia
18. Ensure adequate airway; administer supplemental oxygen as indicated; if responsive and able to swallow, give the patient food that contains glucose (juice with sugar) or glucose gel.
19. True
20. Right; left
21. 1) Occlusion of blood vessels to the brain (thrombus or embolus); and 2) hemorrhage (rupture of cerebral artery)
22. Fever

23. 5 to 30
24. Protect the patient from further injury; provide emotional support; avoid rigid restraints; loosen all restrictive clothing and position the patient in a recovery position (on his or her side) to help keep the airway clear
25. False
26. Dementia
27. Delirium
28. A term for a group of acute and chronic mental disorders with associated brain damage or impaired cerebral function
29. Alzheimer's disease
30. CNS depression; respiratory depression; and constricted pupils
31. Stimulants
32. Nervousness, agitation, and hyperactivity
33. Delusions and alterations of self awareness, mood, and thought
34. Accumulation of toxins in the blood affect the brain.
35. A: alert; V: responds to verbal stimuli; P: responds only to painful stimuli; U: unresponsive

Chapter Quiz

1. B	6. A	11. D	16. B
2. A	7. A	12. D	17. A
3. C	8. C	13. B	18. A
4. A	9. D	14. D	
5. D	10. A	15. A	

Case Scenario

1. Has the patient eaten today? Does the patient take insulin? If so, has she taken her insulin today? These questions can be included as part of the SAMPLE history.
2. The patient is most likely suffering from hypoglycemia.
3. Place the patient on high-flow oxygen; if the patient is able to swallow, give her juice with sugar in it or oral glucose based on medical control directives; perform a thorough assessment; transport the patient to the hospital and consider ALS rendezvous.

18

Allergies

Reading Assignment: Chapter 18 pages 335–342.

DOT Objectives
••

Upon successful completion of the EMT-Basic training program, the EMT-Basic should be able to do the following:

- Recognize the patient experiencing an allergic reaction.
- Describe the emergency medical care of the patient with an allergic reaction.
- Establish the relationship between the patient with an allergic reaction and airway management.
- Describe the mechanisms of allergic response and the complications for airway management.
- State the generic and trade names, dose, administration, action, and contraindications for an epinephrine auto-injector.
- Evaluate the need for medical direction in the emergency medical care of the patient with an allergic reaction.
- Differentiate between the general category of those patients having an allergic reaction and those patients having an allergic reaction requiring immediate medical care, including immediate the use of an epinephrine auto-injector.
- Demonstrate the emergency medical care of the patient experiencing an allergic reaction.
- Demonstrate the use of an epinephrine auto-injector.
- Demonstrate the assessment and documentation of patient response to an epinephrine injection.
- Demonstrate proper disposal of equipment.
- Demonstrate completing a prehospital care report for patients with allergic emergencies.

Supplemental Objectives
••

- Distinguish an anaphylactic reaction from a simple allergic reaction.
- Define allergic reaction.
- Describe and identify urticaria.
- List the antigens that most commonly cause anaphylaxis.
- List the indications for assisting a patient with the administration of epinephrine.
- Describe the use of an epinephrine auto-injector.

Key Terms
••

1. A substance that causes the formation of an antibody and reacts specifically with that antibody is called a(n) _____.

2. The system responsible for recognizing foreign invaders and eliminating them from the body is the _____ system.

3. The chemical released from white blood cells in response to a hypersensitive reaction to an antigen, causing vasodilation is called _____.

4. An exaggerated, life-threatening, hypersensitivity reaction to an antigen is called _____ _____.

5. Protective proteins that circulate and are used to fight off foreign material in the body are called _____.

6. The medical term for hives is _____.

7. An abnormal, high-pitched, musical sound caused by an obstruction in the trachea or larynx is called _____.

8. A response of the body's immune system when challenged by a foreign substance is commonly called a(n) _____.

Content Review

1. Death can occur within minutes of the onset of an allergic reaction.
   A. True
   B. False

2. What are the three most common antigens that cause anaphylaxis?

3. Raised, blanched, irregularly shaped lesions with surrounding redness are called _____ _____.

4. Tissue swelling and bronchospasm are responsible for the clinical signs of an anaphylactic reaction.
   A. True
   B. False

5. Of the patients who die from anaphylaxis, _____% are from anaphylactic shock and _____% are from respiratory problems.

6. The most dangerous complication of a severe allergic reaction is _____ _____.

7. The presence of stridor means what?

8. Stridor is caused by an obstruction of the _____ airway. Wheezing is caused by an obstruction of the _____ airway.

9. List the signs and symptoms associated with anaphylaxis.

10. What is the mechanism of action of epinephrine?

11. What are the side effects of epinephrine?

12. Epinephrine should be used cautiously in patients over _____ years of age.

13. The form of epinephrine available to the EMT is a(n) _____.

14. A preloaded auto-injector contains how much epinephrine?

15. A pediatric dose auto-injector is available with what dose of epinephrine?

16. How is epinephrine administered?

17. If epinephrine is not available, how should the EMT care for the patient suffering from a severe allergic reaction?

Chapter Quiz
• •

1. The most common type of allergic reaction that requires transport to the hospital is a(n):
   A. Chronic hypersensitivity reaction
   B. Immediate hypersensitivity reaction
   C. Latent hyposensitivity reaction
   D. Immediate hyposensitivity reaction

2. Which of the following are common types of antigens associated with an immediate hypersensitivity reaction:
   A. Insect venom and antibiotics
   B. Injected penicillin and nuts
   C. Shellfish and strawberries
   D. All of the above

3. Hypersensitivity reactions cause the release of what chemical?
   A. Antihistamine
   B. Histamine
   C. Hemoglobin
   D. Glucose

4. What effects are due to the release of histamine?
   A. Vasodilation and leaking blood vessels
   B. Vasoconstriction and leaking blood vessels
   C. Vasoconstriction and high blood pressure
   D. Vasoconstriction and vomiting

5. Vasodilation of the peripheral blood vessels causes:
   A. Hives
   B. Urticaria
   C. A rash
   D. All of the above

6. Hives are characterized by:
   A. Raised, blanched, irregularly shaped lesions
   B. Redness
   C. Severe itching
   D. All of the above

7. Generalized vasodilation may lead to hypotension and shock.
   A. True
   B. False

8. Histamine can cause all of the following *except:*
   A. Bronchodilation
   B. Watery eyes and a runny nose
   B. Hives and vomiting
   C. Difficulty breathing and shock

9. Which of the following are signs and symptoms of an anaphylactic reaction?
   A. Difficulty breathing
   B. Shock
   C. Rapid deterioration
   D. All of the above

10. What percentage of anaphylactic patients die from shock and what percentage die from respiratory problems?
    A. Shock—45%; respiratory—55%
    B. Shock—55%; respiratory—45%
    C. Shock—25%; respiratory—75%
    D. Shock —5%; respiratory—95%

11. Which of the following information would be important concerning an anaphylactic patient?
    A. History of reaction and substance exposed to
    B. Mode of exposure, effects, and interventions
    C. Progression of the effects and a time period of symptoms
    D. All of the above

12. What is the most dangerous complication of a severe allergic reaction?
    A. High blood pressure
    B. Slow pulse rate
    C. Kidney failure
    D. Respiratory distress

13. Swelling of the tissues of the oropharynx and larynx can lead to airway obstruction, which will be evident by the presence of stridor.
    A. True
    B. False

14. Which of the following would be the best warning signs to indicate swollen vocal cords?
    A. Swelling in the mouth or tongue
    B. Swollen hands
    C. Swollen abdomen
    D. Swollen ankles

15. What causes wheezing in the lungs with an anaphylactic patient?
    A. Swelling and spasm of the tongue
    B. Swelling and spasm of the smaller airway passages
    C. Swelling and spasm of the large airway passages
    D. Swelling and spasm of the pharynx

16. Which of the following are indications to assist a patient in administering his or her epinephrine?
    A. Shock
    B. Respiratory difficulty
    C. Rapidly progressing symptoms
    D. All of the above

17. Early endotracheal intubation should be a consideration for the anaphylactic patient because:
    A. All allergic reactions should be controlled with ET intubation
    B. The EOA is effective in most allergic reactions
    C. The ET should be placed while the patient is conscious
    D. Increasing laryngeal edema may make it more difficult to accomplish later

18. What are the effects of epinephrine?
    A. Potent vasodilation and bronchodilation
    B. Potent vasoconstriction and bronchodilation
    C. Potent vasodilation and bronchoconstriction
    D. Potent vasoconstriction and bronchoconstriction

19. Which of the following is *not* a side effect of ephinephrine?
    A. Bradycardia
    B. Angina
    C. Hypertension
    D. Myocardial ischemia

20. What is the preloaded dose of epinephrine in the Epi-Pen?
    A. 0.3 mg
    B. 3.0 mg
    C. 0.5 mg
    D. 1.0 mg

21. Epinephrine is administered in which layer of tissue?
    A. Transdermal
    B. Subcutaneous
    C. Intravenous
    D. Intramuscular

22. What should be done for the anaphylactic patient, if he or she has no medication prescribed?
    A. Give the patient an antihistamine by mouth
    B. No intervention is necessary
    C. Transport the patient in the shock position
    D. Use an Epi-Pen from the ambulance

23. What is the primary drug treatment for anaphylaxis?
    A. Norepinephrine
    B. Epinephrine
    C. Diphenhydramine
    D. Glucose

Case Scenario

You are dispatched to the scene for a patient in respiratory distress. En route to the scene, dispatch informs you that the patient is a 10-year-old boy who was stung by a bee. The mother states that he is having a very hard time breathing.

1. What is your general impression of the situation? Is it serious?

You arrive on the scene to find the boy sitting on the couch, leaning forward, gasping for air, with audible wheezing. You note the patient's face has a bright red, flushed appearance and there is considerable edema around the neck and face. The patient exhibits signs and symptoms of rapidly progressing shock. His blood pressure begins to drop and his heart rate is tachycardic at 140 bpm.

You ask the mother if her son has any allergies. She is not aware of any, and she does not recall him ever being stung by a bee before. He has been healthy.

2. How would you care for this patient?

3. Can you administer epinephrine to this patient?

Skill Sheet #27

· ·

EPINEPHRINE AUTO-INJECTOR

Start Time: _____

Stop Time: _____   **Date:** _____

Candidate's Name: _____

Evaluator's Name: _____

	Points Possible	Points Awarded
Takes, or verbalizes, body substance isolation precautions	1	
Obtains order from medical direction either on-line or off-line	1	
Obtains patient's epinephrine auto-injector	1	
Assures auto-injector is prescribed for this patient	1	
Checks medication for expiration date	1	
Removes safety cap from auto-injector	1	
Selects appropriate injection site (thigh or shoulder)	1	
Pushes injector firmly against site until injector activates	1	
Holds injector firmly against site until medication is injected	1	
Properly discards auto-injector in biohazardous container	1	
Records activity and time	1	
Verbalizes continued reassessment and monitoring of the patient during transport	1	
Total:	12	

Critical Criteria

_____ Did not take, or verbalize, body substance isolation precautions

_____ Did not contact medical direction for authorization

_____ Did not use an appropriate injection site

_____ Used the injector against the injection site for ten (10) seconds or longer

_____ Did not discard the auto-injector into an appropriate container

_____ Did not verify prescription label

_____ Did not reassess patient after administration of medication

Answer Key

· ·

Key Terms
1. Antigen
2. Immune
3. Histamine
4. Anaphylaxis
5. Antibodies
6. Urticaria
7. Stridor
8. Allergic reaction

Content Review
1. True
2. Insect venom, antibiotics (especially injected penicillin), and foods (nuts, shellfish, strawberries)
3. Hives
4. True
5. 25; 75
6. Respiratory distress
7. Swelling of the tissues of the oropharynx and larynx, which can lead to airway obstruction
8. Upper; lower
9. Urticaria (hives); wheezing or stridor; hypotension (from vasodilation); abdominal cramping and vomiting; severe itching; respiratory compromise; shock
10. A potent vasoconstrictor and bronchodilator that counteracts the effects of histamine
11. Tachycardia, hypertension, angina, and mycocardial ischemia
12. 50
13. Epi-Pen
14. 0.3 mg
15. 0.15 mg
16. Subcutaneous injection at a 90 degree angle
17. Transport immediately in a shock position with supplemental oxygen; request ALS rendezvous en route; DO NOT delay transport.

Chapter Quiz

1. B	6. D	11. D	16. D	21. B
2. D	7. A	12. D	17. D	22. C
3. B	8. A	13. A	18. B	23. B
4. A	9. D	14. A	19. A	
5. D	10. C	15. B	20. A	

Case Scenario

1. This patient is having a severe allergic reaction to the bee sting. This is very serious since it is causing a compromised airway and respiratory distress.
2. Place the patient supine with his legs elevated; attempt to assist with ventilations with a BVM and 100% oxygen; and transport immediately to the closest hospital. If you are far from the hospital, request that ALS personnel meet you en route since this patient needs immediate definitive care that can be provided by ALS personnel.
3. No. This patient does not have a history of allergies and does not have a prescribed Epi-Pen; therefore the EMT can not administer that medication. An EMT can only assist a patient in taking his or her prescribed epinephrine. It is not carried on the ambulance.

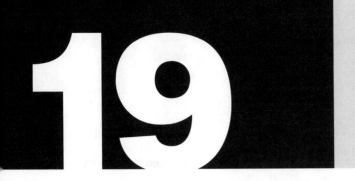

Reading Assignment: Chapter 19 pages 343–354.

DOT Objectives
•••

Upon successful completion of the EMT-Basic training program, the EMT-Basic should be able to do the following:

- List various ways that poisons enter the body.
- List signs/symptoms associated with poisoning.
- Discuss the emergency medical care for the patient with a possible overdose.
- Describe the steps in emergency medical care for the patient with suspected poisoning.
- Establish the relationship between the patient suffering from poisoning or overdose and airway management.
- State the generic and trade names, indications, contraindications, medication form, dose, administration, actions, side effects, and re-assessment strategies for activated charcoal.
- Recognize the need for medical direction in caring for the patient with poisoning or overdose.
- Demonstrate the steps in emergency medical care for the patient with possible overdose.
- Demonstrate the steps in emergency medical care for the patient with suspected poisoning.
- Perform the necessary steps required to provide a patient with activated charcoal.
- Demonstrate the assessment and documentation of patient response.
- Demonstrate completing a prehospital care report for patients with a poisoning/overdose emergency.

Supplemental Objectives
•••

- Define poison.
- Describe the appropriate interaction with the poison control center.
- Explain the various effects of poisons on the body.
- List the forms of activated charcoal that are available.
- Identify the appropriate circumstances in which to use activated charcoal.
- List the contraindications of activated charcoal.
- Define substance abuse.
- Discuss various types of abused substances and their effects.
- Discuss warning signs of substance abuse.
- Discuss the management of toxic emergencies.

Key Terms

• •

1. A government prescribed form describing the actions and toxicities of substances used in the workplace is called a(n) _____.

2. A material specially formulated to bind to substances and used to prevent absorption of swallowed substances from the intestine is called _____.

3. A regional organization that provides telephone information about poisonings and gives advice to patients and healthcare workers is the _____.

4. An agent that directly blocks or reverses the effect of a poison is called a(n) _____.

5. Define poisoning.

Content Review

• •

1. Identify the two age groups where poisoning most commonly occur.

   1)
   2)

2. What agent causes most poisonings of toddlers?

3. How do poisonings of adolescents most commonly occur?

4. All poisons exert their effect after being absorbed into the body.
   A. True
   B. False

5. What is the prehospital management of poisoning patients?

6. Ipecac is used as a method of limiting absorption of a poison in the field.
   A. True
   B. False

7. What are the four ways in which poisons are generally absorbed into the body?

    1)
    2)
    3)
    4)

8. What are the signs and symptoms that would indicate a poisoning by ingestion?

9. Identify two ways in which poisons are absorbed by the body.

    1)
    2)

10. What information at the scene can help the EMT determine the agent used in a poisoning?

11. Assessment of vision can be distinguished in four general categories. What are they?

    1)
    2)
    3)
    4)

12. What is the emergency care for respiratory poisonings?

13. How should the EMT care for a patient with dermal or ocular exposure of a liquid?

14. What can the EMT use for irrigation?

15. Irrigation of the eye or skin should be performed for a minimum of _____ minutes.

16. The EMT can use Narcan to reverse the effect of narcotic overdose.
    A. True
    B. False

17. The most significant problem the EMT usually encounters as a result of narcotic overdose is _____ _____.

18. What is the normal dosage of activated charcoal for an adult and child?

19. What are the contraindications of activated charcoal?

20. An overdose can be intentional or accidental.
    A. True
    B. False

21. What are the commonly abused narcotics?

22. What are some street names of narcotics?

23. What are the signs and symptoms of narcotic overdose?

24. What are some commonly abused benzodiazepines?

25. Benzodiazepines cause pupils to constrict.
    A. True
    B. False

26. What are the signs and symptoms of benzodiazepine overdose?

27. Examples of Barbiturates include _____ and _____.

28. What are the signs and symptoms of amphetamine overdose.

29. What are the signs and symptoms of cocaine overdose?

30. What are the signs and symptoms of phencyclidine use and overdose?

31. LSD causes emotional swings and unpredictable behavior.
    A. True
    B. False

32. Cannabis can be eaten or smoked.
    A. True
    B. False

33. What are the signs and symptoms of cannabis use?

Skill Sheet #28

. . . .

ACTIVATED CHARCOAL ADMINISTRATION

Start Time: _____

Stop Time: _____   **Date:** _____

Candidate's Name: _____

Evaluator's Name: _____

	Points Possible	Points Awarded
Takes, or verbalizes, body substance isolation precautions	1	
Obtains an order from medical direction (either on-line or off-line)	1	
Assures right medication, right patient, right route, & patient alert enough to use inhaler	1	
Checks the expiration date of the activated charcoal	1	
Shakes the container thoroughly	1	
Persuades the patient to drink the medication. Provides a covered container and straw to prevent the patient from seeing the medication and improve patient compliance, if necessary.	1	
Re-shakes the medication, if necessary. If patient does not drink the medication immediately, the charcoal will settle.	1	
Records the name, dose, route, time, and results of administration of the medication	1	
Total:	8	

Critical Criteria

_____ Did not take, or verbalize, body substance isolation precautions

_____ Did not check the medication for expiration date

_____ Did not administer the correct dosage

_____ Did not shake the medication

_____ Did not properly record administration

Chapter Quiz

....

1. Poisoning occurs by:
   A. Inhalation
   B. Absorption
   C. Ingestion
   D. All of the above

2. In cases of ingestion, medical control may recommend the use of activated charcoal to bind the poison in the intestine to prevent absorption into the bloodstream.
   A. True
   B. False

3. The medication most often used to induce vomiting is:
   A. Ipecac
   B. Benadryl
   C. Activated charcoal
   D. Dramamine

4. Activated charcoal is always used for poisonings involving ingestion.
   A. True
   B. False

5. The greatest risk to the patient who has had a narcotic overdose is:
   A. Addiction
   B. Respiratory arrest
   C. Cardiac arrest
   D. Dependence

6. The most common substances involved in the poisoning of children in the 2-year-old age group include:
   A. Duraspan and Spectracide
   B. Household cleaning agents and medications
   C. Gasoline and kerosene
   D. Ammonium nitrate and diesel fuel

7. Poisoning by ingestion occurs when a poison is taken into the patient's:
   A. Mouth
   B. Eyes
   C. Veins
   D. Skin

8. Most absorption from ingested poisons takes place in the:
   A. Small intestine
   B. Upper stomach
   C. Large intestine
   D. Descending colon

9. Some poisons are irritating or corrosive to the tissue that lines the mouth and esophagus. A person who ingests one of these poisons may experience:
   A. Burning
   B. Swelling of the soft tissues of the mouth
   C. Discomfort
   D. All of the above

10. If the concentration of the poisoning agent is high or if the exposure is prolonged, your primary concern as the attending EMT would be:
    A. Potential compromise to the upper airway
    B. Pain or discomfort
    C. Hyperactivity
    D. Restlessness and anxiety

11. A specific antidote for narcotic overdose is:
    A. Syrup of ipecac
    B. Activated charcoal
    C. Narcan
    D. Adenosine

12. In the prehospital field, thorough assessment of poisoned patients is necessary for medical direction, poison control, or both, to determine whether field intervention is appropriate.
    A. True
    B. False

13. If a poison's container is present at the scene and can be safely transported, it is helpful to bring it with the patient because:
    A. The quantity of material is important information
    B. Emergency physicians may do a pill count on bottles to estimate the number ingested
    C. Hospital staff may anticipate a higher risk to the patient and undertake more aggressive treatment if they have more specific information
    D. All of the above are true

14. Central nervous system symptoms may include all of the following *except:*
    A. Dizziness
    B. Headache
    C. Altered mental status
    D. Abdominal pain

15. The acceptable dosing for activated charcoal administration is:
    A. Usually 0.5 to 1 grams/kg of body weight
    B. Usual adult dose of 15 to 30 grams/kg of body weight
    C. Pediatric doses of 1.5 to 2 grams/kg of body weight
    D. Pediatric doses of 10 to 15 grams/kg of body weight

16. Poisoning by injection includes:
    A. Substance abuse and envenomation by animals
    B. Carbon monoxide and nitrogen
    C. Carbon dioxide and ammonia
    D. Lime and organophosphate powder

17. Which of the following drugs is a stimulant?
    A. Amphetamines
    B. Methaqualones
    C. Barbiturates
    D. Cannabis

Case Scenario

You are dispatched to a residence for a sick person. On your arrival, you are greeted by a hysterical mother stating that her 2-year-old may have swallowed some detergent. She states that she "only left him alone for a minute," but when she went back into the kitchen he was sitting in from of the sink with a bottle of detergent sitting next to him with the cap off. You approach the child who is running around the room, something the mother states is normal behavior.

1. What symptoms should you be looking for?

2. What questions might you ask the mother to better understand the potential severity of this event?

3. How should you go about treating this patient?

4. How might activated charcoal help in this situation?

Answer Key

Key Terms
1. Material Safety Data Sheet (MSDS)
2. Activated charcoal
3. Poison control center
4. Antidote
5. The adverse effects that foods, plants, chemicals, or drugs have on the body.

Content Review
1. 1) Toddlers to preschool; and 2) adolescents to young adult
2. Household cleaning agents and medications to which the toddler is accidentally exposed
3. Drugs ingested as a form of suicidal behavior
4. True
5. Assessment and stabilization of the ABCs; decontamination to reduce poison at the scene in the patient, or both (as necessary); and providing emotional support
6. False
7. 1) Absorption; 2) ingestion; 3) inhalation; and 4) injection
8. Burning and swelling of the soft tissues of the mouth
9. 1) Dermal (skin) exposure and 2) ocular (eye) exposure
10. Containers; unusual odors at the scene; material safety data sheet (at an industrial site)
11. 1) No vision; 2) ability to distinguish light and dark; 3) ability to count fingers at a distance of several feet; and 4) ability to read letters or numbers on paperwork or an IV bag
12. Removal of the patient from further exposure; high-flow oxygen; early transport (if unresponsive or in respiratory distress) be prepared to assist ventilations with BVM if necessary
13. Large-volume clear water irrigation of the skin or eyes continuously until arrival at hospital

14. Tap water or normal saline; can use dextrose solution if water or saline is not available.
15. 20
16. False
17. Depressed respiratory and mental status
18. 0.5 to 1 g per kilogram of body weight; adults: 25 to 50 g; pediatrics: 12.5 to 25 g
19. Patient with altered mental status; ingestion of acids or alkalies; patient who cannot or will not swallow the solution
20. True
21. Morphine, heroin, codeine, demerol, dilaudid, talwin, percodan, fentanyl
22. Big M, Birdie, powerer, Dreamer dust, Gungk, Happy Medicine, Morph, MS, Sweet morpheus, and witch
23. Altered LOC, constricted pupils, respiratory depression, decreased in pulse rate and blood pressure, cool and clammy skin
24. Valium, Librium, Xanax, and Ativan
25. False
26. Slurred speech, disorientation, depressed ventilations, clammy skin, dilated pupils
27. Phenobarbitol, Seconal
28. Restlessness, dizziness, agitation, irritability, weakness, tremor, nausea, dilated pupils, irregular heart rates, chest pain, hallucinations, convulsions, coma
29. Agitation, belligerence, dilated pupils, hyperthermia, severely elevated blood pressure, slurred speech, lethargy
30. Illusions, hallucinations, altered perception of time; overdose: severe agitation, belligerence, paranoia, hyperthermia, and increased blood pressure
31. True
32. True
33. Relaxation and decreased user inhibition; paranoia

Chapter Quiz

1. D	6. B	10. A	14. D
2. A	7. A	11. C	15. A
3. A	8. A	12. A	16. A
4. B	9. D	13. D	17. A
5. B			

Case Scenario

1. Burns around the mouth; unusual odor on the breath; unusual behavior; lethargy; nausea or vomiting; uncoordinated movements; abnormal vital signs
2. What was the detergent? How much was in the bottle before her son obtained the bottle (to determine how much may have been ingested)? Does her son have any medical conditions or is he taking any medications?
3. Contact Medical Direction who will contact the Poison Control Center for recommendations specific to the chemical ingested; retrieve the bottle of detergent and transport it with the patient to the hospital; if ordered by the Medical Director, administer activated charcoal.
4. Activated Charcoal binds to the poison to limit its absorption.

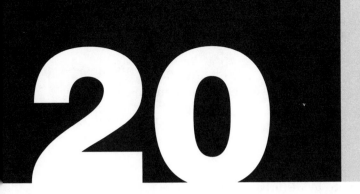

Behavioral Emergencies

Reading Assignment: Chapter 20 pages 335–371.

DOT Objectives

Upon successful completion of the EMT-Basic training program, the EMT-Basic should be able to do the following:

- Demonstrate the assessment and emergency medical care of the patient experiencing a behavioral emergency.
- Demonstrate techniques to safely restrain a patient with a behavioral problem.
- Define behavioral emergency.
- List risk factors of potential suicide.
- State the medicolegal considerations involved with behaviorally and mentally ill patients including those of consent and restraint.
- Describe assessment of the potentially violent patient, including considerations of past history, posture, vocal activity, and physical activity.
- Discuss the general factors that may cause an alteration in a patient's behavior.
- State the various reasons for psychological crisis.
- Discuss the special considerations for assessment of a patient with behavioral problems.
- Discuss methods to calm behavioral emergency patients.
- Describe management and emergency medical care of a patient undergoing a behavioral emergency.

Supplemental Objectives

- State the questions to be considered in assessing a behavioral emergency.
- List three major causes of behavioral emergencies.
- Describe the steps to conduct a mental status assessment.
- Describe the steps to conduct an initial assessment of a patient undergoing a behavioral emergency.
- List the warning signs of potential suicide.

Key Terms

1. How a person functions or acts is called _____.

2. The activities usually accomplished during a normal day, such as eating, dressing, and washing are termed _____.

3. Symptoms or illness caused by mental or psychic factors as opposed to organic ones are called _____ _____.

4. Define mental disorder.

5. Transient or permanent dysfunction of the brain, caused by disturbances of physiologic functioning of brain tissue is called _____.

Content Review

1. List those situations involving behavioral emergencies that the EMT needs to immediately recognize that require emergency medical care.

2. List some causes of various types of behavioral emergencies.

3. The process of adapting to a variety of situations involving activities of daily living is called _____ _____.

4. Define behavioral emergency.

5. A mental disorder is characterized by symptoms and/or impairment in functioning.
   A. True
   B. False

6. Identify questions to consider in assessing a patient with a behavioral emergency.

7. In order for the EMT to adequately care for a patient who is experiencing a behavioral emergency, it is necessary for him or her to determine the exact cause of the current crisis.
   A. True
   B. False

8. Identify questions or factors that will help the EMT assess a patient's "interview behavior."

9. Identify questions or factors that will help the EMT assess a patient's "motor behavior."

10. Identify questions or factors that will help the EMT assess a patient's "thought content."

11. Identify questions or factors that will help the EMT assess a patient's "speech."

12. Identify questions or factors that will help the EMT assess a patient's orientation, affect, and proficiency.

    Orientation:

    Affect:

    Proficiency:

13. Words that have no logical connection to one another such as: "the street next year March moon and I love hate the beach" is called _____.

14. List the seven basic categories of mental disorders.

    1)
    2)
    3)
    4)
    5)
    6)
    7)

15. List the risk factors of suicide.

16. What are the signs and symptoms of paranoia?

17. How does the EMT obtain consent for emergency care from a patient who is not mentally competent?

18. Who has the legal authority to restrain a patient?

19. Why should the EMT involve police intervention when handling a psychiatric crisis?

20. What is the general rule regarding the use of force when dealing with a psychiatric crisis?

21. What are the four principal determinants of violence or potentially violent behavior?

    1)
    2)
    3)
    4)

22. The primary factor indicating potential violence is _____.

23. Identify other factors of potential violence.

24. How should the EMT care for a patient experiencing a psychiatric emergency?

25. What is the least confrontational position for the EMT to stand when talking with a patient experiencing a psychiatric emergency?

26. What should the EMT do if he or she is caring for a patient and encounters a dangerous weapon?

Chapter Quiz
· ·

1. If the EMT encounters a patient who is experiencing a behavioral emergency and threatening violence, the EMT should:
   A. Restrain the patient
   B. Leave the immediate area and call the police
   C. Call another EMS unit for assistance
   D. Not interfere

2. You and your crew arrive at a scene where a patient is threatening to kill himself. After talking with the patient, he states that he was only joking and will be fine now. What should you do?
   A. Accept that the patient has dealt with the emergency
   B. Wait until a friend or loved one arrives and then leave the scene
   C. Assume control of the scene and restrain the patient
   D. Encourage the patient to be transported for physician evaluation

3. Irrational behaviors may be the result of:
   A. Sudden illness or trauma
   B. Drug or alcohol intoxication
   C. Acute organic brain syndrome
   D. All of the above

4. Abnormal or disturbing behavior may indicate some types of mental illness.
   A. True
   B. False

5. When caring for a patient undergoing a behavioral emergency who will not respond to questions, the EMT should observe the patient's emotional state via assessment of:
   A. Facial expressions, posture, and gestures
   B. Pulse and ventilatory rates
   C. Tears, sweating, or blushing
   D. All of the above

6. In assessing a patient involved in a behavioral emergency, the same initial principles apply as for any other patient.
   A. True
   B. False

7. Assessment of a behavioral emergency includes consideration of the patient's:
   A. Orientation and memory
   B. Patient responses
   C. Level of distraction
   D. All of the above

8. Assessment and emergency care of a patient suffering from a behavioral emergency requires that the EMT determine the cause of the current crisis.
   A. True
   B. False

9. A behavioral emergency is a reaction to an event that interferes with the daily activities of living.
   A. True
   B. False

10. Patients who are anxious, reluctant, suspicious, and show unnatural fears of what most people would consider normal activities (e.g., walking outside) may be categorized as:
    A. Chronically depressed
    B. Phobic
    C. Suicidal
    D. Homicidal

11. The most significant factor contributing to suicide that transcends any other marker is:
    A. Depression
    B. Phobia
    C. Paranoia
    D. Anxiety

12. Suicide threats indicate that a person is in a crisis that he or she cannot handle and requires thorough, immediate care.
    A. True
    B. False

13. Risk factors of suicide have been identified as all of the following *except:*
    A. Depression at any age
    B. Male sex and over 40 years of age
    C. Intact, strong emotional bonds
    D. Recent loss of spouse or family member

14. If, during the initial assessment of a patient, you think that suicide is a possibility, you should:
    A. Not hesitate to ask the patient questions that may lead to a preliminary assessment
    B. Discount the feelings, realizing that the patient is just depressed
    C. Ignore it, if vague and offered in a joking context
    D. Not bring the subject up because it may give the patient ideas

15. A critical warning sign that a patient has a specific suicide plan includes:
    A. Recently preparation of a will
    B. Advising friends what to do with significant possessions
    C. Arranging for funeral services
    D. All of the above

16. Management of a suicidal patient includes:
    A. Doing nothing either to frighten the patient or to arouse suspicion
    B. Not risking your life or the lives of your crew
    C. Police intervention
    D. All of the above

17. A standard of care must be carefully adhered to since the patient experiencing a behavioral emergency may not have the ability to make rational decisions about his or her emergency medical care.
    A. True
    B. False

18. Most states have statutory provisions that provide _____ with the authority to place mentally ill and drug-dependent persons in protective custody so that emergency care can be rendered.
    A. Mental health workers
    B. Human resource agents
    C. Law enforcement officers
    D. Emergency medical officers

19. In emergency situations, the implied consent rule that "if an emergency exists and the patient is unable to give consent, the EMT is able to provide care" applies to the mentally ill patient.
    A. True
    B. False

20. When assessing the violent patient, the most obvious factors to look for are:
    A. Eye contact
    B. Voice
    C. Posture
    D. Crying

Case Scenario

• •

You respond to an apartment complex in response to a call from police for assistance with a reported suicide attempt. On your arrival, you are met at the door by a police officer who advises you that they have a 32-year-old male subject who called 911 earlier and said he was going to commit suicide by slashing his wrists. When police arrived, they found the man sitting in the bathroom with a kitchen knife, which he had used to cut his left wrist. There was a moderate amount of blood on the floor and the patient was crying. He offered no resistance, and asked the police to "please help me, I'm so scared."

Initial assessment reveals a conscious, alert, and oriented patient crying softly while holding a towel on his wrist. The towel is partially soaked with blood. The patient appears to be in no distress. He looks at you and asks for help. He states that he lost his job, his wife, his home, and that he has been unable to find work. He decided today, after another day of unsuccessful job hunting, to end his life. The patient has the smell of alcohol on his breath, but he does not speak with slurred speech or appear uncoordinated in his movements.

After several minutes of conversation, he agrees to let you look at his wrist. He has a small cut on the inner aspect of his wrist that does not appear to have gone deep enough to cut the artery. The bleeding is mostly under control and you apply a sterile dressing and bandage. The patient's radial pulse is strong, and he has normal ventilations. After approximately 15 minutes, the patient agrees to go with you to be evaluated and helped by hospital personnel. A police officer agrees to ride in the ambulance with you. The ride to the hospital is uneventful.

1. What types of questions would you want to ask this patient to help determine his state of mind at this event?

2. What are the major causes of a behavioral emergency such as this one?

3. If this patient had refused to be transported to the hospital, what options would you have had?

4. What are the signs that the EMT should look for in assessing a patient with a behavioral emergency to determine the possibility of violence or aggressive behavior?

Answer Key

Key Terms
1. Behavior
2. Activities of daily living (ADL)
3. Psychogenic
4. An illness with psychologic or behavioral manifestations and/or impairment in functioning due to social, psychologic, genetic, physiologic, chemical, or biologic disturbances
5. Organic brain syndrome

Content Review
1. Overdose (drug or other chemical); suicidal or self-destructive behavior; and homicidal behavior
2. Sudden illness or trauma; drug or alcohol intoxication; sudden grief; organic brain syndrome; physiologic disturbance of the brain; psychogenic or mental illness
3. Adjustment
4. Any reaction to events that interferes with the activities of daily living
5. True
6. Is the patient's perception of reality compromised or distorted? Is there inadequate cerebral oxygenation? Are drugs or alcohol involved? Are circumstances of a psychogenic nature involved (i.e., major life change, death of a loved one)? Is there a history of mental illness? Is the patient suffering from severe depression? Has the patient made any suicidal threats?
7. False
8. How does the patient relate to you (friendly or hostile)? Are statements coherent? Is the patient aware you are questioning him or her? How is the patient's general appearance and grooming (is the patient reasonably cleaned and dressed under the circumstances)?
9. Is the patient moving in a coordinated way? Are movements jerky or smooth? Is the patient hyperactive or hypoactive? Do the patient's movements have purpose or are they aimless? Are the patient's facial expressions appropriate for the circumstances? Do the patient's facial expressions change with the subject being discussed?
10. Try to determine what is bothering the patient. What is the patient thinking? Note the patient's inability to respond or evade answers. Is the patient preoccupied? Check responses to several simple questions
11. Is the patient's speech and voice quality normal for the situation? Is the patient's voice too loud or too soft? Is the patient's voice flat and dreary or unrestrained? Is the patient's speech very slow or very fast?
12. Orientation: does the patient speak naturally or reluctantly? Affect: is the patient attentive, apathetic, or indifferent to what is going on around him? Are emotional reactions appropriate to the subject? Proficiency: does the patient maintain mental status or go in and out?
13. Word salad
14. 1) Acute anxiety; 2) phobias; 3) depression; 4) suicide (self-destructive acts); 5) paranoia; 6) disorientation; and 7) disorganization
15. Depression at any age; male 40 years and older; lack of strong emotional bonds; recent loss of spouse, significant other, or family member; chronic debilitating illness; financial setback or loss of job; previous suicide attempt; family history of suicide; substance abuse; child of alcoholic parent; mental disorder (e.g., paranoia)
16. Distrust, jealousy, seclusiveness, hostile behavior, or uncooperativeness
17. Implied consent exists
18. Law enforcement personnel
19. To provide the appropriate back-up that is often needed in managing the crisis and to provide necessary legal authority to restrain patients

20. Apply only the force necessary to keep a patient from causing injury or harm to himself or herself or to others
21. 1) Past history of hostile, overly aggressive, or violent behavior; 2) posture; 3) vocal activity (loud, obscene, erratic, and bizarre speech pattern); or 4) physical activity (agitation, pacing or protection of personal space)
22. Physical activity
23. Poor impulse control; instability of family structure; inability to keep a steady job; substance abuse; functional disorder (hallucinations, paranoia); and depression
24. Have a definite plan of action; calmly identify yourself; speak in a low, calm voice; be direct and state your intentions; assess the scene; stay with the patient; do not let the patient leave the area; encourage purposeful movement; avoid challenging the patient's personal space; avoid fighting with the patient or getting into a power struggle; be honest with and interested in the patient
25. Squatting at a 45° angle
26. Withdraw from the scene and seek immediate law enforcement assistance

Chapter Quiz

1. B	6. A	11. A	16. D
2. D	7. D	12. A	17. A
3. D	8. B	13. C	18. C
4. A	9. A	14. A	19. A
5. D	10. B	15. D	20. C

Case Scenario

1. The EMT should ask questions that will help determine the patient's state of mind and whether they are a threat to themselves or others. Questions to ask include: "How are you feeling today?"; "What is bothering you?"; "Can I do anything to help you?"; "Do you want to hurt yourself or someone else?"; "Have you tried to hurt yourself today?"
2. Most suicide calls involve patients who have become overwhelmed with the day to day tasks of living. Often a personal or professional loss is involved such as major life interruption, death of a loved one, or loss of a job. Other causes include: diabetes, particularly lack of glucose; trauma, including blood loss and poisoning; hallucinogens or other drugs or alcohol.
3. Each state or local jurisdiction will have rules governing the transport against their will of patients suffering a behavioral emergency. In some states, the police can invoke protective custody and have the patient transported. In other states, legislation has been passed that provides for medical transport of a patient, with or without their consent, if the EMT believes the patient cannot make an informed decision.
4. Specific things to look for include: the patient's posture; movement, voice, facial expressions, threatening statements, or evidence of weapons.

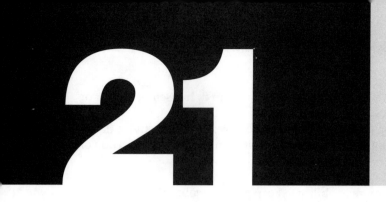

Reading Assignment: Chapter 21 pages 372–400.

DOT Objectives

Upon successful completion of the EMT-Basic training program, the EMT-Basic should be able to do the following:

- Describe the function of the following structures: uterus, vagina, fetus, placenta, umbilical cord, amniotic sac, amniotic fluid, and perineum.
- Demonstrate the use of personal protection precautions when dealing with the obstetric and gynecologic patient.
- Identify and describe the use of the equipment in an obstetric kit.
- Identify and describe appropriate care for patients with predelivery and gynecologic emergencies.
- Identify indications for imminent delivery, and state the steps necessary in the predelivery preparation of the mother.
- Identify and describe the care needed for a normal vaginal delivery, a multiple birth delivery, a breech delivery, a prolapsed cord delivery, a limb delivery, a meconium delivery, and a premature delivery.
- Describe the necessary steps for the care of the infant as the head appears.
- Describe the technique and appropriate time to cut the umbilical cord and the indications and steps necessary for the delivery and transport of the placenta.
- Differentiate between the emergency medical care provided to a patient with predelivery emergencies and that provided to a patient with a normal delivery.
- Differentiate among the special considerations for multiple births.
- Describe special considerations of meconium.
- Describe special considerations of a premature infant.
- List the steps in the emergency medical care of the mother after delivery.
- Summarize neonatal resuscitation procedures.
- State the steps to assist in the delivery.
- Discuss the emergency medical care of a patient with a gynecologic emergency.
- Demonstrate the steps to assist in the normal delivery.
- Demonstrate infant neonatal procedures.
- Demonstrate post delivery care of an infant.
- Demonstrate how and when to cut the umbilical cord.
- Attend to the steps in the delivery of the placenta.
- Demonstrate the post-delivery care of the mother.
- Demonstrate the steps in the emergency medical care of the mother with excessive bleeding.
- Demonstrate completing a prehospital care report for patients with obstetrical/gynecologic emergencies.

Key Terms

....

1. Match the following terms with their definitions.

   _____ Contractions that occur at irregular intervals but do not increase in pain intensity

   _____ The expulsion of an embryo or fetus from the uterus before the 20th week

   _____ A "natural" or spontaneous abortion

   _____ An increase in blood pressure with resultant seizure activity in a pregnant patient

   _____ The periodic sloughing of the uterine lining

   _____ Sudden separation of the placenta from the wall of the uterus

   _____ A condition where the placenta implants itself either on or near the opening of the cervix

   _____ Regular uterine contractions that increase in frequency and intensity and propel the fetus from the uterus

   _____ The monthly release of a mature egg from the ovary

   A. Abortion
   B. Abruptio placentae
   C. Braxton Hicks
   D. Eclampsia
   E. Labor
   F. Menstruation
   G. Miscarriage
   H. Ovulation
   I. Placenta previa

2. The opening to the uterus is called the _____.

3. The fertilized egg up through the first 8 weeks of pregnancy is called a(n) _____.

4. The fibrous sac filled with fluid that protects the fetus is called the _____.

5. A birth in which the presenting part of the fetus is either the buttocks, foot, or leg is called a(n) _____.

6. The space located between the vaginal opening and the anal opening is called the _____ _____.

7. The muscular organ that houses the fetus during fetal development is the _____.

8. Another term for the navel is the _____.

9. Bulging of the perineum when birth is imminent is called _____.

10. The fluid that acts as a shock absorber and maintains a uniform pressure for the fetus is called _____ _____.

11. The tightening and hardening of the uterus that expels the fetus is called _____.

12. The developing unborn offspring from eight weeks after conception until birth is called the _____ _____.

13. Paired canals that connect the ovary to the uterus are called _____.

14. The permanent absence of menstruation is called _____.

15. The branch of medicine that deals with management of women during pregnancy, childbirth, and 42 days after expulsion of all contents of pregnancy is called _____.

16. The study of the diseases of women's reproductive organs is called _____.

17. Fetal intestinal contents that stain the amniotic fluid green or black is called _____ _____.

18. Contractions that occur at irregular intervals but do not increase in pain intensity, also known as Braxton Hicks contractions, are called _____.

19. The paired, almond-shaped organs that release a mature egg once a month are called _____ _____.

20. An accumulation of mucus that acts as a protective barrier between the cervix and vagina for the length of pregnancy is called the _____.

21. Pregnancy in which the fertilized egg implants in the fallopian tube is called a(n) _____ _____.

22. The highly vascular disk-shaped structure that links the tissue of the mother with that of the fetus is called the _____.

23. A three-month period during pregnancy is called a(n) _____.

24. The part of the fetus that protrudes initially during the birthing process is called the _____ _____.

25. Premature expulsion of the umbilical cord is called a(n) _____.

Content Review

1. Identify the structures that develop and fill the pelvic/abdmoninal cavity as a result of pregnancy.

2. Identify the following anatomical structures of a pregnant woman.

Amniotic sac	Rectum	Urethra
Cervix	Umbilical cord	Vagina
Placenta		

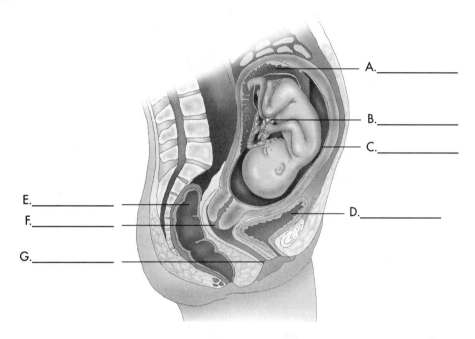

A._____

B._____

C._____

D._____

E._____

F._____

G._____

3. The normal time-span for a pregnancy averages _____ weeks or _____ trimesters.

4. There are _____ stages of labor.

5. The first stage of labor begins with _____ and ends with _____ _____.

6. The cervix can dilate to a maximum diameter of _____ cm.

7. The amniotic sac usually ruptures during the _____ stage of labor

8. The average time for the first stage of labor is _____ hours.

9. The second stage of labor starts with _____ and ends with _____ _____.

10. Contractions occur in regular intervals lasting _____ minutes during the first stage of labor and _____ minutes during the second stage of labor.

11. The third stage of labor starts _____ and ends with _____ _____.

12. It is normal for a woman to lose _____ mL of blood during delivery of the placenta.

13. List the contents that should be included in an OB delivery kit.

14. What are the signs and symptoms of a spontaneous abortion?

15. What is the appropriate emergency care for a patient bleeding during the last 3 months of pregnancy?

16. Describe and list the signs and symptoms of abruptio placentae.

17. Describe and list the signs and symptoms of placenta previa.

18. Describe and list the signs and symptoms of eclampsia.

19. Eclampsia is experienced only during pregnancy.
    A. True
    B. False

20. Eclampsia is equally common in women who are pregnant for the first time as with those pregnant more than once.
    A. True
    B. False

21. Seizures during pregnancy are seen more often in patients without prenatal care.
    A. True
    B. False

22. What are the three most important interventions for the EMT caring for a pregnant woman actively having a seizure?

    1)
    2)
    3)

23. How should a pregnant woman having seizures be transported? Why?

24. Identify the questions to consider in the assessment of a pregnant woman.

25. If contractions are _____ minutes apart, birth of the baby is imminent.

26. The fetus usually needs to be delivered within _____ hours after the membranes have ruptured, even if labor has not started.

27. What are the signs that delivery is imminent?

28. Suctioning of the infant occurs in what order?

29. Immediately after delivery of the infant, what steps should the EMT take?

30. Describe the steps for cutting the baby's umbilical cord.

31. Delivery of the placenta usually occurs an average of _____ minutes after delivery of the infant.

32. How should the EMT care for a newborn?

33. What is a major source of heat loss in an infant?

34. The use of oxygen in an infant can decrease the heart rate for a short period of time.
    A. True
    B. False

35. What does APGAR stand for and how is it assessed?

36. A normal APGAR score for a newborn is _____ at 1 minute after birth.

37. Identify situations in which resuscitation of a newborn may be likely.

38. Resuscitation of a newborn includes what steps?

39. If a patient has spontaneous ventilations, has received supplemental oxygen for 30 seconds and still maintains a heart rate of less than _____ beats per minute, the EMT should begin chest compressions.

40. Identify those situations in which an EMT should place a gloved hand into the mother's vagina.

41. What are the key points in the assessment and management of a pregnant trauma patient?

42. Clothing collected from a sexual assault victim should be transported with her to the hospital in a plastic bag.
    A. True
    B. False

43. Abrasions and superficial wounds on a sexual assault victim should not be cleaned or dressed.
    A. True
    B. False

Chapter Quiz

1. The process in which the lining of the uterus is shed when the egg is not fertilized is known as:
   A. Ovulation
   B. Menstruation
   C. Ministration
   D. Fertilization

2. A sexual assault victim should be discouraged from bathing or changing clothes before being transported to the hospital.
   A. True
   B. False

3. The _____ houses the unborn baby during fetal development.
   A. Vagina
   B. Cervix
   C. Umbilicus
   D. Uterus

4. Lying on the back during the last 3 months of pregnancy can restrict the circulation of blood to the placenta because the uterus will be resting on the mother's:
   A. Inferior vena cava
   B. Superior vena cava
   C. Amniotic sac
   D. Placenta

5. The _____ is a fibromuscular sheath that encloses the lower end of the uterus.
   A. Vagina
   B. Anus
   C. Urethra
   D. Orifice

6. The umbilical cord is a fibrous, whitish tube that connects the baby to the:
   A. Placenta
   B. Amniotic opening
   C. Umbilical vessels
   D. Uterus

7. Once the embryo is imbedded in the uterus, a protective covering called the _____ completely surrounds the embryo.
   A. Amniotic sac
   B. Mucous plug
   C. Umbilicus
   D. Placenta

8. The _____ stage of labor begins with the full dilation of the cervix and ends with the delivery of the baby.
   A. First
   B. Second
   C. Third
   D. Fourth

9. Visualization of the presenting part during delivery is commonly referred to as:
   A. Posturing
   B. Condensing
   C. Crowning
   D. Contracting

10. The contents of a delivery kit should include all of the following *except:*
    A. Surgical scissors, hemostats, cord clamps
    B. Umbilical tape, bulb syringe, towels
    C. Gauze sponges, forceps, nonsterile gloves
    D. Baby blankets, sanitary napkins, plastic bag

11. One type of late vaginal bleeding is known as _____ and is caused by the sudden separation of the placenta from the wall of the uterus.
    A. Abruptio placentae
    B. Vaginal hemorrhage
    C. Placenta previa
    D. Placenta implantation

12. Treatment for patients with abruptio placentae and placenta previa consists of:
    A. Maintaining an open airway
    B. Administering high-flow oxygen via a nonrebreather mask
    C. Placing the patient in a supine position and elevating her legs
    D. All of the above

13. During delivery, BSI must be maintained and includes protective eyewear.
    A. True
    B. False

14. All of the following are signs that the EMT must prepare to deliver a baby *except:*
    A. The beginning of one contraction to the beginning of the next contraction is between 6 and 9 minutes
    B. Contractions are regular and last from 45 to 60 seconds
    C. The woman wants to go to the bathroom to move her bowels
    D. The mother wants to bear down or push

15. Each patient (mother and baby) should have at least one EMT.
    A. True
    B. False

16. During delivery, if the looped umbilical cord cannot be slipped over the infant's head, the EMT should:
    A. Clamp the umbilical cord in three places
    B. Place ties between the clamps
    C. Clamp the umbilical cord in two places
    D. Leave the cord around the infant's neck

17. The average time for the delivery of the placenta is approximately _____ minutes after delivery of the infant.
    A. 10
    B. 20
    C. 30
    D. 45

18. If the mother is in shock, she should be treated with:
    A. Supplemental oxygen
    B. Proper positioning
    C. Rapid transport
    D. All of the above

19. The EMT should treat a newborn who needs resuscitation by:
    A. Drying and warming the infant
    B. Positioning and suctioning the infant
    C. Stimulating the infant
    D. All of the above

20. It is important to clear the infant's airway of meconium immediately after birth in order to prevent severe _____ problems from occurring.
    A. Cardiovascular
    B. Circulatory
    C. Respiratory
    D. Hepatic

21. Situations in which the EMT should insert a gloved hand into the vagina includes:
    A. A prolapsed cord
    B. Lower body or leg breech delivery
    C. Shoulder or hand delivery
    D. All of the above

22. A patient delivering twins should have _____ EMTs at the scene.
    A. 2
    B. 4
    C. 3
    D. 1

23. Multiple births are at risk for premature deliveries.
    A. True
    B. False

24. Premature babies are always at risk for:
    A. Rapid heart rate
    B. Rapid body heat loss
    C. Slow body heat loss
    D. Rapid dehydration

25. A pregnant trauma victim should be transported to the hospital even though an injury may appear to be minor.
    A. True
    B. False

Case Scenario

You are dispatched to a residence for a pregnant patient. En route to the scene, dispatch notifies you that the husband states that his wife is bleeding. On your arrival, you find a 36-year-old female patient in her 39th week of pregnancy. This is her first pregnancy. The patient states that she noticed bright red vaginal bleeding that started approximately 20 minutes earlier. She is obviously anxious and upset. She denies any pain.

On initial assessment and physical examination, you find the patient is pale and her skin moist and cool. On visual inspection, you note a moderate amount of bright red blood oozing from the vaginal opening. Vital signs reveal BP: 90/60; pulse: 130; ventilations: 32 and shallow. Lungs are clear and equal bilaterally.

1. What do this patient's vital signs reveal?

2. How would you care for this patient?

3. What is most likely wrong with this patient?

4. Differentiate between placenta previa and abruptio placentae.

skill sheet #29

OB/GYN EMERGENCIES—Normal Delivery

Start Time: _____

Stop Time: _____   Date: _____

Candidate's Name: _____

Evaluator's Name: _____

	Points Possible	Points Awarded
Takes, or verbalizes, body substance isolation precautions including gloves, mask, gown, and eye protection	1	
Has mother lie with knees drawn up and spread apart	1	
Elevates buttocks—with blankets or pillow	1	
Creates a sterile field around the vaginal opening with sterile towels or paper barriers	1	
When the infant's head appears during crowning, places fingers on the bony part of the skull (not the fontanelle or face) and exerts very gentle pressure to prevent explosive delivery; uses caution to avoid fontanelle	1	
If the amniotic sac does not break or has not broken, uses a clamp to puncture the sac and push it away from the infant's head and mouth as they appear	1	
As the infant's head is being born, determines if the umbilical cord is around the infant's neck; slips over the shoulder or clamps, cuts and unwraps	1	
After the infant's head is born, supports the head, suctions the mouth two or three times and the nostrils; uses caution to avoid contact with the back of the mouth	1	
As the torso and full body are born, supports the infant with both hands	1	
As the feet are born, grasps the feet	1	
Wipes blood and mucus from the mouth and nose with sterile gauze; suctions mouth and nose again	1	
Wraps infant in a warm blanket and places on its side, with the head slightly lower than the trunk	1	
Keeps infant level with vagina until the cord is cut	1	
Assigns partner to monitor infant and complete initial care of the newborn	1	
Clamps, ties, and cuts umbilical cord (between the clamps) as pulsations cease approximately 4 fingers width from patient	1	
Observes for delivery of placenta while preparing mother and infant for transport	1	
When delivered, wraps placenta in towel and puts it in a plastic bag; transports placenta to hospital with mother	1	
Places sterile pad over vaginal opening, lowers mother's legs, helps her hold them together	1	
Records time of delivery and transports mother, infant, and placenta to hospital	1	
Reassesses mother and infant en route	1	
Total:	20	

• •

Critical Criteria

_____ Did not take, or verbalize, body substance isolation precautions

_____ Did not assess for imminent delivery

_____ Did not suction newborn's mouth and nose appropriately

_____ Did not check for umbilical cord around infant's neck during delivery

_____ Did not clamp and cut umbilical cord appropriately

_____ Did not dry and warm the infant

_____ Did not assess the mother for excessive bleeding or shock after delivery

_____ Did not assess and care for both the mother and infant after delivery

Answer Key

Key Terms
1. C, A, G, D, F, B, I, E, H
2. Cervix
3. Embryo
4. Amniotic sac
5. Breech birth
6. Perineum
7. Uterus
8. Umbilicus
9. Crowning
10. Amniotic fluid
11. Contractions
12. Fetus
13. Fallopian tubes (or oviducts)
14. Menopause
15. Obstetrics
16. Gynecology
17. Meconium
18. False contractions
19. Ovaries
20. Mucous plug
21. Tubal pregnancy
22. Placenta
23. Trimester
24. Presenting part
25. Prolapsed cord

Content Review

1. Fetus, placenta, umbilical cord, amniotic sac, amniotic fluid, and mucous plug
2. A. Placenta
   B. Umbilical cord
   C. Amniotic sac
   D. Urethra
   E. Rectum
   F. Cervix
   G. Vagina
3. 40; 3
4. 3
5. Onset of the first true contraction; the complete dilation of the cervix
6. 10
7. First
8. 8-12
9. Full dilation of the cervix; delivery of the baby
10. 5 to 15; 2 to 4
11. After delivery of the infant; delivery of the placenta
12. 300 to 500
13. Surgical scissors; hemostats or cord clamps; umbilical tape or sterilized cord; bulb syringe; towels; gauze sponges; sterile gloves, eye goggles, and mask for BSI; baby blanket; sanitary napkins; and plastic bag
14. Vaginal bleeding (mild to profuse) and cramp like pain or back pain
15. Administer high-concentration oxygen; treat for shock; apply sanitary pad on perineum to absorb and document blood loss; rapidly transport in Trendelenberg position.
16. It is the sudden separation of the placenta from the wall of the uterus and presents with sudden, severe low abdominal pain with or without vaginal bleeding.
17. It is the tearing away of the placenta when the cervix begins to dilate during early stages of labor and presents with profuse red blood without pain.
18. It is seizure activity that occurs after the 20th week of pregnancy and presents with progressive increase in blood pressure, fluid retention in ankles and face, persistent headache, visual disturbances, protein in urine, and periods of confusion.
19. True
20. False
21. True
22. Protect the patient from injury; maintain an airway; provide high-concentration oxygen.
23. She should be transported on her left side to relieve the weight of the fetus on the mother's inferior vena cava.
24. When was the patient's last menstrual period? When is the patient's due date? How many times has the patient been pregnant? How many children does the patient have? Does the patient have back pain or contractions? Does the patient have a history of OB/GYN problems? What is the frequency and duration of any contractions? Is the patient's abdomen rigid and hard (if it disappears the patient has had a contraction)? Has the patient's membrane ruptured? Does the patient have vaginal bleeding or discharge? Does the patient feel like she needs to move her bowels or bear down? Is the baby crowning?
25. 1 to 2
26. 24
27. Contractions (from the beginning of one to the beginning of the next) is between 1 to 2 minutes; contractions are regular and last 45 to 60 seconds each; the woman wants to go to the bathroom to move her bowels; the mother wants to bear down; crowning is present.
28. Mouth then nose
29. Dry off the infant; wrap the infant in a warm blanket; keep the infant at the level of the vagina until the umbilical cord is cut; cut the cord and examine for oozing blood.

30. Fasten one clamp approximately 4 inches from the infant's belly; fasten the second clamp approximately 2 inches from the first clamp toward the placenta; with sterilized scissors, cut between the two clamps and pat the ends with sterilized gauze, examine both sides of the cut umbilical cord for oozing blood.
31. 20
32. Keep the infant dry and warm; suction the airway as necessary; and provide mild stimulation.
33. The head
34. True
35. A: appearance; P: pulse; G: grimace; A: activity; R: respirations. Each characteristic is assigned a value of 0, 1, or 2 and the numbers are then added for a total APGAR score.
36. 8 to 10
37. Multiple births; a mother who is drug dependent; a mother who delivers before the seventh month of pregnancy; prolonged delivery; delivery in which the head is not the presenting part; presence of meconium stained anmiotic fluid; an infant with slow, shallow, or nonexistent breathing; an infant whose heart rate is 100 beats per minute or less; or an infant whose chest and abdomen are cyanotic
38. Warm, dry, position, suction, and stimulate the infant; apply oxygen for the breathing infant with signs of distress; apply oxygen by bag-valve-mask at 100% for a non-breathing infant; in no pulse or inadequate pulse, perform chest compressions.
39. 80
40. Prolapsed cord; lower body or leg breech delivery; upper shoulder or hand delivery
41. Management of shock; immobilization on backboard if spinal injury is suspected; resuscitation efforts as needed to maintain circulation to the infant
42. False
43. True

Chapter Quiz

1. B	6. A	11. A	16. C	21. D
2. A	7. A	12. D	17. B	22. C
3. D	8. B	13. A	18. D	23. A
4. A	9. C	14. A	19. D	24. B
5. A	10. C	15. A	20. C	25. A

Case Scenario

1. The patient's vital signs reveal compromised circulation with a high index of suspicion of impending shock based on her BP and pulse rate. The patient is breathing without distress and does not have an altered mental status at this point; and the patient appears to have adequate perfusion to the brain. Her pulse rate is rapid, which could be a compensatory mechanism for coping with blood loss and in response to her anxiety level.
2. Take BSI precautions; realize that vaginal bleeding in the third trimester is serious; perform a visual examination of the patient's perineal area; place the patient on high-flow oxygen via a non-rebreather mask; place the patient on her left side; transport the patient to the hospital as quickly as possible, meeting ALS personnel en route if possible; notify the hospital of your ETA so they can be prepared for your arrival and summon the patient's obstetrician to attend to the patient.
3. The patient is most likely presenting with placenta previa, which is a true emergency for both mother and child.
4. In abruptio placentae, there is more likely to be pain related to the bleeding. Bright red blood is more characteristic of placenta previa. The passage of dark blood is more common with abruptio placentae. It is not important to distinguish between the two conditions in the field, because all cases of third-trimester bleeding should be considered a medical emergency with the patient treated accordingly.

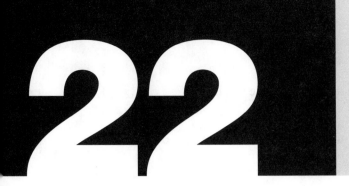

Kinematics of Trauma

Reading Assignment: Chapter 22 pages 403–441.

DOT Objectives

None identified for this chapter.

Supplemental Objectives

- Define energy and force as they relate to trauma.
- Define the laws governing motion.
- Describe the role increased speed plays in causing injuries.
- Describe each type of auto impact and its effect on unrestrained victims (e.g., down-and- under, up-and-over, compression, shear).
- Describe the injuries produced in the head, spine, thorax, and abdomen that result from the various types of automobile collisions.
- Describe the kinematics of penetrating injuries.
- Describe the mechanism of energy exchange and the factors that affect speed reduction for a moving body.
- List the motion and energy considerations of mechanisms other than motor vehicle crashes.
- Define the role of kinematics as an additional tool for patient assessment.

Key Terms

1. The process of surveying an injury scene to determine what injuries might have resulted from the forces and motion involved is called _____.

2. What is Newton's first law of motion?

3. The energy of motion is called _____.

4. The process in which tissue in the human body is knocked out of its normal position, creating a cavity, is called _____.

5. The type of collision that occurs when a slow-moving or stationary object is struck from behind is called a _____ collision.

6. The type of collision that occurs when a vehicle is struck from the side is called a _____ _____ collision.

7. The type of collision that occurs when one corner of a car strikes an immovable object is called a _____ collision.

Content Review

1. What are the two most important factors determining the extent of bodily injury?

   1)

   2)

2. Energy cannot be created or destroyed, but it can be changed in form.
   A. True
   B. False

3. Kinetic energy is a function of an object's _____ and _____.

4. The relationship between weight and speed as it affects kinetic energy is defined how?

5. An increase in mass increases the rate of production of kinetic energy more than an increase in the velocity.
   A. True
   B. False

6. What is Newton's second law of motion?

7. An unrestrained driver will be more severely injured than a restrained driver because the restraint system, rather than the body, absorbs a significant portion of the energy of deceleration.
   A. True
   B. False

8. What are the two factors that control the energy exchange in cavitation?

   1)

   2)

9. Describe the two types of cavities produced by cavitation.

   1)

   2)

10. Automobile collisions can be divided into what five types?

    1)
    2)
    3)
    4)
    5)

11. During a motor vehicle collision, there are three separate events or impacts that occur. What are they?

    1)

    2)

    3)

12. An occupant of a motor vehicle collision receives force from the same direction as the vehicle.
    A. True
    B. False

13. A patient in a head-on collision will follow one of two possible paths. What are they?

    1)

    2)

14. What is the most common lead point in a down-and-under collision path?

15. What is the most common lead point in an up-and-over front end collision?

16. A lateral impact collision affects what three parts of the body?

    1)
    2)
    3)

17. What injuries may occur if the chest receives the impact of a side collision?

18. Because of body positioning within the vehicle, drivers involved in a side-impact collision are more vulnerable to rupture of the _____, whereas front seat occupants are more vulnerable to injuries of the _____.

19. What are the two forces involved in blunt trauma impact?

    1)

    2)

20. Diagonal seat belt straps worn alone can produce severe neck injuries, including decapitation.
    A. True
    B. False

21. Air bags may cause what type of injuries?

22. What injuries are commonly associated with an angular-impact motorcycle collision?

23. A motorcyclist involved in a head-on collision will most likely suffer from what type of injuries?

24. There are two injury patterns commonly seen in pedestrian/motor vehicle collisions. Describe each.

    Adult:

    Child:

25. Describe the three phases involved in a pedestrian/motor vehicle collision.

    1)

    2)

    3)

26. To properly assess a fall victim, what factors should the EMT analyze?

27. In general, falls from _____ the height of the victim are considered severe.

28. Describe the injuries that occur in the three phases of an explosion.

Chapter Quiz

1. _____ first law of motion states that a body at rest will remain at rest and a body in motion will remain in motion unless acted on by some outside force.
   A. Morton's
   B. Pavlov's
   C. Newton's
   D. Einstein's

2. One principle of physics states that:
   A. Energy cannot be created
   B. Energy cannot be destroyed
   C. Energy can be changed in form
   D. All of the above

3. Energy may change into a form of all of the following types *except:*
   A. Mechanical
   B. Extrinsic
   C. Thermal
   D. Chemical

4. Kinetic energy is the energy of _____ and is a function of an object's weight and speed.
   A. Sound
   B. Light
   C. Motion
   D. Heat

5. The factor that is considered the most influential when calculating the amount of injury that will be caused by a moving object is the object's:
   A. Mass
   B. Weight
   C. Height
   D. Speed

6. A small child and adult are different in size and weight, and if they are both in a vehicle traveling 65 mph, the most vital determinant of the amount of force that will be applied to them in a crash is their:
   A. Common speed, not their weight difference
   B. Weight difference, not their common speed
   C. Height and weight difference, not their common speed
   D. Height difference, not their common speed

7. An unrestrained driver will be more severely injured compared to a restrained driver, because the restraint system absorbs a significant portion of the energy of deceleration.
   A. True
   B. False

8. Loss of motion of a moving object can translate into tissue damage to the victim.
   A. True
   B. False

9. Energy exchange is directly related to the density and size of the frontal area at the point of contact between the object and the victim's body.
   A. True
   B. False

10. Shear force, which tears organs or their supporting structures, comes into place with:
    A. Deceleration
    B. Acceleration
    C. Penetrating injuries
    D. A and B

11. In the management of trauma patients, one of the most critical determinates of the outcome is the time from onset of the injury to:
    A. Transport
    B. Initial assessment
    C. Definitive care
    D. Dispatch

12. If a patient has followed a down-and-under path during a frontal collision, the EMT should have a high index of suspicion of all of the following injuries *except:*
    A. Shoulder dislocation
    B. Knee dislocation
    C. Femur injury
    D. Hip dislocation

13. In the up-and-over motion of a frontal collision, the _____ is usually the lead body portion.
    A. Chest
    B. Abdomen
    C. Head
    D. Pelvis

14. A victim involved in an up-and-over motion of a frontal collision may have compression injuries to the anterior chest, which may include:
    A. Broken ribs
    B. An anterior flail chest
    C. A pulmonary contusion
    D. All of the above

15. Fractures of the spine are more common with lateral collisions than with rear collisions.
    A. True
    B. False

16. Shear injury to abdominal organs at the point of attachment to the mesentery can occur in which of the following?
    A. Kidneys
    B. Small intestine
    C. Spleen
    D. All of the above

17. One of every thirteen ejection victims suffers a:
    A. Spinal fracture
    B. Hip fracture
    C. Pelvic fracture
    D. Skull fracture

18. Air bags are extremely effective in the first collision of head-on impacts, but they are not effective in multiple-impact collisions.
    A. True
    B. False

19. In pedestrian collisions, children are initially struck higher on the body than adults.
    A. True
    B. False

Case Scenario

You are dispatched to a motor vehicle collision. On your arrival at the scene, you find a one car crash with the vehicle sustaining moderate damage to the front driver's side, which hit a telephone pole.

The driver was the only occupant in the car. He is still in the driver's seat. The patient admits that he was not wearing a seat belt, and his car is not equipped with air bags. The steering column is bent, and you note a starburst pattern on the windshield.

On assessment, you determine the patient is conscious and alert but very anxious. His vital signs are as follows: BP, 86/64; pulse, 132; ventilations, 28.

1. Considering the kinematics, what injuries would you expect this patient may have suffered?

2. What do the patient's vital signs reveal?

3. What would you expect is causing this patient's hypotension?

4. Is this patient a candidate for rapid extrication and transport? Why?

Answer Key

•••

Key Terms
1. Kinematics
2. A body at rest will remain at rest, and a body in motion will remain in motion unless acted on by some outside force.
3. Kinetic energy
4. Cavitation
5. Rear-impact
6. Lateral- (side) impact
7. Rotational impact

Content Review
1. 1) The amount of force (energy) the body absorbs; and 2) the anatomical structures involved in the energy exchange
2. True
3. Weight (mass); speed (velocity)
4. Kinetic energy = $\dfrac{Mass \times Velocity^2}{2}$
5. False
6. Force is required to put an object in motion and to stop it. Force equals mass times acceleration. [Mass × Acceleration = Force = Mass × Deceleration]
7. True
8. 1) The density of the material or tissue through which the missile is passing or that it impacts; and 2) the frontal area of the impacting object
9. 1) *Temporary* cavity—forms at the time of impact and is caused by stretching; but tissue returns to previous position and the cavity cannot be seen when the patient is later examined; 2) *Permanent* cavity—caused by impact and compression of tissue; can be seen later.
10. 1) Head-on or frontal impact; 2) rear impact; 3) lateral or side impact; 4) rotational impact; and 5) rollover
11. 1) The vehicle crashes into an object; 2) the unrestrained occupant collides with the inside of the vehicle; and 3) the occupant's internal organs collide with one another or with the wall of the cavity.
12. True
13. 1) Down-and-under; and 2) up-and-over
14. The knee against the dashboard
15. The head striking the windshield and/or the chest or abdomen colliding with the steering wheel
16. 1) Chest, 2) pelvis, and 3) cervical spine
17. Compression fracture of the ribs; flail chest; pulmonary contusion; pneumothorax; and ruptured liver or spleen
18. Spleen; liver
19. 1) Shear (change of speed); and 2) compression
20. True

21. Abrasions of the arms, chest, and face; and injuries caused by the occupant's eyeglasses; neck injuries in children

22. Crushing injuries of the lower leg that causes open fractures of the tibia or fibula and dislocation of the ankle.

23. Injury to the head, chest, or abdomen, depending on what part of the anatomy strikes the handlebars; and bilateral femur fractures, if the rider's feet remain in the pegs and the thighs hit the handlebars

24. *Adult:* When adults see an oncoming vehicle, they try to protect themselves by turning away, therefore injuries are frequently lateral or posterior on the body.
   Child: children face oncoming vehicles and, therefore, suffer injuries to the anterior part of the body.

25. 1) Initial impact to the legs of an adult and sometimes to the hips, abdomen, or chest of a child; 2) the torso rolls onto the hood of the automobile; 3) the victim falls off the automobile and onto the asphalt, usually head first, with possible cervical spine trauma

26. The height of the fall; the surface on which the victim landed; and which part of the body struck first

27. Greater than three times

28. *Primary:* Caused by the pressure wave of the blast, usually occur in gas-containing organs and may include pulmonary bleeding, pneumothorax, air emboli, perforation of the GI organs, or burns.
   Secondary: Occur when the victim is struck by flying glass, falling mortar, or other debris from the blast and usually include lacerations, fractures, and burn injuries.
   Tertiary: occur when the victim becomes a missile and is thrown against some object causing injuries at the point of impact with the force of the blast being transferred to other body organs as energy of the impact is absorbed.

Chapter Quiz

1. C	6. A	11. C	16. D
2. D	7. A	12. A	17. A
3. B	8. A	13. C	18. A
4. C	9. A	14. D	19. A
5. D	10. D	15. A	

Case Scenario

1. Head: possible skull fracture(s), cerebral contusion, or other head injury.
   Spine: possible spine or spinal cord injury.
   Chest: possible rib fracture(s), flail chest, cardiac contusion, pneumothorax, and pulmonary contusion.
   Abdomen: laceration or rupture of the liver and/or spleen with possible associated injury to the pancreas.
   Extremities: dislocation or fracture of the knee, fracture of the femur, or dislocation of the hip.

2. The patient is exhibiting signs and symptoms of shock and is in need of rapid treatment and transport.

3. The hypotension is most likely due to laceration of the liver and/or spleen resulting in hemorrhage into the patient's abdomen.

4. Yes. This patient is hypotensive and requires definitive treatment in the operating room.

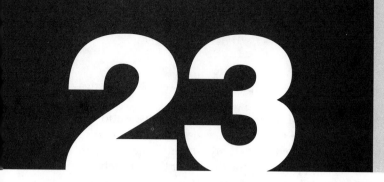

Soft-Tissue Injury and Bleeding Control

Reading Assignment: Chapter 23 pages 442–459.

DOT Objectives

Upon successful completion of the EMT-Basic training program, the EMT-Basic should be able to do the following:

- Describe the anatomy and physiology of the skin.
- List the types and describe the emergency medical care of closed and open soft tissue injuries, including control of hemorrhage.
- Describe and contrast the emergency medical care considerations for a penetrating chest injury and an open abdominal wound.
- Describe the purpose and function of dressings and bandages, and outline the steps in the application of a pressure dressing.
- Describe the effects of improperly applied dressings, splints, and tourniquets.
- Describe the emergency medical care of a patient with an impaled object or a traumatic amputation.
- Establish the relationship between body substance isolation (BSI) and soft tissue injuries.
- State the types of open soft tissue injuries.
- Differentiate the care of an open wound to the chest from that for an open wound to the abdomen.
- Establish the relationship between airway management and the patient with chest injury, and blunt and penetrating injuries.
- Demonstrate the steps in the emergency medical care of closed soft tissue injuries.
- Demonstrate the steps in the emergency medical care of open soft tissue injuries.
- Demonstrate the steps in the emergency medical care of an impaled object.
- Demonstrate the steps in the emergency medical care of a patient with an amputation.
- Demonstrate the steps in the emergency medical care of an amputated part.
- Demonstrate completing a prehospital care report for patients with soft tissue injuries.

Supplemental Objectives

- Describe compartment syndrome and its complications.
- Describe estimation of blood loss at the scene.

Key Terms

••

1. Material that holds a dressing in place is called a(n) _____.

2. The measured area of a body involved, usually when dealing with burns, is called the _____ _____.

3. Sterile material placed directly on a wound is called a(n) _____.

4. The abnormal accumulation of fluid that causes swelling in tissues in response to an injury is called _____.

5. The middle layer of the skin that contains the blood vessels, glands, hair follicles, and nerve endings is called the _____.

6. The outermost layer of the skin is called the _____.

7. A system for measuring the percentage of body surface area (BSA) involved in a burn is called the _____.

8. The deepest layer of the skin is called the _____.

9. Match the following terms with their appropriate description.

_____ Injury where organs protrude from the abdominal cavity through a wound in the abdominal wall	A. Abrasion
_____ Damage to the epidermis and dermis from shearing forces	B. Amputation
_____ Minor damage in the dermal layer causing discoloration from blood leaking into the surrounding tissue	C. Compartment syndrome
	D. Contusion
_____ Injuries resulting when skin is pierced by a sharp object	E. Crush injury
_____ A condition that can result in complete death of an extremity if not stopped by surgical intervention	F. Evisceration
	G. Hematoma
_____ Injury where limb or other body part is torn completely from the body	H. Laceration
_____ Damage resulting from a body part being compressed between two surfaces	I. Penetrating wound
_____ A break in the skin from a forceful impact with a sharp object	
_____ Damage to tissue where larger blood vessels are torn causing a collection of blood in deep tissues	

Content Review

1. What are the functions of the skin?

2. Identify whether each of the following injuries are closed (C) or open (O).

   _____ Abrasion
   _____ Amputation
   _____ Avulsion
   _____ Bruise
   _____ Contusion
   _____ Crush injury
   _____ Hematoma
   _____ Impaled object
   _____ Laceration
   _____ Puncture
   _____ Penetrating wound

3. A hematoma may contain 1 liter or more of blood.
   A. True
   B. False

4. A hematoma may result in shock.
   A. True
   B. False

5. An injury that occurs when a part of the body is caught between two compressing surfaces is called a(n) _____ injury.

6. An injury in which a flap of skin or tissue is torn loose or pulled completely off is called a(n) _____ _____.

7. What should the EMT do with an amputated or avulsed body part?

8. The preferred method of controlling bleeding is _____.

9. Avulsed or amputated body parts should be kept directly on ice during transport to the hospital.
   A. True
   B. False

10. Identify three complications of soft tissue injuries.

    1)
    2)
    3)

11. Why should an EMT not use a wet dressing?

12. How can the EMT help to decrease contamination and help prevent further injury to damaged tissue?

13. A fractured femur can cause up to _____ liter(s) of blood loss into the thigh and a broken humerus can bleed _____ liter(s) of blood into the upper arm.

14. Bleeding does not need to be visible to the EMT to be severe.
    A. True
    B. False

15. The key component of assessment of a patient with soft tissue injuries is to determine the _____ _____.

16. What are the signs and symptoms of a crush injury?

17. Materials placed over dressings to hold them in place are called _____.

18. Identify the different types of bandages.

19. A bandage that forms an air-tight seal is called a(n) _____ bandage.

20. An open chest wound should be treated with what type of dressing?

21. What should the EMT do if a patient with an open chest wound exhibits signs of respiratory status deterioration?

22. An abdominal wound where organs protrude through the wound is called a(n) _____ _____.

23. How should the EMT treat a patient with an abdominal evisceration?

24. Why is an abdominal evisceration covered with a moistened dressing?

25. When should an impaled object be removed in the field?

26. How should an EMT care for a patient with an impaled object?

27. The EMT should not soak an amputated part in water or saline, place it directly on ice or ice packs, or cool it with dry ice.
    A. True
    B. False

28. What are two possible complications of a neck wound?

    1)
    2)

29. How should the EMT care for a patient with a neck wound?

30. Describe the different ways to control bleeding.

31. When necessary, a tourniquet should be placed as close as possible to the point of injury and tightened only until blood loss is reduced to a controllable state with dressings.
    A. True
    B. False

32. The potential for successful re-attachment of a traumatic amputation is significantly reduced when a tourniquet is applied.
    A. True
    B. False

Chapter Quiz

1. If a dressing becomes saturated with blood:
   A. Nothing else can control the bleeding
   B. It should be replaced with a new dressing
   C. A new dressing should be placed on top of it
   D. A tourniquet should be applied

2. When bleeding is evident in an extremity, lowering the extremity may work to slow blood flow to the area and reduce the amount of blood loss.
   A. True
   B. False

3. Pulse-point pressure should be used to control bleeding when:
   A. Direct pressure and/or elevation has not been effective
   B. There is venous bleeding
   C. There is capillary bleeding
   D. All of the above

4. The use of a tourniquet is:
   A. The best method to control a venous bleed
   B. A last resort treatment for control of bleeding
   C. Always used to control bleeding from an amputation
   D. Best applied by ALS personnel

5. What are the layers of the skin?
   A. Epidermis, dermis, and subcutaneous tissue
   B. Outer dermis, dermis, and subcutaneous tissue
   C. Epidermis, dermis, and muscle tissue
   D. Endodermis, dermis, and muscle tissue

6. The dermis contains:
   A. Blood vessels and lymphatic vessels
   B. Nerve endings and hair follicles
   C. Sweat glands and sebaceous glands
   D. All of the above

7. The deepest layer of the skin is composed of:
   A. Fatty tissue
   B. Fibrous tissue
   C. Elastic tissue
   D. All of the above

8. Which of the following is a function of the skin:
   A. Protection from invading microorganisms
   B. Prevention of fluid loss
   C. Maintenance of normal body temperature
   D. All of the above

9. The palm of the patient's hand is equal to about _____% body surface area.
   A. 3
   B. 9
   C. 1
   D. 6

10. Which of the following is *not* a closed soft tissue injury?
    A. Contusion
    B. Avulsion
    C. Hematoma
    D. Crush injury

11. Which of the following are open soft tissue injuries?
    A. Abrasions and lacerations
    B. Avulsions and penetrating wounds
    C. Puncture wounds and amputations
    D. All of the above

12. Contusions are commonly called:
    A. Lacerations
    B. Bruises
    C. Abrasions
    D. Avulsions

13. When part of the body is caught between two compressing surfaces, a _____ injury results.
    A. Penetrating
    B. Crush
    C Push and pull
    D. Shear

14. Forceful impact with a sharp object producing a break in the skin of varying depth is called a(n):
    A. Abrasion
    B. Crush
    C. Laceration
    D. Contusion

15. An injury where flaps of skin or tissue are torn loose or pulled completely off is called a(n):
    A. Avulsion
    B. Amputation
    C. Laceration
    D. Contusion

16. The preferred method to control blood loss is:
    A. Direct pressure
    B. Tourniquet
    C. Elevation
    D. Indirect pressure

17. Massive hemorrhage of up to 1 or 2 liters of blood loss can occur with all of the following injuries *except:*
    A. Liver laceration
    B. Pelvic fracture
    C. Femur fracture
    D. Radial fracture

18. Most closed soft tissue injuries do not require treatment in the field by the EMT.
    A. True
    B. False

19. Proper management of open soft tissue injuries includes which of the following?
    A. Application of a sterile dressing
    B. Immediate control of severe external hemorrhage
    C. Preventing hypothermia
    D. All of the above

20. Proper management of an evisceration includes:
    A. Pushing the organ back into the body cavity
    B. Placing a dry, sterile dressing over the injury
    C. Placing a moist dressing over the injury
    D. All of the above

21. Treatment modalities common to both chest and abdominal injuries include all of the following *except:*
    A. Estimating BSA
    B. Supplemental oxygen
    C. Assessment of airway, breathing, and circulation
    D. Expeditious transport to the hospital

22. Which of the following is the purpose of dressings and bandages?
    A. Prevention of further contamination
    B. Protection from additional injury
    C. Decreased fluid loss from the disrupted skin
    D. All of the above

23. Which of the following is true concerning open wounds to the neck?
    A. Severe hemorrhage is possible
    B. An air embolism is possible
    C. A sterile occlusive dressing should be applied
    D. All of the above

24. When applying a pressure dressing, it should be placed tightly enough to ensure that blood flow distal to the wound is occluded.
    A. True
    B. False

Case Scenario

• •

You are dispatched to a local bar for an injured person involved in an altercation. On your arrival, you are directed to a 28-year-old male patient with multiple injuries. The patient is alert and oriented and very agitated. He has an obvious odor of alcohol on his breath. There is no sign of the other victim.

1. What are your initial concerns?

After ensuring that law enforcement is on the scene and that the scene is safe, you begin to examine the patient. You note a 2-inch laceration on the patient's left upper arm that is oozing blood and a 1-inch laceration just above his left wrist that is bleeding profusely. There is a 3-inch laceration on the lower part of his abdomen with the intestines protruding and he has contusions on his face, arms, and chest. His vital signs reveal: BP, 100/70; pulse, 128; ventilations, 26. Lungs are clear and equal bilaterally.

2. What BSI precautions are appropriate when caring for this patient?

3. Based on MOI and assessment, how would you care for this patient?

4. What is the medical term for the patient's abdominal condition?

5. What type of dressing should you apply to the patient's abdomen?

6. If blood from the wrist laceration soaks the dressing, what should the EMT do?

7. If bleeding of the wrist is not controlled by direct pressure, how should the EMT control the bleeding?

Answer Key

●●

Key Terms
1. Bandage
2. Body surface area (BSA)
3. Dressing
4. Edema
5. Dermis
6. Epidermis
7. Rule of nines
8. Subcutaneous tissue
9. F, A, D, I, C, B, E, H, G

Content Review
1. To prevent bacteria from invading the body; to prevent fluid loss from the body; to maintain normal body temperature; and to detect environmental dangers
2. O, O, O, C, C, C, C, O, O, O, O
3. True
4. True
5. Crush
6. Avulsion
7. Wrap the part in a sterile dressing and place it in a plastic bag; keep the part cooled, not frozen; and transport it with the patient to an appropriate facility as quickly as possible.
8. Direct pressure
9. False
10. Infection, shock from fluid loss, and hypothermia
11. Wet dressings cause heat to evaporate from damaged tissues that are no longer able to regulate their own temperature.
12. Apply a sterile dressing
13. 2; 1
14. True
15. Mechanism of injury
16. Painful, swollen, deformed extremity; contusion; signs and symptoms of shock
17. Bandages
18. Gauze rolls, elastic bandages, triangular bandages, adhesive tape, air splints
19. Occlusive
20. Air-tight (occlusive) petroleum jelly gauze foil package covering the wound and taped on three sides
21. Remove one corner of the occlusive dressing to allow air to escape from the chest and then reapply the dressing
22. Evisceration
23. Cover the area with a moistened sterile dressing as soon as possible; secure the dressing in place; do not touch the organs or push them back into the abdomen; flex the patient's hips and knees for comfort.
24. It prevents drying and further injury to the exposed organs and reduces evaporation and heat loss.
25. If it interferes with necessary chest compressions, establishment of an airway, or transport of the patient.
26. Stabilize the object with bulky dressings; manage the airway; treat for shock as necessary; and transport quickly to an appropriate facility.
27. True

28. 1) Bleeding to death from uncontrolled hemorrhage; 2) air embolism from air sucked into the blood vessels; 3) loss of airway; 4) aspirations of blood; 5) aspiration of GI content.
29. Apply a sterile occlusive dressing to prevent air from entering the circulation; apply direct pressure to control bleeding; compress the carotid artery only if necessary to control bleeding and only on one side.
30. Elevation of the injured part; direct pressure; pulse point pressure; and a tourniquet
31. True
32. True

Chapter Quiz

1. C	5. A	9. C	13. B	17. D	21. A
2. B	6. D	10. B	14. C	18. A	22. D
3. A	7. D	11. D	15. A	19. D	23. D
4. B	8. D	12. B	16. A	20. C	24. B

Case Scenario

1. The primary concern should be for scene safety. The consumption of alcohol by the victim may increase violence tendencies. Where is the other person involved in the fight? Is he dangerous? Are there any weapons around? Is the scene safe for you and your crew to provide emergency care?
2. Gloves. If blood is spattering or the patient's actions place the EMT at risk for increased exposure of blood of body fluids, consider the use of a mask, gown, and eye protection.
3. Take BSI precautions; administer high-flow supplemental oxygen via a nonrebreather mask; control bleeding by applying direct pressure to lacerations using gauze pads; secure dressings in place with tape; cover the abdominal wound with a moistened sterile dressing; keep the patient warm; monitor the patient for signs of shock and treat accordingly; and transport the patient, with his hips and knees flexed for comfort, to a trauma center.
4. Abdominal evisceration
5. A sterile dressing moistened with sterile saline solution
6. Apply a second dressing on top of the first.
7. Apply pulse-point pressure to the brachial artery.

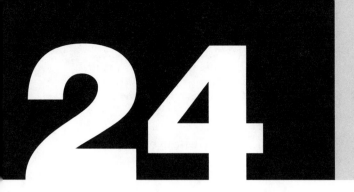

Head Trauma

Reading Assignment: Chapter 24 pages 460–475.

DOT Objectives

None identified for this chapter.

Supplemental Objectives

Upon successful completion of the EMT-Basic training program, the EMT-Basic should be able to do the following:

- List the structures of the head and describe the function of each structure.
- Describe the relationship of mechanism of injury to potential injuries of the head.
- Discuss the importance of the meninges.
- Define and draw a "potential space."
- Name the three divisions of the brain and give a brief description of the function of each.
- Discuss the importance of cerebrospinal fluid (CSF).
- Discuss why the scalp is more prone to blood loss.
- Discuss bleeding control for open and closed head injuries.
- Discuss brain edema and its consequences.
- Discuss intracranial pressure (ICP).
- Discuss the importance of frequent assessment of level of consciousness (LOC).

Key Terms

1. The three highly vascular membranes that separate the cranium from the brain are called the _____ _____.

2. Immobile, interlocking joints that connect the cranial bones are called _____.

3. A potential space located between the skull and dura mater is called the _____.

4. Accumulation of blood in the space between the dura mater and the arachnoid membrane is called a(n) _____.

5. The fluid that circulates around and protects the brain and spinal cord is called _____ _____.

6. The pressure that builds up inside the cranial cavity due to fluid accumulation is referred to as _____
   _____ .

7. A phenomenon seen with increased intracranial pressure, presenting as an increase in blood pressure, decrease in pulse, and change in respirations, is called _____ .

8. Match the following anatomical terms with their appropriate description.

   _____ The opening at the base of the skull
   _____ The outermost layer of the meninges
   _____ The second membrane of the meninges
   _____ The innermost layer of the meninges
   _____ The portion of the brain divided into two hemispheres
   _____ The portion of the brain responsible for coordination of movement
   _____ The part of the brain responsible for consciousness
   _____ A structure located in the brainstem and responsible for vital functions of the body

   A. Arachnoid membrane
   B. Brainstem
   C. Cerebellum
   D. Cerebrum
   E. Dura mater
   F. Foramen magnum
   G. Medulla
   H. Pia mater

9. Match the following assessment terms with their appropriate description.

   _____ Bruising around the eyes associated with basilar skull fractures
   _____ Discoloration behind the ears found with skull fractures
   _____ An assessment of mental function
   _____ A standardized rating system used to evaluate the degree of consciousness impairment based on three areas
   _____ Characterized by a period of slow and shallow respirations, followed by deep ventilations, then repeated
   _____ Flexion of the upper extremities with the lower extremities rigid and extended
   _____ Extension of the upper extremities with the lower extremities rigid and extended

   A. Battle's sign
   B. Cheyne-Stokes
   C. Decerebrate
   D. Decorticate
   E. GSC
   F. LOC
   G. Racoon's eyes

Content Review

....

1. A subdural hematoma involves arterial blood and manifests signs and symptoms within hours.
   A. True
   B. False

2. An epidural hematoma involves venous bleeding and may not manifest signs and symptoms for several hours or days after the traumatic injury.
   A. True
   B. False

3. The survival rate is worse with a subdural hematoma than with an epidural hematoma.
   A. True
   B. False

4. Increased intracranial pressure can come from what two sources?

   1)
   2)

5. When brain cells swell, they can expand into what three places?

   1)
   2)
   3)

6. Identify the following bones of the skull.
   Frontal   Maxilla   Orbital
   Mandible   Nasal   Zygomatic

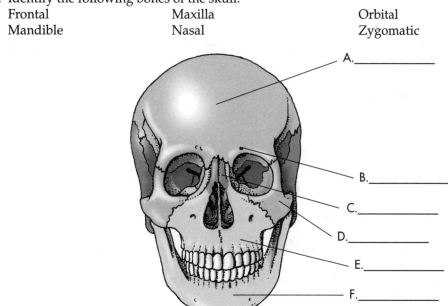

A._____

B._____

C._____

D._____

E._____

F._____

7. How can the EMT determine if blood contains CSF?

8. What are the signs of increased intracranial pressure?

9. What are the three major complications associated with skull fractures?

   1)
   2)
   3)

10. What type of injury causes Battle's sign?

11. Battle's sign may not develop until 24–36 hours after a traumatic injury.
    A. True
    B. False

12. The medical term for a "black eye" is _____.

13. If an EMT finds a patient with blood accumulated around the tissue of only one eye, he or she should assume it was caused by local trauma rather than a fracture at the base of the skull.
    A. True
    B. False

14. What acronym should the EMT use to assess a patient's level of consciousness?

15. A patient who is "alert and oriented x 4" can answer what questions?

16. The Glasgow coma scale assesses a patient's LOC by assigning numbers to what three categories?

17. How should the EMT manage a patient with a head injury?

Chapter Quiz

• •

1. Altered mental status is the single most important sign of a head injury.
   A. True
   B. False

2. Regarding the head-injured patient, all of the following statements are true *except:*
   A. Mental status must be evaluated critically and continually.
   B. Assessment information must be documented for medical and legal reasons.
   C. It is essential to fully apprize hospital staff of any change in the patient's condition.
   D. If the patient is ambulatory at the scene, spinal precautions are not necessary.

3. Knowledge of the mechanism of injury is very useful in assisting the EMT to identify the injuries that a patient may have sustained.
   A. True
   B. False

4. The _____ is the outermost part of the head.
   A. Cranium
   B. Brain
   C. Scalp
   D. Meninges

5. Because the head is very vascular, the scalp tends to bleed heavily, but this bleeding is easily controlled.
   A. True
   B. False

6. The most efficient method for handling bleeding from the scalp is:
   A. Pressure points
   B. Tourniquets
   C. Direct pressure
   D. Pressure dressings

7. Bones of the cranium are joined by immobile interlocking joints called:
   A. Joints
   B. Sutures
   C. Fistulas
   D. Foramens

8. The opening at the base of the skull through which the brainstem and spinal cord pass is called the:
   A. Foramen magnum
   B. Calcaneus
   C. Circle of Willis
   D. Inferior orifice

9. The membranes that separate the cranium and the brain are collectively known as the:
   A. Meninges
   B. Ventricles
   C. Foramen
   D. Cerebrum

10. An epidural hematoma is a condition in which blood leaks into the epidural space.
    A. True
    B. False

11. When evaluating the mechanism of injury, the EMT should do all of the following *except:*
    A. Use bystanders as a source of information
    B. Evaluate the evidence at the scene and look at the vehicle
    C. Rely only on information provided by the patient
    D. Examine entrance and exit wounds

12. The medulla is located in the brainstem and is responsible for which of the following body functions:
    A. Heart rate
    B. Respirations
    C. Blood pressure
    D. All of the above

13. Cerebrospinal fluid (CSF) is produced in the brain and found within the:
    A. Subarachnoid space
    B. Dural space
    C. Potential space
    D. Formenal space

14. Cerebrospinal fluid serves as a:
    A. Shock absorber for the brain
    B. Mechanism for leakage to the outside
    C. Deterrent to bacteria entering the brain
    D. Place for the production of red blood cells

15. Complications of open head injuries not associated with closed head injuries include all of the following *except:*
    A. Increased intracranial pressure
    B. Leakage of CSF
    C. Bacterial contamination of the brain
    D. Herniation of the brain through the skull

16. All of the following are signs of Cushing's triad *except:*
    A. Increased blood pressure
    B. Change in respiratory effort
    C. Increase in pulse rate
    D. Decrease in pulse rate

17. Head trauma is the leading cause of traumatic death in blunt trauma, with most resulting from motor vehicle collisions.
    A. True
    B. False

18. Periorbital ecchymosis is caused by blood accumulating in the tissue around the eye, a condition known as:
    A. Kernig's sign
    B. Battle's sign
    C. Raccoon's eyes
    D. Horner's sign

19. Level of consciousness is an indirect measurement of cerebral oxygenation.
    A. True
    B. False

Case Scenario

You are dispatched to Route I-95, mile marker 235 for an automobile crash. On your arrival, you find a two car collision. The driver of the first vehicle is walking around uninjured. The driver of the second car is still in his vehicle. The car sustained a spider crack in the windshield. The patient was not wearing a seatbelt, however, there was an air bag, which did deploy.

On initial assessment and physical examination, you determine that the patient is in an altered state of consciousness. He cannot remember the crash and does not know the year or where he is, but he does know his name. He has a large contusion above his left eye and complains of a headache and pain in his neck. His vital signs reveal: BP, 160/98; pulse, 48; ventilations, 14 shallow and irregular. Pupils are constricted but reactive to light.

1. What is most likely wrong with this patient?

2. What leads you to this conclusion?

3. How would you care for this patient?

4. What signs and symptoms should you watch for that would indicate an increase in ICP or deterioration of the patient's condition?

Answer Key

Key Terms
1. Meninges
2. Sutures
3. Epidural space
4. Subdural hematoma
5. Cerebrospinal fluid (CSF)
6. Intracranial pressure (ICP)
7. Cushing's triad
8. F, E, A, H, D, C, B, G
9. G, A, F, E, B, D, C

Content Review
1. False
2. False
3. True
4. 1) Lesions such as a blood clot or brain tumor; or 2) increased fluid accumulation in and around brain cells
5. 1) The space around the cell itself; 2) out of the cranium into the spinal cord through the foramen magnum; or 3) out of an open fracture of the skull
6. A. Frontal
   B. Orbital
   C. Nasal
   D. Zygomatic
   E. Maxilla
   F. Mandible
7. It appears as a "halo" or yellowish fluid surrounding the blood when separated onto a sheet or gauze.
8. Increased blood pressure; change in respiratory effort; decreased pulse; change in pupillary size, equality, and reaction time; and a change in mental status
9. 1) Injury to the brain beneath the fracture (laceration or compression); 2) hemorrhage from open ends of the bone; and 3) leakage of CSF
10. Occipital or basilar skull fractures
11. True

12. Periorbital ecchymosis
13. True
14. AVPU (alert, responds to verbal stimuli, responds only to painful stimuli, or is unresponsive)
15. Questions indicating that he knows his name (person); where he is (place); what happened (situation); and day, date, or year (time)
16. Ability to open eyes; motor response; and verbal response
17. Take BSI precautions; perform an initial assessment; maintain spinal in-line immobilization; maintain a patent airway; administer high-flow oxygen at 15 liters via a non-rebreather mask; assist with ventilations as necessary (under 12 or over 30 breaths per minute); control bleeding (do not exert too much pressure to an open or depressed skull injury); assess for CSF leakage; dress and bandage open wounds; and continually assess for changes in status.

Chapter Quiz

1. A	6. C	11. C	16. C
2. D	7. B	12. D	17. A
3. A	8. A	13. A	18. C
4. C	9. A	14. A	19. A
5. B	10. A	15. A	

Case Scenario

1. A closed head injury with possible skull fracture and increased intracranial pressure; a possible cervical spine injury.
2. The mechanism of injury; damage to the vehicle (specifically the windshield); the patient's complaints of a headache and pain in the neck; the contusion on his forehead; and his vital signs of an increased BP, decreased pulse, irregular breathing pattern, and constricted pupils.
3. Initiate in-line cervical spine stabilization; ensure the patient's adequate airway; administer high-concentration oxygen via a non-rebreather mask at 15 liters per minute; be prepared to assist with ventilations if the patient's breathing falls below 12 or above 29 breaths per minute; apply a cervical collar; watch for signs of shock and treat accordingly; immobilize on a long spine board; and transport quickly to a trauma center.
4. Decorticate or decerebrate posturing and/or possible seizure activity

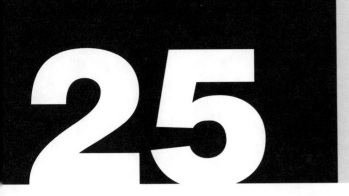

Chest Trauma

Reading Assignment: Chapter 25 pages 476–492.

DOT Objectives

Upon successful completion of the EMT-Basic training program, the EMT-Basic should be able to do the following:

- Demonstrate the steps in the emergency medical care of a patient with an open chest wound.

Supplemental Objectives

- Describe the physiology associated with breathing.
- Describe the anatomy of the chest cavity.
- Describe the relationship of the anatomy of the chest cavity to the ventilatory process.
- Describe why ventilation (breathing) is not respiration.
- Describe the adverse outcome of pulmonary contusion, pneumothorax, hemothorax, and flail chest.
- Describe pneumothorax (simple and tension), hemothorax, flail chest, fractured ribs, and sources of blood contributing to the hemothorax.
- Describe sheer injury to the aorta.
- Describe pulmonary contusion.
- Describe the breathing process.
- Describe the prehospital assessment and management of chest injuries.
- Describe the trauma center and the benefit of taking patients to a properly staffed and equipped hospital for the management of traumatic injuries.

Key Terms

1. The dome-shaped muscle that separates the thoracic cavity from the abdominal cavity is the _____ _____.

2. The lower third of the pharynx is called the _____.

3. A condition where the patient has a shortage of oxygen at the cellular level is called _____ _____.

4. The muscles located between the ribs are called _____.

5. A vertical line on a standing patient that runs from the center of the clavicle on either side is called the _____.

6. Movement of the chest where one section of the rib cage moves in an opposite direction from the rest of the rib cage, indicating that a section has been broken is called _____ _____.

7. Match the following terms with their appropriate definition.

_____ Accumulation of blood and fluid in the pleural cavity
_____ Collapsed alveoli in the lung
_____ Increased pressure collapsing the lung on an affected side and pushing it toward the other
_____ Damage in the dermal layer of the skin causing discoloration from blood leaking into surrounding tissue
_____ A collection of air in the pleural space
_____ A condition in which the patient has a shortage of oxygen at the cellular level

A. Atelectasis
B. Contusion
C. Hemothorax
D. Hypoxia
E. Pneumothorax
F. Tension pneumothorax

Content Review

1. What are the three major conditions that affect the expansion of the chest wall?

2. A patient with paradoxic motion of the chest wall is most likely suffering from _____ _____.

3. Pain associated with fractured ribs reduces a patient's ventilatory effort.
   A. True
   B. False

4. What are the signs and symptoms of hypoxia?

5. Bleeding into the chest cavity, which causes a hemothorax, can come from what three sources?

   1)
   2)
   3)

6. Approximately _____ % of patients with exsanguination of the aorta die within the first hour of a traumatic event.

7. Blunt cardiac trauma causes what injuries?

8. Hemorrhage associated with penetrating cardiac trauma falls into what two categories?

   1)

   2)

9. The difference between systolic and diastolic blood pressures is called the _____

   _____.

10. Assessment of thoracic injuries begins with suspicion from _____.

11. Describe the steps for assessing the thoracic cavity.

12. What are the signs of tension pneumothorax?

13. Tracheal deviation is the most visible sign the EMT will find in the prehospital environment indicating a tension pneumothorax.
    A. True
    B. False

14. Management of a thoracic injury in the field includes what techniques (basic and advanced)?

15. What steps should the EMT take to manage a patient with fractured ribs?

16. Collapse of alveoli or part of the lung is called _____.

17. Stabilization of a fractured rib during transport is done using a(n) _____.

18. List the four consequences of a flail chest.

    1)

    2)

    3)

    4)

19. The key technique to managing a flail chest is _____

    _____.

20. Emergency care of a patient with a pneumothorax includes:

21. What is the first step of managing an open pneumothorax?

22. An open pneumothorax is sealed by using what type of dressing?

Chapter Quiz

1. The most common site of intrathoracic blood loss, producing a hemothorax, is the:
   A. Intercostal arteries
   B. Bronchial arterioles
   C. Pericardial sac
   D. Xiphoid process

2. Which of the following symptoms is most serious?
   A. Decreased systolic pressure and decreased diastolic pressure
   B. Decreased systolic pressure and normal diastolic pressure
   C. Increased systolic pressure and decreased diastolic pressure
   D. Normal systolic pressure and decreased diastolic pressure

3. The difference between systolic and diastolic pressures is called the _____.
   A. Pulse
   B. Blood pressure
   C. Pulse rhythm
   D. Pulse pressure

4. It is often difficult to identify a tension pneumothorax in the field.
   A. True
   B. False

5. Possible complications of a fractured rib include all of the following *except:*
   A. Hypovolemia
   B. Pneumothorax
   C. Perforated ulcer
   D. Atelectasis

6. Fractured ribs should be stabilized by taping the area around the chest.
   A. True
   B. False

7. Deep, full ventilations and coughing for a patient with fractured ribs should be encouraged, despite the associated pain.
   A. True
   B. False

8. Emergency care of a patient with a flail chest includes all of the following *except:*
   A. Endotracheal intubation
   B. Sand bags to prevent movement
   C. Positive-pressure ventilation
   D. High-concentration oxygen

9. Positive-pressure ventilations in a patient with a pneumothorax may increase the possibility of a tension penumothorax.
   A. True
   B. False

10. Taping only three sides of a dressing over an open pneumothorax is preferred to a complete occlusive dressing.
   A. True
   B. False

11. The collapse of alveoli in the lungs is called:
   A. Atelectasis
   B. Hemothorax
   C. Pneumothorax
   D. Diaphragmatic herniation

12. Accumulation of blood in the pleural cavity is called:
   A. Atelectasis
   B. Spontaneous pneumothorax
   C. Tension pneumothorax
   D. Hemothorax

13. A patient with paradoxic motion of the chest wall is most likely suffering from:
   A. Pneumothorax
   B. Fractured ribs
   C. Tension pneumothorax
   D. Atelectasis

14. The small air sacs in the lungs where the exchange of gas takes place are called:
   A. Glands
   B. Alveoli
   C. Capillaries
   D. Venules

Case Scenario

You are dispatched to 525 Park Drive (the Dunvey Manufacturing Plant) for an injured person. On your arrival, police direct you to a warehouse where you find the patient lying supine on the floor. Co-workers explain that the patient was driving a forklift when it hit a rock and rolled over. The driver was ejected and the lift landed on his chest, abdomen, and pelvis. Co-workers lifted the forklift and pulled the patient free prior to arrival of the ambulance.

On initial assessment and physical examination, you find the patient is cyanotic around the lips and nail beds. His skin is pale and diaphoretic, and he has a large contusion on his sternum. He complains of a crushing pain in his chest during ventilation and has paradoxic movement with ventilations. He appears responsive but dazed and confused. Vital signs reveal: BP, 90/60 mm Hg; pulse, 120 bpm; ventilations, 14 and shallow; pupils, PEARLA. Breath sounds are diminished but equal on both sides.

1. What is most likely wrong with this patient?

2. How would you care for this patient?

Answer Key

....

Key Terms
1. Diaphragm
2. Hypopharynx
3. Hypoxia
4. Intercostal muscles
5. Midclavicular line
6. Paradoxic motion
7. C, A, F, B, E, D

Content Review
1. Nerve supply (the ability to contract and relax intercostal muscles from stimuli from the brain); 2) bony stability of the thoracic cage; and 3) pain
2. A flail chest
3. True
4. Dyspnea, restlessness, confusion, lethargy, and poor skin color
5. 1) Intrathoracic blood loss from intercostal arteries; 2) the lung and bronchial vessels; and 3) the aorta
6. 80
7. Damage to the electrical system causing abnormal rhythms; damage to the wall of the heart causing compression, contusion, traumatic edema, bruising, intramuscular hemorrhage, or vascular damage; or rupture of the wall
8. 1) Injury in which the hole in the myocardium is so large that rapid blood loss causes instant death; and 2) blood loss into the pericardial sac reducing the ability of the heart to expand and fill causing a decrease in cardiac output
9. Pulse pressure
10. Kinematics of the incident (mechanism of injury)
11. Inspect the chest wall for deformities, paradoxical chest wall motion, rapid breathing pattern, asymmetry of chest wall, asymmetry of chest wall expansion, or abdominal breathing; palpate the chest wall to locate abnormal movement of ribs, pain produced by pressure on ribs, broken bones moving across each other, or subcutaneous air in tissues; and listen to breath sounds to identify absent sounds.
12. Tracheal deviation, distended neck veins, cyanosis, and decreased breath sounds on injured side
13. False
14. Airway control, assisted ventilations, decompression of tension pneumothorax, volume replacement, and rapid transport to an appropriate facility
15. Splint the area to reduce pain, reassure the patient, anticipate complications (pneumothorax and hypovolemia), provide high-concentration oxygen, and provide ventilatory assistance as necessary.
16. Atelectasis
17. Sling and swathe

18. 1) A decrease in vital capacity proportional to the size of the flail segment; 2) an increase in labor of breathing; 3) pain produced by fractured ribs, limiting the amount of thoracic cage expansion; and 4) contusion of the lung beneath the flail segment
19. Assisting the patient's ventilatory effort with positive-pressure ventilations via a bag-valve- mask.
20. Placing the patient in a position of comfort; providing a high concentration of oxygen; assisting with ventilations, if ventilatory rate is below 12 or above 20 per minute or if patient displays signs of hypoxia; rapid transport; and careful monitoring for signs of tension pneumothorax
21. Closing the hole in the chest
22. Occlusive (vaseline gauze covered with sterile gauze secured with tape) or plastic or aluminum foil taped on three sides.

Chapter Quiz

1. A	6. B	11. A
2. A	7. A	12. D
3. D	8. B	13. B
4. A	9. A	14. B
5. C	10. A	

Case Scenario

1. This patient is most likely suffering from a flail chest with possible pulmonary contusions bilaterally with the potential for a pneumothorax and possible cardiac contusion.
2. Assist the patient with a positive-pressure ventilations using a bag-valve-mask with 100% oxygen; be prepared to intubate; immobilize the patient on a long spine board; watch for increasing signs and symptoms of shock and treat accordingly; transport immediately to a trauma center; and request ALS rendezvous en route if ETA to the hospital is prolonged.

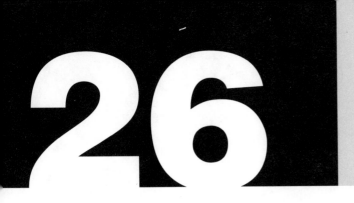

Abdominal Emergencies

Reading Assignment: Chapter 26 pages 493–503.

Supplemental Objectives

Upon successful completion of the EMT-Basic training program, the EMT-Basic should be able to do the following:

- Describe the anatomy of the abdominal cavity and the retroperitoneal space.
- Describe the physiology of the major abdominal organs.
- Describe the pathophysiology of traumatic injuries to the abdominal organs.
- Describe the pathophysiology of significant conditions seen in the prehospital period that require assessment and management from the field.

Key Terms

1. The serous membrane covering the organs and lining the abdominal cavity is called the _____ _____.

2. A digestive enzyme produced in the pancreas is called _____.

3. A wormlike organ extending from the cecum is called the _____.

4. Acute or chronic inflammation of the gallbladder is called _____.

5. The portion of the large intestine that extends from the cecum to the rectum is called the _____ _____.

6. The first subdivision of the small intestine is the _____.

7. An abnormal passage from an internal organ to the body surface is called a(n) _____.

8. Inflammation of the peritoneum is called _____.

9. The term for behind the peritoneum is _____.

10. A crater like lesion on the skin or mucous membrane is called a(n) _____.

Content Review

1. Identify the major organs located in each of the following quadrants.

    RUQ:
    RLQ:
    LUQ:
    LLQ:

2. Identify the following structures of the abdomen.

    Appendix   Gallbladder   Spleen
    Ascending colon   Liver   Stomach
    Descending colon   Pancreas   Transverse colon
    Duodenum

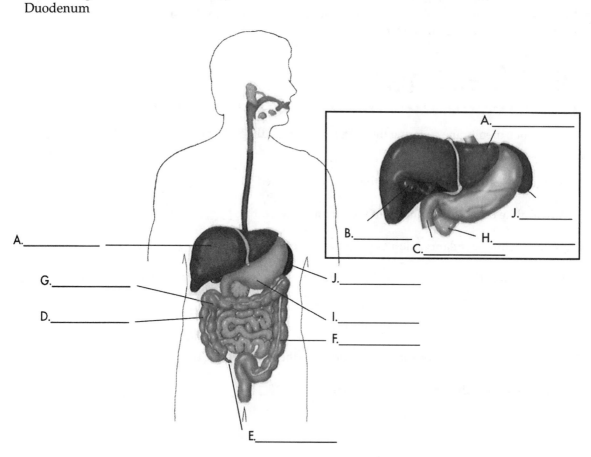

3. The gland located posterior in the abdominal cavity over the twelfth vertebral body, and which is particularly vulnerable to blunt trauma, is the _____.

4. The abdominal cavity can hide _____ liters of blood loss in a short period of time.

5. Abdominal organs that can cause massive hemorrhage if injured include the _____ _____ and _____.

6. In blunt trauma, the most frequently injured organ in the abdominal cavity is the _____.

7. Injury to the spleen will result in more blood loss quicker than injury to the liver.
   A. True
   B. False

8. Identify six complications that can occur with the GI tract.

   1)
   2)
   3)
   4)
   5)
   6)

9. How should the EMT care for a patient with a GI illness or injury?

10. Tightening the overlying abdominal muscles in an attempt to resist abdominal pain is called _____ _____.

11. Guarding is generally described based on severity in what terms?

12. A recurrent condition that is associated with eating fatty foods, producing excessive flatulence, belching, and LUQ or epigastric pain is called _____.

13. A stone that prevents the outflow of bile through the cystic duct, common duct, and into the duodenum is called a _____.

14. What are the two functions of the pancreas?

15. Inflammation of the tissue surrounding the pancreas is called _____.

16. What are the symptoms of pancreatitis?

17. A patient who presents with pain around the umbilicus migrating to the RLQ over a period of 6 to 8 hours is most likely suffering from _____.

18. A patient history should include what areas?

19. Identify symptoms that require immediate transport.

Chapter Quiz
. . . .

1. A penetrating injury from any direction has the potential of entering the GI tract.
   A. True
   B. False

2. The liver is located primarily in the _____.
   A. RUQ
   B. LUQ
   C. RLQ
   D. LLQ

3. In blunt trauma the most frequently injured organ in the abdominal cavity is the:
   A. Pancreas
   B. Liver
   C. Spleen
   D. Abdominal aorta

4. Solid organs contained in the abdominal cavity include the:
   A. Spleen and transverse colon
   B. Pancreas and spleen
   C. Spleen and intestines
   D. Gallbladder and stomach

5. Hollow organs contained in the abdominal cavity include the:
   A. Spleen and pancreas
   B. Stomach and gallbladder
   C. Liver and intestines
   D. Kidneys and gallbladder

6. Organs in the retroperitoneal space include the:
   A. Spleen and pancreas
   B. Stomach and gallbladder
   C. Liver and kidney
   D. Kidney and pancreas

7. A patient complains of severe pain in the RUQ of the abdomen. She states that the pain started shortly after dinner and that she has noticed an increase in burping. She is most likely suffering from:
   A. Gastritis
   B. Appendicitis
   C. Cholecystitis
   D. Peritonitis

8. A patient complains of severe flank pain radiating to the groin, with irritability and restlessness. He is most likely suffering from:
   A. Appendicitis
   B. Kidney stones
   C. Gallstones
   D. Genital injury

9. Organs in the LLQ include the:
   A. Descending colon, appendix, and right ovary
   B. Right kidney, stomach, and pancreas
   C. Ascending colon, small intestine, and right fallopian tube
   D. Spleen, pancreas, and colon

10. The tightening of overlying abdominal muscles in an attempt to resist abdominal pain is called:
    A. Minimizing
    B. Guarding
    C. Transferring
    D. Transcending

Case Scenario

You are dispatched to 402 South Matlack Street, "Joe's Bar," for a sick person. On your arrival, police direct you to the back of the bar where a fight had occurred. You find the patient lying unconscious on the floor with a knife impaled in the RUQ of his abdomen. His girlfriend is hysterical. She is screaming that "he was sitting at the bar minding his own business when this idiot spills his beer on me. My boyfriend stood up and yelled at him and next thing you know the guy whips out this knife and jabs it into his stomach."

On initial assessment and physical examination, you find the patient is unconscious, pale, cool, and moist, with cyanosis noted around his lips and nail beds. There is blood oozing from the laceration in the abdomen where the knife is still impaled. The abdomen shows rigidity. Vital signs reveal: BP, 84/60 mm Hg; pulse, 122 bpm; ventilations, 26, shallow, and labored. Pupils equal but sluggish.

1. What is most likely wrong with this patient?

2. Should you remove the impaled knife? Why?

3. How should you care for this patient?

Answer Key

•••

Key Terms
1. Peritoneum
2. Amylase
3. Appendix
4. Cholecystitis
5. Colon
6. Duodenum
7. Fistula
8. Peritonitis
9. Retroperitoneum
10. Ulcer

Content Review
1. RUQ: liver, gallbladder, part of the colon; RLQ: appendix and part of the colon; LLQ: part of the colon and part of small intestine; LUQ: stomach, spleen, part of the colon, and part of the small intestine.
2. A: Liver
   B: Gallbladder
   C: Duodenum
   D: Ascending colon
   E: Appendix
   F: Descending colon
   G: Transverse colon
   H: Pancreas
   I: Stomach
   J: Spleen
3. Pancreas
4. 3 to 5
5. Liver; spleen
6. Liver
7. True
8. 1) Ulcers; 2) perforation; 3) hemorrhage; 4) abscess; 5) inflammation; and 6) fistula
9. Administer oxygen; treat for shock as indicated; and transport to the hospital quickly.
10. Guarding
11. Minimal, moderate, severe, or rigid
12. Acute cholecystitis
13. Gallstone
14. Produce insulin and provide enzymes to assist in the digestion of foods (especially fats)
15. Pancreatitis
16. Back pain and epigastric pain associated with nausea and vomiting

17. Appendicitis
18. Length of the illness; length of time since onset; factors that might have influenced the onset (foods eaten what, where, when, did others eat and become sick); recent trauma to the abdomen; associated conditions (pregnancy, sexual trauma, or assault); drugs or medications; and recent hospitalizations
19. Signs of shock (hypotension and tachycardia); tachypnea; fractured pelvis; lower rib fractures; abdominal tenderness; abdominal guarding; or abdominal distention

Chapter Quiz

1. A	6. D
2. A	7. C
3. B	8. B
4. B	9. C
5. B	10. B

Case Scenario

1. Laceration of the liver with subsequent hemorrhage
2. No. Removal of the knife may cause further injury and may increase the amount of bleeding. It should be secured in place using bulk dressings.
3. Take proper BSI precautions; ensure an adequate airway; insert an oral airway or intubate as per local protocol; administer high concentration oxygen via a non-rebreather mask; monitor ventilation and be prepared to ventilate for the patient if necessary; immobilize the impaled object using bulky dressings, and taping them in place; transport as quickly as possible to a trauma center with the feet elevated; request to meet ALS personnel en route if ETA to hospital is prolonged; and consider the use of PASG below the site of the injury.

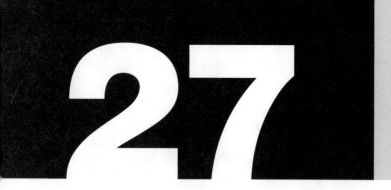

Spinal Trauma

Reading Assignment: Chapter 27 pages 504-528.

DOT Objectives

- Describe the central nervous system.
- Describe the peripheral nervous system.
- Define the structure of the skeletal system as it relates to the nervous system.
- Relate mechanism of injury to potential injuries of the head and spine.
- Describe the implications of not properly caring for potential spinal injuries.
- State the signs and symptoms of a potential spinal injury.
- Describe the method of determining if a responsive patient may have a spinal injury.
- Relate the airway emergency medical care techniques to the patient with a suspected spinal injury.
- Describe how to stabilize the cervical spine.
- Discuss indications for sizing and using a cervical spine immobilization device.
- Establish the relationship between airway management and the patient with head and spinal injuries.
- Describe a method for sizing a cervical spine immobilization device.
- Describe how to logroll a patient with a suspected spinal injury.
- Describe how to secure a patient to a long spine board.
- List instances when a short spine board should be used.
- Describe how to immobilize a patient using a short spine board.
- Describe indications for the use of rapid extrication.
- List steps in performing rapid extrication.
- State the circumstances when a helmet should be left on a patient.
- Discuss the circumstances when a helmet should be removed.
- Identify different types of helmets.
- Describe the unique characteristics of sports helmets.
- Explain the preferred methods for removal of a helmet.
- Discuss alternative methods for removal of a helmet.
- Describe how the patient's head is stabilized to remove the helmet.
- Differentiate how the head is stabilized with a helmet compared to without a helmet.
- Demonstrate opening of the airway in a patient with suspected spinal cord injury.
- Demonstrate evaluation of a responsive patient with a suspected spinal cord injury.
- Demonstrate stabilization of the cervical spine.
- Demonstrate the four-person logroll for a patient with a suspected spinal cord injury.
- Demonstrate how to logroll a patient with a suspected spinal cord injury using two people.
- Demonstrate securing of a patient to a long spine board.
- Demonstrate use of the short board immobilization technique.
- Demonstrate the procedure for rapid extrication.
- Demonstrate preferred methods for stabilization of a helmet.
- Demonstrate helmet removal techniques.
- Demonstrate alternative methods for stabilization of a helmet.
- Demonstrate completion of a prehospital care report for patients with head and spinal injuries.

Supplemental Objectives

- Name the five sections of the spinal column.
- Define Newton's law of motion.
- Describe the importance of determining mechanism of injury.
- Define *lateral bending.*
- Describe the importance of in-line stabilization.
- Describe the steps of nervous system assessment.
- Describe the methods of assessing the nervous system.

Key Terms

1. The part of the nervous system that regulates involuntary vital functions and consists of the sympathetic and parasympathetic nervous systems is called the _____ _____.

2. The part of the nervous system that consists of the brain and spinal cord is the _____ _____.

3. The padding between vertebrae is called a(n) _____.

4. The movement technique used to position a patient on a long spine board is called a(n) _____ _____.

5. Paralysis of the lower limbs and trunk is called _____.

6. A nerve that carries responses from the central nervous system to an organ or muscle is called a(n) _____.

7. An injury in which the spine is pulled apart is called a(n) _____.

8. A fracture of a bone resulting from a force from above and below the bone is called a(n) _____ _____.

9. Nerves that carry impulses from the sensory receptors to the central nervous system are called _____.

10. Paralysis affecting all four extremities is called _____.

11. The part of the nervous system that is voluntary is called the _____ nervous system.

12. The part of the nervous system consisting of all the nerves that extend from the brain and spinal cord is the _____ nervous system.

Content Review

1. Identify the five regions of the spinal column in the diagram below and state the number of vertebrae included in each region.

   Cervical   Lumbar   Thoracic
   Coccyx   Sacral

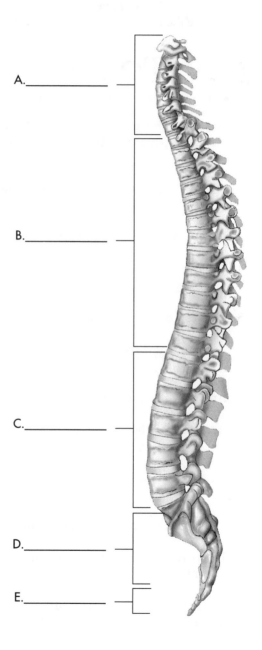

A._____

B._____

C._____

D._____

E._____

2. The nervous system is divided into two parts: the _____ and the
   _____.

3. The peripheral nervous system has what two functions?

   1)

   2)

4. The physical law that states that an object in motion will stay in motion until acted on by an outside
   force is called _____.

5. The autonomic nervous system is divided into the _____ and
   _____ nervous systems.

6. An EMT must maintain a high index of suspicion of spinal injury during which types of emergency
   situations?

7. Compression fractures are often seen in which types of situations?

8. Bending of the spine from side to side is called _____.

9. An injury where a ligament and muscles are overstretched and/or torn is called a(n) _____
   _____.

10. An unstable spine can only be ruled out by x-ray.
    A. True
    B. False

11. Up to 20% of patients who require surgical repair of spinal injuries are found ambulatory.
    A. True
    B. False

12. The best time to control the spine is _____.

13. Spinal immobilization should be maintained until _____.

14. Complete the following components of the McSwain-Paturas Spinal Assessment System (MPSAS).

    S:
    P:
    I:
    N:
    E:

15. The position in which a patient is found may indicate the possibility of spinal injury.
    A. True
    B. False

16. What situations require the rapid extrication of a patient?

17. When should an EMT remove a helmet from a patient?

18. How should an EMT immobilize an infant or child involved in a motor vehicle collision?

19. Once in-line immobilization is initiated, it must not be relieved until _____
    _____.

Chapter Quiz
· ·

1. The nervous system is divided into two parts, the central nervous system and the:
   A. Core nervous system
   B. Superficial nervous system
   C. Peripheral nervous system
   D. Primary nervous system

2. The spinal column is composed of 33 bones called:
   A. Disks
   B. Vertebrae
   C. Meninges
   D. Phalanges

3. The EMT must maintain a high index of suspicion for head and spinal injuries when any of the following has occurred *except:*
   A. Motor vehicle collisions
   B. Falls or blunt trauma
   C. Motorcycle or bicycle crashes
   D. Distal extremity lacerations

4. If the MOI suggests that a patient may have spinal trauma, the EMT should initiate spinal precautions, regardless of physical findings.
   A. True
   B. False

5. Signs and symptoms associated with spinal injuries include all of the following *except:*
   A. Quadriplegia
   B. Paraplegia
   C. Hypoglycemia
   D. Point enderness

6. The patient's ability to walk should not alter the EMT's suspicion regarding the possibility of spinal injuries.
   A. True
   B. False

7. The appropriate time to control the spine is:
   A. When assessing the airway
   B. After assessing the air circulation
   C. During transport to the hospital
   D. After placement on the stretcher

8. Spinal immobilization should be maintained until spinal injury has been completely ruled out.
   A. True
   B. False

9. The EMT must put the patient's head in a _____ in-line position to open the airway.
   A. Flexed
   B. Neutral
   C. Hyperextended
   D. Pronate

10. To establish a patent airway on an unresponsive patient who has a suspected spinal injury, the EMT should use the:
    A. Head-tilt chin-lift technique
    B. Modified jaw-thrust
    C. Head-tilt neck-lift technique
    D. Jaw-thrust lift with head tilt

11. An improperly fitted immobilization device may do more harm than good.
    A. True
    B. False

12. Responsibilities of the EMT who is maintaining in-line immobilization of the spine include all of the following *except:*
    A. Maintaining constant, in-line control of the spine
    B. Maintaining cervical spine control only when logrolling the patient
    C. Providing continual airway assessment
    D. Maintaining stabilization until the patient is secured to the long spine board

13. Short back boards may be used:
    A. To immobilize seated, noncritical patients with suspected spinal injuries
    B. As a long spine board for a pediatric patient
    C. Both A and B
    D. None of the above

14. Initial steps used in applying the short back board include:
    A. The first EMT initiates manual spinal immobilization and performs the initial assessment
    B. The second EMT performs the focused assessment and prepares to apply the cervical collar and short spine board
    C. The second EMT positions the device behind the patient
    D. All of the above

15. Indications for rapid extrication of a patient include all of the following *except:*
    A. An unsafe scene
    B. A patient with a life-threatening condition requires immediate transport
    C. A family member or friend prevents the EMT from providing care
    D. The police are present and in control of the scene and the patient is stable

16. Sports helmets typically open in the:
    A. Left side
    B. Back
    C. Front
    D. Right side

17. Two types of helmets most likely to be seen in the prehospital environment are the sports helmet and the:
    A. Motorcycle helmet
    B. Stater's helmet
    C. Flight helmet
    D. Military helmet

18. Consideration regarding whether to remove a helmet includes all of the following *except:*
    A. The fit of the helmet
    B. Impending airway or breathing problems
    C. Transport time to definitive care
    D. Ability to provide proper spinal immobilization

19. When considering methods for helmet removal, the EMT should remember that a minimum of _____ EMTs should participate in the technique.
    A. 1
    B. 2
    C. 3
    D. 4

20. Small children and infants not found in a car seat can be immobilized on a short spine board, providing the legs do not hang over the edge.
    A. True
    B. False

Case Scenario

• •

You are dispatched to the Sugardale Farm for an equestrian accident. On your arrival, you find a single victim lying in the field. The patient is conscious but agitated and disoriented. He states that he was trying out the arena and making routine jumps on his horse but assumes that the horse threw him. He does not remember the crash. He is complaining of a headache and tenderness to the cervical spine and chest area with pain on deep inspiration. He cannot feel his legs.

On initial assessment and physical examination, you note a 1-inch laceration on the patient's forehead and abrasions to his face and hands. There is tenderness to the area of the fourth cervical vertebrae on palpation and tingling of the fingers of the patient's left hand. The patient is unable to move his lower extremities. Vital signs reveal: BP, 140/88 mm Hg; pulse, 116 bpm; ventilations, 24 and normal. Breath sounds are clear and equal bilaterally; and pupils are unequal but reactive to light. The patient's skin is pale, cool, and moist.

1. What do your assessment findings tell you?

2. What is most likely wrong with this patient?

3. Is this patient a candidate for rapid transportation? Why?

4. How would you care for this patient?

Answer Key

Key Terms
1. Autonomic nervous system
2. Central nervous system
3. Intervertebral disk
4. Diagonal slide
5. Paraplegia
6. Motor nerve
7. Distraction injury
8. Compression fracture
9. Sensory nerves
10. Quadriplegia
11. Somatic
12. Peripheral

Content Review
1. A. Cervical (7)
   B. Thoracic (12)
   C. Lumbar (5)
   D. Sacral (5)
   E. Coccyx (4)
2. Central; peripheral

3. 1) Sensory—to carry impulses from sensory receptors in the skin, muscles, or organs to the CNS or to the spinal cord and then to the brain; 2) Motor— to carry responses from the CNS to organs or muscles
4. Newton's first law of motion
5. Parasympathetic; sympathetic
6. Motor vehicle collisions; pedestrian versus vehicle collisions; falls; blunt trauma; motorcycle or bicycle crashes; hangings; diving injuries; and unresponsive trauma victims
7. MVAs with an unrestrained occupant striking the windshield; falls; diving incidents; and ejection from a motorcycle or automobile
8. Lateral bending
9. Distraction injury
10. True
11. True
12. When assessing the airway
13. Spinal injury has been completely ruled out
14. S: suspicion of injury (kinematics); P: pain in any part of the spine; I: immobilization of any part of the spine by the patient; N: neurological examination of all extremities; E: examine the patient again after placement on the long board.
15. True
16. An unsafe scene or a life-threatening patient condition
17. If it does not fit well or if the EMT cannot assess or reassess the patient's airway and breathing or intervene if necessary
18. If the patient is found in a child seat, immobilize in the seat, apply a cervical spine immobilization device, then use tape to secure the child in the seat. If not found in a child seat, immobilize on a short spine board that does not allow the legs to hang over the edge. Pad the child from shoulders to heels to maintain neutral immobilization.
19. The patient is secured onto a long spine board and head immobilized in place

Chapter Quiz

1. C	6. A	11. A	16. C
2. B	7. A	12. B	17. A
3. D	8. A	13. C	18. C
4. A	9. B	14. D	19. B
5. C	10. B	15. D	20. A

Case Scenario

1. The patient's vital signs are stable. He is breathing and has an adequate heart beat. He does not appear to be in shock and is not having any difficulty with ventilations. He has unequal pupils, which may indicate a head injury.
2. This patient is most likely suffering from a head injury and a cervical spine injury. The tingling sensation in his fingers, inability to feel his legs, and tenderness in the area of the fourth vertebra indicate trauma to the cervical spine that requires extreme care.
3. No. This patient is not in immediate distress. His vital signs are stable and there is a greater risk of damage by rapid transport. The EMT should take time to ensure that every cervical spine stabilization precaution is taken and package the patient well prior to transport. Care should also be taken during transport to ensure a smooth ride, avoiding bumps or jolting of the patient.
4. Establish and maintain in-line stabilization; carefully apply a cervical collar; apply a long spine board and CID; pad all open areas to ensure adequate immobilization. Place the patient on high-flow oxygen via a non-rebreather mask; monitor vital signs; and transport cautiously to a trauma center.

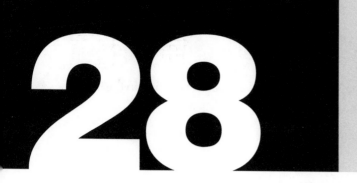

Musculoskeletal Trauma

Reading Assignment: Chapter 28 pages 529–559.

DOT Objectives

Upon successful completion of the EMT-Basic training program, the EMT-Basic should be able to do the following:

- Describe the functions of the muscular system.
- Describe the functions of the skeletal system.
- List the major bones or bone groupings of the spinal column; the thorax; the upper extremities; and the lower extremities.
- Differentiate between an open and a closed painful, swollen, deformed extremity.
- State the reasons for splinting.
- List the general rules of splinting.
- List the complications of splinting.
- List the emergency medical care for a patient with a painful, swollen, deformed extremity.
- Demonstrate the emergency medical care of a patient with a painful, swollen, deformed extremity.
- Demonstrate completion of a prehospital care report for patients with musculoskeletal injuries.

Supplemental Objectives

- Define the signs and symptoms of a fracture, a dislocation, and a sprain.

Key Terms

1. A fracture in which the skin integrity has not been compromised is called a _____ fracture.

2. Separation of two pieces of bone at the joint is called a(n) _____.

3. A fracture in which the skin's integrity is broken is called a(n) _____ fracture.

4. An injury in which ligaments are stretched or partially torn is called a(n) _____.

5. A condition in which nerves, arteries, or veins are compromised due to increased swelling in the interstitial space is called _____.

6. A soft tissue injury that occurs around a joint, also known as a muscle pull, is called a(n) _____ _____.

7. A sound or feeling made by bones grating against each other is called _____.

Content Review

1. Identify the following components of the skeletal system.

Femur   Ribs
Tibia   Fibula
Sacrum   Ulna
Humerus   Scapula
Vertebral column Radius
Skull

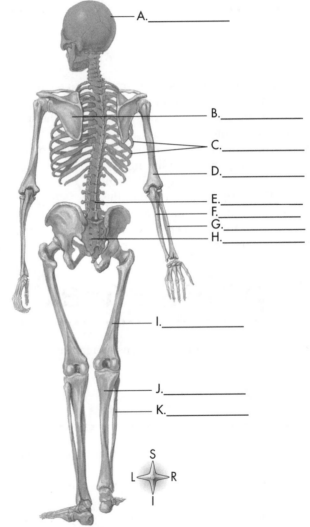

A._____

B._____

C._____

D._____

E._____
F._____
G._____
H._____

I._____

J._____

K._____

2. To adequately immobilize a fracture, the EMT should splint the joint _____ the site of the injury.

3. If a patient is suspected of having a fracture, as well as a life-threatening emergency, should the EMT immobilize the fracture? If so, how?

4. The bones of the hand include the _____, _____ and _____.

5. The bones of the feet include the _____, _____ and _____.

6. What are the functions of muscles?

7. Muscles are attached to bone by _____.

8. The heart is made up of what type of muscle?

9. The structures that connect bone to bone across a joint are called _____.

10. What are the three forces that cause bone and joint injuries?

11. What are the possible complications associated with open fractures?

12. What is the most significant complication of a closed fracture?

13. What are the signs and symptoms of a musculoskeletal injury?

14. List the eleven general guidelines for splinting a possible fracture.

    1)
    2)
    3)
    4)
    5)
    6)
    7)
    8)
    9)
    10)
    11)

15. If a commercial device is not available to splint a long bone fracture, what can the EMT use?

16. If a triangular bandage is not available, what can the EMT use as a swathe?

17. What can the EMT use to immobilize a possible fractured wrist or ankle?

18. What type of splint is used to manage a possible fracture of the femur?

Chapter Quiz

1. The medical term for a broken bone is a:
   A. Fracture
   B. Dislocation
   C. Displacement
   D. Sprain

2. A strain is also known as a:
   A. Fracture
   B. Muscle pull
   C. Stint
   D. Sprain

3. Determining the mechanism of injury is important because it may help to determine the nature and extent of injuries.
   A. True
   B. False

4. The bones of the upper extremities include all of the following *except:*
   A. Scapula
   B. Clavicle
   C. Femur
   D. Humerus

5. A painful, swollen, deformed extremity, in which the skin integrity has been compromised is called a(n) _____ injury.
   A. Open
   B. Closed
   C. Vertical
   D. Compromised

6. If the determination has been made that the patient has a life-threatening injury, painful, swollen, deformed extremities should be splinted using an anatomical splint, such as a long spine board.
   A. True
   B. False

7. Crepitus:
   A. Is a sound bones can make when they are broken
   B. Is the feeling caused by grating of bone ends against each other
   C. Can cause further damage if improperly manipulated
   D. All of the above

8. Bones of the lower extremities include all of the following *except:*
   A. Pelvis
   B. Femur
   C. Scapula
   D. Tibia

9. Common complications of painful, swollen, deformed extremities include all of the following *except:*
   A. Edema
   B. Hemorrhage
   C. Discoloration
   D. Proper alignment

10. The dislodging of a bone from its normal position in a joint is called a(n):
    A. Dislocation
    B. Strain
    C. Sprain
    D. Avulsion

11. Signs and symptoms to look for when assessing a painful, swollen, deformed extremity include:
    A. Deformity and crepitus
    B. Swelling and discoloration
    C. Pain and loss of sensation or movement
    D. All of the above

12. Complications of splinting may include all of the following *except:*
    A. Ulceration
    B. Decreased circulation
    C. Muscle damage
    D. Nerve damage

13. Injuries to muscles are more common than injuries to bones.
    A. True
    B. False

14. It is not the responsibility of an EMT to differentiate between a muscle injury and a bone injury.
    A. True
    B. False

15. A _____ is a soft tissue injury or muscle spasm that occurs around a joint anywhere in the musculature.
    A. Strain
    B. Sprain
    C. Lacertion
    D. Contusion

16. If no life-threatening conditions are evident, the EMT should splint a patient's injury before moving him.
    A. True
    B. False

17. Traction splints are indicated for possible fractures of the:
    A. Ankle
    B. Elbow
    C. Hip
    D. Thigh

18. If a severe deformity exists or the distal extremity is cyanotic or pulseless, the EMT should align the bones with gentle traction before splinting.
    A. True
    B. False

19. The extremity should be supported while being splinted, thus splinting requires two people.
    A. True
    B. False

20. Painful, swollen, deformed extremities must be supported while being splinted.
    A. True
    B. False

Case Scenario

You are dispatched to 415 Willowdale Drive for a person injured from a fall. On your arrival, you find a 34-year-old male patient who lost his balance and fell approximately 12 feet from the roof, landing on the driveway.

On initial assessment and physical examination you find the patient to be conscious but agitated. He is complaining of severe pain in the right thigh and pain to his right elbow with a tingling sensation down his right forearm. There is a contusion with deformity to the right elbow and a 2-inch laceration on the right femur with protruding bone ends. There is a radial pulse in the right arm. The right pedal pulse is absent. The patient's skin is warm and dry. Vital signs reveal: BP, 110/70 mm Hg; pulse, 120 bpm; ventilations, 26 and normal; pupils, PEARLA

1. What is most likely wrong with this patient?

2. What do the vital signs reveal about this patient?

3. What are the seven signs and symptoms to look for when assessing a possible fracture?

4. What are the possible complications of an open fracture to the femur?

5. How would you care for this patient?

Skill Sheet #30

•••

IMMOBILIZATION SKILLS
Long Bone Injury

Start Time: _____

Stop Time: _____   **Date:** _____

Candidate's Name: _____

Evaluator's Name: _____

	Points Possible	Points Awarded
Takes, or verbalizes, body substance isolation precautions	1	
Directs application of manual stabilization of the injury	1	
Assesses motor, sensory, and circulatory function in the injured extremity	1	
Note: The examiner acknowledges "motor, sensory, and circulatory functions are present and normal."		
Measures the splint	1	
Applies the splint	1	
Immobilizes the joint above the injury site	1	
Immobilizes the joint below the injury site	1	
Secures the entire injured extremity	1	
Immobilizes the hand/foot in the position of function	1	
Reassesses motor, sensory and circulatory function in the injured extremity	1	
Note: The examiner acknowledges "motor, sensory, and circulatory function are present and normal."		
Total:	10	

Critical Criteria

_____ Grossly moves the injured extremity

_____ Did not immobilize the joint above and the joint below the injury site

_____ Did not reassess motor, sensory, and circulatory function in the injured extremity before and after splinting

Skill Sheet #31

● ●

IMMOBILIZATION SKILLS
Joint Injury

Start Time: _____

Stop Time: _____   **Date:** _____

Candidate's Name: _____

Evaluator's Name: _____

	Points Possible	Points Awarded
Takes, or verbalizes, body substance isolation precautions	1	
Directs application of manual stabilization of the shoulder injury	1	
Assesses motor, sensory, and circulatory function in the injured extremity	1	
Note: The examiner acknowledges "motor, sensory, and circulatory functions are present and normal."		
Selects the proper splinting material	1	
Immobilizes the site of the injury	1	
Immobilizes the bone above the injured joint	1	
Immobilizes the bone below the injured joint	1	
Reassesses motor, sensory, and circulatory function in the injured extremity	1	
Note: The examiner acknowledges "motor, sensory, and circulatory function are present and normal."		
Total:	8	

Critical Criteria

_____ Did not support the joint so that the joint did not bear distal weight

_____ Did not immobilize the bone above and below the injured site

_____ Did not reassess motor, sensory, and circulatory function in the injured extremity before and after splinting

Skill Sheet #32

• •

IMMOBILIZATION SKILLS—TRACTION SPLINTING

Start Time: _____

Stop Time: _____   **Date:** _____

Candidate's Name: _____

Evaluator's Name: _____

	Points Possible	Points Awarded
Takes, or verbalizes, body substance isolation precautions	1	
Directs application of manual stabilization of the injured leg	1	
Directs the application of manual traction	1	
Assesses motor, sensory, and circulatory function in the injured extremity	1	
Note: The examiner acknowledges "motor, sensory, and circulatory function are present and normal."		
Prepares/adjusts splint to the proper length	1	
Positions the splint next to the injured leg	1	
Applies the proximal securing device (e.g., ischial strap)	1	
Applies the distal securing device (e.g., ankle hitch)	1	
Applies mechanical traction	1	
Positions/secures the support straps	1	
Re-evaluates the proximal/distal securing devices	1	
Reassesses motor, sensory, and circulatory function in the injured extremity	1	
Note: The examiner acknowledges "motor, sensory, and circulatory function are present and normal."		
Note: The examiner must ask the candidate how he/she would prepare the patient for transportation.		
Verbalizes securing the torso to the long board to immobilize the hip	1	
Verbalizes securing the splint to the long board to prevent movement of the splint	1	
Total:	14	

Critical Criteria

_____ Loss of traction at any point after it was applied

_____ Did not reassess motor, sensory, and circulatory function in the injured extremity before and after splinting

_____ The foot was excessively rotated or extended after the splint was applied

_____ Did not secure the ischial strap before taking traction

_____ Final immobilization failed to support the femur or prevent rotation of the injured leg

_____ Secured the leg to the splint before applying mechanical traction

Note: If the Sagar splint or the Kendricks Traction Device is used without elevating the patient's leg, application of manual traction is not necessary. The candidate should be awarded one (1) point as if manual traction were applied.

Note: If the leg is elevated at all, manual traction must be applied before elevating the leg. The ankle hitch may be applied before elevating the leg and used to provide manual traction.

Skill Sheet #33

● ●

SPINAL IMMOBILIZATION
Seated Patient

Start Time: _____

Stop Time: _____   **Date:** _____

Candidate's Name: _____

Evaluator's Name: _____

	Points Possible	Points Awarded
Takes, or verbalizes, body substance isolation precautions	1	
Directs assistant to place/maintain head in the neutral in-line position	1	
Directs assistant to maintain manual immobilization of the head	1	
Reassesses motor, sensory, and circulatory function in each extremity	1	
Applies appropriately sized extrication collar	1	
Positions the immobilization device behind the patient	1	
Secures the device to the patient's torso	1	
Evaluates torso fixation and adjusts as necessary	1	
Evaluates and pads behind the patient's head as necessary	1	
Secures the patient's head to the device	1	
Verbalizes moving the patient to a long board	1	
Reassesses motor, sensory, and circulatory function in each extremity	1	
Total:	12	

Critical Criteria

_____ Did not immediately direct, or take, manual immobilization of the head

_____ Released, or ordered relsease of, manual immobilization before it was maintained mechanically

_____ Patient manipulated, or moved excessively, causing potential spinal compromise

_____ Device moved excessively up, down, left, or right on the patient's torso

_____ Head immobilization allows for excessive movement

_____ Torso fixation inhibits chest rise, resulting in respiratory compromise

_____ On completion of immobilization, head is not in the neutral position

_____ Did not assess motor, sensory, and circulatory function in each extremity after voicing immobilization to the long board

_____ Immobilized head to the board before securing the torso

Skill Sheet #34

· ·

SPINAL IMMOBILIZATION
Supine Patient

Start Time: _____

Stop Time: _____ **Date:** _____

Candidate's Name: _____

Evaluator's Name: _____

	Points Possible	Points Awarded
Takes, or verbalizes, body substance isolation precautions	1	
Directs assistant to place/maintain head in the neutral in-line position	1	
Directs assistant to maintain manual immobilization of the head	1	
Reassesses motor, sensory, and circulatory function in each extremity	1	
Applies appropriately sized extrication collar	1	
Positions the immobilization device appropriately	1	
Directs movement of the patient onto the device without compromising the integrity of the spine	1	
Applies padding to voids between the torso and the board as necessary	1	
Immobilizes the patient's torso to the device	1	
Evaluates and pads behind the patient's head as necessary	1	
Immobilizes the patient's head to the device	1	
Secures the patient's legs to the device	1	
Secures the patient's arms to the device	1	
Reassesses motor, sensory, and circulatory function in each extremity	1	
Total:	14	

Critical Criteria

_____ Did not immediately direct, or take, manual immobilization of the head

_____ Released, or ordered relsease of, manual immobilization before it was maintained mechanically

_____ Patient manipulated, or moved excessively, causing potential spinal compromise

_____ Patient moves excessively up, down, left, or right on the patient's torso

_____ Head immobilization allows for excessive movement

_____ On completion of immobilization, head is not in the neutral position

_____ Did not assess motor, sensory, and circulatory function in each extremity after immobilization to the device

_____ Immobilized head to the board before securing the torso

Answer Key

• •

Key Terms
1. Closed
2. Dislocation
3. Open
4. Sprain
5. Compartment syndrome
6. Strain
7. Crepitus

Content Review
1. A. Skull
   B. Scapula
   C. Ribs
   D. Humerus
   E. Vertebral column
   F. Ulna
   G: Radius
   H: Sacrum
   I: Femur
   J: Tibia
   K. Fibula
2. Above and below
3. Yes; with complete body immobilization on a long backboard. Treatment of life-threatening injuries always take precedence over caring for a fracture. However, as time permits, complete body immobilization is a quick way to immobilize all possible fractures so the EMT can concentrate of life-threatening conditions.
4. Carpals; metacarpals; phalanges
5. Tarsals; metatarsals; phalanges
6. Provide the body with its shape; protection of internal organs, blood vessels, and nerves near the bone; and to provide movement via the skeletal system
7. Tendons
8. Cardiac muscle
9. Ligaments
10. Direct force; indirect force; and twisting force
11. External hemorrhage; and contamination
12. Hemorrhage resulting in compartment syndrome and/or blood volume loss; further damage to muscles and nerves
13. Deformity; crepitus; swelling; discoloration; pain; interruption of pulse, movement, or sensation to injured areas
14. (1) Assess pulse, motor and sensation distal to the injury prior to and following splinting application and record findings; (2) support the area of injury; (3) remove or cut away clothing; (4) cover open wounds with a sterile dressing and control external hemorrhage; (5) if a severe deformity exists or the distal extremity is cyanotic or lacks pulses, align with gentle traction before splinting; (6) do not intentionally replace a protruding bone, but if they return within the skin while aligning and immobilizing the fracture it is okay; (7) pad each splint to prevent pressure and discomfort to the patient; (8) when feasible, splint the patient's injury before moving the patient if no life-threatening conditions are evident; (9) if the patient shows signs and symptoms of shock, align the patient in a supine position on the long back board, treat for shock, and transport immediately; (10) if the extremity is deformed, gently attempt to restore alignment; (11) when the patient has multiple injuries or is in shock, immobilizing the patient to a long backboard will immobilize all the fractures at the same time.

15. A piece of wood, rolled newspaper, or cardboard long enough to reach above and below the site of the injury.
16. Roller gauze
17. A pillow splint, air splint, or padded board splint
18. A traction splint

Chapter Quiz

1. A	6. A	11. D	16. A
2. B	7. D	12. A	17. D
3. A	8. C	13. A	18. A
4. C	9. D	14. A	19. A
5. A	10. A	15. A	20. A

Case Scenario
1. This patient is most likely suffering from a fractured femur and a fractured or dislocated elbow with possible cervical spinal injury based on the mechanism of injury.
2. The vital signs are within normal limits with the exception of an increased pulse rate. The pulse rate may be caused by anxiety or a sign of another condition. The blood pressure is normal, indicating that the patient is either not in shock or is in compensated shock. Lack of distal pulses in the leg indicate decreased circulation to the lower leg most likely as a result of the fractured femur.
3. Deformity, crepitus, swelling, discoloration, pain, loss of sensation or movement, and/or interruption of blood supply
4. Severe hemorrhage, contamination, edema, and further damage to muscles and nerves
5. Establish and maintain cervical-spine immobilization and apply a cervical collar; administer high-flow oxygen via a non-rebreather mask; immobilize the elbow with a padded board splint; carefully control bleeding of the laceration and apply a dressing and bandage to the open wound; immobilize the leg with a traction splint; closely monitor the patient's vital signs, and transport to a trauma center. Do not delay transport of this patient.

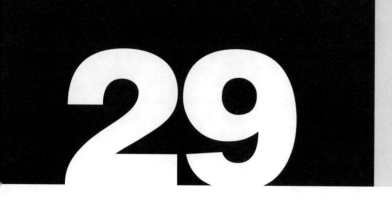

Environmental Emergencies

Reading Assignment: Chapter 29 pages 560–582.

DOT Objectives

Upon successful completion of the EMT-Basic training program, the EMT-Basic should be able to do the following:

- Describe the ways the body maintains and/or loses heat.
- List the signs and symptoms of general and local exposure to cold.
- List the signs and symptoms of general and local exposure to heat.
- Detail the steps of emergency care for the patient exposed to cold or heat.
- Identify the signs and symptoms of water-related emergencies.
- Describe the complications of near drowning.
- Describe the emergency medical treatment of bites and stings.
- List the classifications of burns.
- Define superficial burn.
- List the characteristics of a superficial burn.
- Define partial-thickness burn.
- List the characteristics of a partial-thickness burn.
- Describe the emergency medical care of the patient with a superficial burn.
- Describe the emergency medical care of the patient with a partial-thickness burn.
- Describe the emergency care for a chemical burn.
- Describe the emergency care for an electrical burn.

Supplemental Objectives

- Describe the difference between an allergic reaction and anaphylaxis

Key Terms

1. The outside or environmental air temperature that surrounds the body is called the _____ _____ temperature.

2. The temperature in the center of the body is called the _____ temperature.

3. Match the following heat-related terms with their appropriate definitions.

_____ Heat exchange that occurs when air currents move across an exposed surface
_____ Heat exchange that occurs when a liquid is changed into a gas
_____ Direct heat exchange that occurs when two or more surfaces come into contact
_____ Heat exchange that occurs when heat is transmitted through air or water

A. Conduction
B. Convection
C. Evaporation
D. Radiation

4. Match the following environmental emergency with their descriptions.

_____ The loss of the protective lining within the lungs that caused by aspiration of water, causing alveoli to collapse and fluid to accumulate in lungs
_____ Injury to the skin caused by a prolonged exposure to the cold (skin cells freeze)
_____ A condition in which the core body temperature falls below 95° F
_____ Burn involving all skin layers
_____ Injury from prolonged exposure to cold affecting only the topmost layers of the skin
_____ Asphyxia following submersion with at least temporary survival
_____ The most minor of thermal injuries involving the epidermis
_____ To be completely soaked in a wet substance
_____ Burns associated with blisters and intense pain
_____ A form of heat exposure that occurs within the body that causes profuse perspiration
_____ A condition in which the core body temperature exceeds normal limits and starts to malfunction
_____ A life-threatening condition that results from heat exposure where critical body functions deteriorate
_____ The first and mildest form of heat exposure caused by excessive loss of body fluids and salts
_____ Death resulting from asphyxiation following submersion in a liquid

A. Frostbite
B. Frostnip
C. Full-thickness burn
D. Heat cramps
E. Heat exhaustion
F. Heat stroke
G. Hyperthermia
H. Hypothermia
I. Immersion
J. Near drowning
K. Partial-thickness burn
L. Secondary drowning
M. Superficial burn
N. Drowning

5. A measurement of the amount of water or moisture in the air is called _____.

6. A measurement of the combined effect of temperature and humidity on the apparent temperature is called the _____.

7. A system of measuring the percent of body substance area (BSA) involved in a burn is the _____ _____.

8. A noxious or poisonous substance is called a(n) _____.

9. A measurement of the combined effect of ambient temperature plus wind velocity on exposed surface is called the _____.

10. The ability of the skin to change from a lighter color to a normal color after slight pressure is applied to the area is called _____.

Content Review

....

1. How is heat generated?

2. The normal oral body temperature for a healthy person is _____.

3. When the amount of heat gained is greater than the amount given off, _____ exists.

4. When the amount of heat gained is less than the amount given off, _____ exists.

5. List the five ways in which the body can give off heat:

    1)
    2)
    3)
    4)
    5)

6. How does the body react to exposure to cold?

7. What factors can predispose a patient to hypothermia?

8. How should the EMT care for a patient of generalized cold exposure?

9. The EMT should not massage the extremities of a patient with generalized cold exposure.
    A. True
    B. False

10. If a hypothermic patient is unresponsive, the EMT should assess the pulse for _____ seconds before initiating CPR.

11. Localized cold injuries most often involve the skin surface of what body areas?

12. Cold injury characterized by discoloration, blanching of skin, and loss of sensation is called _____ _____.

13. What is the emergency care for frostnip?

14. When caring for a patient with frostbite, it is appropriate for the EMT to gently rub or massage the affected area.
    A. True
    B. False

15. When caring for a patient with frostnip, the EMT should apply direct heat to the affected area.

16. When rewarming a frostbitten area, the affected body part should be immersed in water that is _____ ° F.

17. An affected extremity should be rewarmed until:

18. After rewarming an affected area, what steps should the EMT take?

19. When should frostbitten areas be rewarmed?

20. What are the three categories of localized cold exposure?

    1)
    2)
    3)

21. What are the signs and symptoms of heat cramps?

22. What are the signs and symptoms of heat exhaustion?

23. Heat stroke is a true life-threatening emergency.
    A. True
    B. False

24. What is heat stroke?

25. What are the signs and symptoms of heat stroke?

26. How should the EMT care for a patient with heat cramps?

27. What are the three classifications of burns?

    1)
    2)
    3)

28. What are the signs and symptoms of first-degree burns?

29. A patient with a burn that appears as a reddened area with blisters and localized pain has a _____
    _____ burn.

30. What are the signs and symptoms of a full-thickness burn?

31. When estimating the degree of body surface area involved in a burn, it is estimated that an adult hand
    will cover approximately _____ % BSA of an average adult body.

32. Burns involving more than _____ % BSA partial or full-thickness burns are considered critical.

33. Burns involving which areas of the body are considered critical, if they are more than just superficial?

34. How should the EMT care for a patient with burn injuries?

35. Generally, if the burn area involves less than _____ % total BSA, cover with a clean, dry or moist dressing. If the burn area is greater than _____ %, use a dry dressing only.

36. Any pulseless, non-breathing patient who has been submerged in cold water of _____ °F or less for a realistically limited amount of time should be resuscitated.

37. The longest documented survival without neurological deficit is _____ minutes under water.

38. If a patient is responsive and in the water, a spinal injury should be suspected and the patient secured to a long backboard prior to removal from the water.
    A. True
    B. False

39. An unresponsive patient should be placed in what position?

40. How should the EMT care for a patient who has gastric distention that interferes with the EMTs ability to adequately ventilate?

41. What are the signs and symptoms associated with bites or stings of spiders, snakes, insects, or marine animals?

42. If a patient is stung and the stinger is visible at the injection site, the EMT should remove it by scraping along the skin with the edge of a stiff card.
    A. True
    B. False

Chapter Quiz

· ·

1. Major compensatory mechanisms of the body to release heat include:
   A. Peripheral vasodilation
   B. Sweating
   C. Increased ventilatory rate
   D. All of the above

2. A regular oral body temperature for a healthy individual is:
   A. 99.6° F
   B. 98.6° F
   C. 96.8° F
   D. 39° C

3. Most of the time, the body is cooler than the surrounding air.
   A. True
   B. False

4. When the amount of heat gained is greater than the amount of heat given off, _____ exists.
   A. Hypothermia
   B. Hyperthermia
   C. Hypovolemia
   D. Hypernatremia

5. The body is warmed by the evaporation of sweat.
   A. True
   B. False

6. The direct heat exchange that occurs when two or more different temperature surfaces come into direct contact is called _____.
   A. Convection
   B. Evaporation
   C. Radiation
   D. Conduction

7. High humidity levels hinder the evaporation of sweat from the skin surface.
   A. True
   B. False

8. Exposure to a cold environment can create a condition known as _____.
   A. Hypothermia
   B. Hyperthermia
   C. Hypovolemia
   D. Hypernatremia

9. Factors that can predispose a patient to hypothermia include all of the following *except:*
   A. Age
   B. Medical conditions
   C. Use of drugs or alcohol
   D. Increased heart rate

10. Head and/or spinal cord injury can affect the central nervous system and alter the body's ability to control internal temperature.
    A. True
    B. False

11. Medical conditions that may contribute to the body's ability to regulate its internal temperature include all of the following *except:*
    A. Diabetes
    B. Hypoglycemia
    C. Hypertension
    D. CNS disorders

12. The skin's condition may help show the extent and/or phase of cold exposure, which usually progresses in the following order:
    A. Blue, pale, red
    B. Red, pale, blue
    C. Pale, blue, red
    D. Red, blue, pale

13. Signs and symptoms to look for in possible environmental emergencies include all of the following *except:*
    A. Changes in level of consciousness or mental status
    B. Poor coordination, memory disturbances, and reduced sense of touch or sensation
    C. Mood changes and an increase in the normal level of communication abilities and good judgement
    D. Dizziness and speech difficulties

14. Treatment of localized cold-exposed patients include all of the following *except:*
    A. Remove the patient from the environment as safely and rapidly as possible
    B. Protect the cold injured extremity or tissue from re-freezing
    C. Do not remove restricting clothing
    D. Administer oxygen

15. The most serious category of localized cold exposure is:
    A. Frostnip
    B. Superficial frostbite
    C. Deep frostbite
    D. Internal frostbite

16. A slow heart rate is very common in the hypothermic patient.
    A. True
    B. False

17. All of the following statements regarding heat stroke are true *except:*
    A. It is a true life-threatening emergency.
    B. It results from the failure of the body's heat-regulating mechanisms.
    C. The body is able to cool itself and the core temperature is hypothermic.
    D. Most cases occur on hot, humid days.

18. General characteristics of partial-thickness burns include:
    A. Reddening of the skin
    B. Blisters
    C. Localized pain
    D. All of the above

19. Charring of skin and tissue damage through the skin to underlying tissues are general characteristics of _____ burns.
    A. Full-thickness or third-degree
    B. Superficial or first-degree
    C. Partial-thickness or second-degree
    D. Superficial and partial-thickness

20. _____ is defined as death by asphyxia after submersion.
    A. Drowning
    B. Near drowning
    C. Suffocation
    D. Submersion

21. If it is uncertain whether a patient is known to have had a diving injury, the EMT should always suspect an injury to the spine and take appropriate precautions.
    A. True
    B. False

22. The overall treatment of any near-drowning patient includes all of the following *except:*
    A. Allow the stable patient to go home
    B. Protect and maintain the airway
    C. Ventilate the patient if necessary
    D. Retain body heat and transport

23. Patients who have been submerged and who are now alert and responsive should be evaluated by a physician due to the tremendous potential for complications.
    A. True
    B. False

24. If a stinger is still present in the injection site, the EMT should:
    A. Remove it by scraping along the skin with the edge of a stiff card
    B. Use tweezers or forceps to remove the stinger
    C. Never attempt to remove the stinger in the field
    D. Cover the stinger with a sterile dressing and transport

25. Management of a patient who has been the victim of an animal bite includes which of the following?
    A. Gently washing the area
    B. Removing jewelry from the injured extremity
    C. Placing the bite site below the level of the patient's heart
    D. All of the above

Case Scenario

You are dispatched to an industrial fire where there are multiple victims. On your arrival, you are directed to a 52-year-old male patient who is sitting on the ground, somewhat dazed and confused. The fire started as a result of an explosion in the plant. Your patient suffered burns to his face, chest and anterior portions of both arms.

On assessment, you note that the patient is complaining of pain in his face, chest, and arms. There is some charring of the skin to his right forearm, redness on his chest underneath his clothing, and redness with blisters on his face and arms. You note singed nasal hair and soot around the patient's mouth.

1. What does your assessment indicate?

2. What percentage of body surface area is involved in this burn injury?

3. Are this patient's burns considered critical?

4. How would you care for this patient?

5. Should you use dry or wet dressings on this patient's wounds? Why?

Answer Key

Key Terms
1. Ambient
2. Core
3. B, C, A, D
4. L, A, H, C, B, J, M, I, K, E, G, F, D, N
5. Humidity
6. Heat index
7. Rule of nines
8. Toxin
9. Wind chill
10. Blanching

Content Review
1. Metabolism—conversion of food (sugar) to energy; muscle contractions during activity, exercise, and shivering
2. 98.6° F (37° C)
3. Hyperthermia
4. Hypothermia
5. 1) Breathing; 2) conduction; 3) convection; 4) evaporation; and 5) radiation
6. Constriction of blood vessels, thereby retaining heat in the core and preventing its escape through the surface of the skin
7. The patient's age, medical condition, immersion or submersion, and use of drugs or alcohol

8. Remove the patient from the cold environment to protect him or her against further heat loss; handle the patient gently; do not let the patient exert energy; once in a warm environment, remove all wet clothing and cover the patient with a blanket; administer high-concentration oxygen (warmed and humidified if possible); turn up the heat in the patient compartment of the ambulance; if the patient is alert and responsive, actively rewarm him or her with warm blankets and heat pads in the groin, axillary, and cervical regions; if the patient is unresponsive, passively rewarm him or her with warm blankets.
9. True
10. 30 to 60 seconds
11. Ears, nose, face, and distal extremities (fingers and toes)
12. Superficial frostbite or frostnip
13. Remove the patient from the environment; protect the tissue from further injury; remove all wet or restrictive clothing; gently rewarm skin surface by blowing air on affected part or covering with warm hands; splint and cover extremity if involved; and do not re-expose injured areas to the cold
14. False
15. False
16. 100 to 105
17. The affected part is soft to the touch and color and sensation have returned
18. Pat the area dry (do not rub); place a dry sterile dressing over the area; place dry sterile dressings between the fingers and toes, if involved; protect body parts against re-freezing; be prepared to provide psychological support as needed; and expect the patient to complain of severe pain as the affected area regains sensation.
19. When immediate transport will be delayed or is extremely lengthy and there is no chance of the injured area re-freezing
20. 1) Superficial frostbite (frostnip); 2) frostbite; and 3) deep frostbite
21. Muscle cramps of the legs and abdominal area; exhaustion; dizziness; and periods of near syncope
22. Rapid and shallow ventilations; weak pulses; cool, clammy, pale skin; heavy perspiration; total body weakness; dizziness; and possible unresponsiveness
23. True
24. The inability of the body to cool itself, resulting in core hyperthermia
25. Deep breathing followed by periods of shallow breathing; rapid, strong pulses, followed by rapid weak pulses; dry, hot skin (may be red); large (dilated) pupils; loss of consciousness; and muscle twitching or seizures
26. Remove the patient from heat and place in a cool environment; cool the patient by loosening or removing clothing and fanning the patient; place the patient in the supine position with feet elevated to aid in circulation; administer supplemental oxygen; if patient is responsive, have him or her slowly drink electrolyte solution.
27. 1) Superficial (first-degree); 2) partial-thickness (second-degree); and 3) full-thickness (third-degree)
28. Reddened area; no blisters; localized pain
29. Second-degree (partial-thickness) burn
30. Charring of the skin (black, white, or gray in color); tissue damage through the skin to underlying tissues; minimal to no pain
31. 1
32. 20
33. Face, hands, feet, or genital region
34. Remove the patient from the environment and stop the burning process; remove all clothing from the injured area and remove any burning, smoldering, or heat-retaining materials (jewelry, belt buckle, snaps, etc.); protect the patient from further heat exposure and heat loss; cover the injured area to protect it from further contamination and to help limit the loss of body fluid; administer high-concentration humidified oxygen; monitor the airway (especially with burns of the face and/or inhalation of hot gas or steam from fire).

35. 9; 9
36. 70
37. 66
38. True
39. On the left side providing no spinal injury is suspected
40. Place the patient on his or her left side; have suction ready; place hand over epigastric region of abdomen; and apply gentle pressure to help relieve the distention.
41. Localized pain; fatigue; weakness; dizziness; nausea and vomiting; chills; fever; unresponsiveness; wheezing; localized redness and/or swelling; hives; bite marks; a visible stinger; and/or difficulty breathing
42. True

Chapter Quiz

1. D	6. D	11. C	16. A	21. A
2. B	7. A	12. B	17. C	22. A
3. B	8. A	13. C	18. D	23. A
4. B	9. D	14. C	19. A	24. A
5. B	10. A	15. C	20. A	25. D

Case Scenario

1. The singed nasal hair and soot indicate possible airway damage from an inhalation injury. Assessment further shows that the patient has suffered from first-degree burns to the chest, second-degree burns to the face and arms, and third-degree burns to the right forearm.
2. 27% BSA [head = 9%; anterior portion of both arms = 9%; chest = 9%]
3. Yes. Greater than 20% BSA of partial- or full-thickness burns is considered critical.
4. Remove the patient from the environment and stop the burning process; remove all clothing from the injured area and remove any burning, smoldering, or heat-retaining materials (jewelry, belt buckle, snaps, etc.); protect the patient from further heat exposure and heat loss; cover the injured area with dry dressings to protect from further contamination and help limit loss of body fluid; administer high-concentration humidified oxygen; monitor the airway; and transport to a burn center as quickly as possible.
5. This patient's burns should be dressed in dry dressings. A patient with more than 9% BSA burned will likely experience problems with excess body temperature loss through burned tissue and, therefore, require dry dressings only.

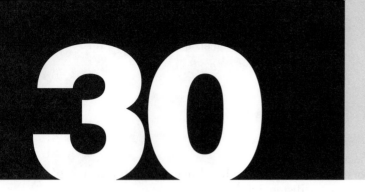

30 Geriatric Patients

Reading Assignment: Chapter 30 pages 585–603.

Supplemental Objectives

- Define the term elderly.
- State the leading causes of death of the elderly.
- Describe the process of gathering patient information for the elderly person.
- List the steps in assessing an elderly patient.
- Describe communication basics used with an elderly patient.
- Describe trauma assessment in the elderly.
- Describe acute illness assessment in the elderly.
- State the nature of the problem of elder abuse.
- List the categories and characteristics of elder abuse.

Key Terms

1. Define elder abuse.

2. The term *elderly* is traditionally given to those persons _____ years of age or older.

3. A high concentration of CO_2 in the blood is called _____.

4. A physician who specializes in treatment of the elderly is called a _____.

5. The state of relative constancy of the internal environment of the body is called _____
   _____.

6. The medical term for "ringing in the ears" is _____.

7. Curvature of the thoracic spine is called _____.

8. The term for a brief lapse of consciousness is _____.

9. The increased porosity of bone is called _____.

10. The medical term for the process of aging is _____.

Content Review

1. The leading cause of death in the elderly is _____.

2. What are the risk factors affecting the death rate in the elderly?

3. The changes in the musculoskeletal system that occur with age make the elderly more likely to suffer from what type of injury?

4. What effect does the aging process have on the skin?

5. What effect does the aging process have on the respiratory system?

6. What effect does the aging process have on the cardiovascular system?

7. What cardiac emergency situations are the most common in the geriatric patient?

8. The elderly may learn more slowly than the young, but once material is learned, retention is good.
   A. True
   B. False

9. The normal biologic aging of the brain is not a predictor for disease of the brain.
   A. True
   B. False

10. Overall, approximately _____ % of elderly persons have hearing problems and _____ % have visual problems.

11. Any impenetrability of light rays (opacity) in the lens of the eye is called a(n) _____.

12. Identify some factors that can result in a hearing deficit.

13. The loss of intellectual abilities, especially those higher order functions measured by memory, judgment, abstract thinking, reasoning, and visual-spatial relations, in the context of perceived alertness, is called _____.

14. Dementia and delirium are the same illness.
    A. True
    B. False

15. Memory loss, asking repeated questions, trouble using words, confusion, and disorientation are all classic indications of _____.

16. What factors lead to underutilization on medication in the elderly?

17. Overdosing on medication occurs in the elderly for what reasons?

18. When assessing an elderly patient, the EMT should:

19. Some conditions that results from chronic hypertension and age and that presents with a patient complaining of severe tearing or ripping chest pain, nausea and vomiting, and diaphoresis is called _____.

20. Drugs associated with syncopal episodes include:

21. Elderly patients at risk of heat stroke include those with:

22. Identify the classic signs of hyperpyrexia.

23. Identify signs of hypothermia in the elderly.

Chapter Quiz
. . . .

1. The leading cause of death in the elderly is:
   A. Cancer
   B. Cardiovascular disease
   C. Diabetes
   D. Traumatic injuries

2. The elderly are considered at high risk for mental health problems.
   A. True
   B. False

3. Patients who are _____ years of age and older are considered elderly.
   A. 45
   B. 50
   C. 65
   D. 70

4. Risk factors affecting the death rate in the elderly include:
   A. Being over 75 years of age
   B. Living alone and being immobile
   C. The recent death of a significant other
   D. All of the above

5. The incidence of _____ is greater in women than in men.
   A. Cardiomyopathy
   B. Osteoporosis
   C. Parkinson's disease
   D. Prostatitis

6. Older women have a greater probability of fractures, particularly of the:
   A. Femur
   B. Wrist
   C. Foot
   D. Spine

7. Osteoarthritis is characterized by:
   A. Stiffness
   B. Deformity and pain
   C. Swelling of the joints
   D. All of the above

8. The cardiac emergencies most consequential in the care of geriatric patients include all of the following *except:*
   A. Acute chest pain
   B. Dysrhythmia
   C. Epiglottitis
   D. Coronary artery disease

9. _____ is the name given to a group of diseases characterized by thickening and loss of elasticity of arterial walls.
   A. Osteoporosis
   B. Arteriosclerosis
   C. Occlusive disorder
   D. Arterioritis

10. A risk associated with narrowing and eventual obstruction of coronary arteries is:
    A. Osteoporosis
    B. Pericarditis
    C. Heart attack
    D. Mesenteric infarction

11. In the prehospital environment, when the elderly are managed for acute illness or trauma, the EMT must be alert to advanced disease states that may cloud initial patient assessment including:
    A. Failure of the heart to provide adequate circulation
    B. Respiratory insufficiency
    C. Auditory and visual loss
    D. All of the above

12. Assessment of the elderly in the prehospital environment often takes longer and may be more difficult to conduct due to communication problems such as:
    A. Visual impairment
    B. Hearing loss
    C. Fatigue
    D. All of the above

13. When assessing an elderly patient, the EMT must be aware of all of the following factors *except:*
    A. The elderly desire more privacy
    B. The elderly make quick decisions
    C. The elderly do not respond to directions requiring them to think quickly
    D. Sequences of assessment of the elderly may need modification because of sensory deficits

14. Ordinarily, dentures should be left in place because maintaining a seal around the mouth with a mask is more difficult without the dentures in place.
    A. True
    B. False

15. Degenerative arthritis of the cervical spine may subject the elderly patient to spinal cord injury while maneuvering the neck, even if there is no injury to the spine.
    A. True
    B. False

16. The extent of elder abuse is not fully known because:
    A. Elder abuse has been a problem largely hidden from society
    B. There are varying definitions of abuse/neglect in the elderly
    C. The reluctance of elders or others to report the problem
    D. All of the above

17. Abuse is defined as any action on the part of an elderly person's family, professional caregiver, or associated persons who have daily household contact or on whom the elderly person is reliant for daily needs who takes advantage of the individual's person, property, or emotional state.
    A. True
    B. False

18. It is important to remember that many patients suffering from abuse are terrorized into making false statements for fear of retribution.
    A. True
    B. False

19. Abuse of the elderly may be:
    A. Physical
    B. Financial
    C. Psychologic
    D. All of the above

Case Scenario

••

You are dispatched to 122 Lincoln Way, the Jamison residence, for a patient in respiratory distress. On your arrival, you are directed to the living room where you find the patient leaning forward in a chair. The patient is fatigued with severe difficulty breathing and audible wheezing. The patient is alert and oriented but has periods of confusion. She complains "I can't catch my breath." She is 83 years old, wears glasses, dentures, and a hearing aid.

On initial assessment and physical examination, you note that the patient's skin is pale and diaphoretic. Her lips and nail beds are cyanotic. You note neck vein distension, a barrel chest, pursed lips, and edema in the hands and ankles. The patient has a history of COPD and is currently on oxygen at 3 L via a nasal cannula; she takes Lasix. She states that she has felt progressively worse over the past few days, but today she "can't even take a step without stopping to catch my breath." When you look at the oxygen tank, you notice it is empty. The prescription bottle for Lasix is empty as well. You ask the patient when she last took her medicine; she cannot answer.

Vital signs reveal: BP, 172/80 mm Hg; pulse, 122; ventilations, 24 and labored; pupils, PEARLA.

1. What communication problems might you expect to find while assessing this patient?

2. How would you assess and care for this patient?

3. What may have caused this patient to run out of oxygen and Lasix?

4. Should you give oxygen to this patient? If so, why and how much?

5. If it becomes necessary to ventilate this patient, what should you do with her dentures?

Answer Key

Key Terms
1. The physical, psychologic, and/or financial mistreatment of the elderly
2. 65
3. Hypercarbia
4. Gerontologist
5. Homeostasis
6. Tinnitus
7. Kyphosis
8. Syncope (or syncopal episode)
9. Osteoporosis
10. Senescence

Content Review
1. Cardiovascular disease
2. Age over 75 years; living alone; recent hospitalization; recent death of a significant other; incontinence; immobility; and/or an unsound mind
3. Muscle fatigue leading to fractures from falls
4. Loss of sweat glands reduce the body's ability to regulate temperature; thinning and drying of skin reduces the ability of the skin to protect the body from invasion by microorganisms; and loss of fatty tissue predisposes the elderly to hypothermia and hyperthermia.
5. The chest cage becomes less pliable with the loss of lung elasticity predisposing the elderly to hypercarbia; the alveoli become smaller, thereby reducing the amount of oxygen exchanged in the lungs; and the number of cilia in the lungs decrease, which may result in more infections and illness associated with inhaled particulate matter
6. Degeneration of heart muscle and less pacemaker cells make the elderly prone to various dysrhythmias; atherosclerosis, arteriosclerosis, and loss of elastic properties of arteries may result in hypertension and increase the risk of heart attack; and changes in the heart itself may reduce the ability of the heart to withstand acute illness or trauma.
7. Acute chest pain, dysrhythmias, coronary artery disease, pericarditis, and thoracic aortic dissection
8. True
9. True
10. 28; 13
11. Cataract
12. Trauma, diabetes, vascular lesions, middle ear disease, barotrauma, hypertension, benign body growths, arteriosclerosis, accumulation of ear wax, and environmental noise
13. Dementia
14. False
15. Alzheimer's disease
16. Confusion, forgetfulness, arthritis of the hands (making it difficult to open bottles), and trying to save money
17. Confusion, visual impairment, arthritis (making it difficult to take the proper dosage); mis- selection of medications, and self-destruction (suicide)
18. Plan for more time to gather information; be patient; be compassionate and empathetic; do not underestimate the patient's intelligence merely because communication may be difficult or absent; ask close relatives to participate in giving information or help validating information; obtain a list of medications the patient is taking; and make sure the patient can hear (stand directly in front of the patient)
19. Myocardial infarction, thoracic aortic dissection, esophagus tear
20. Diuretics, antidysrhythmics, antihypertensives, nitrates, calcium channel blockers, psychotropics, beta-blockers, and digitalis

21. Preexisting febrile illness, infection, skin disease, heat cramps, heat exhaustion, chronic dehydration, taking certain medications (diuretics, antihistamines, and antiparkinsonian medications)
22. Hot, dry skin with no perspiration; high body temperature (100° to 106° F); and altered mental status
23. Body temperature under 95° F; lack of coordination; lethargy; stiffness of muscles; rigidity; shivering (ceases when hypothermia progresses); and altered mental status

Chapter Quiz

1. B	6. A	11. D	16. D
2. A	7. D	12. D	17. A
3. C	8. C	13. B	18. A
4. D	9. B	14. A	19. D
5. B	10. C	15. A	

Case Scenario
1. Confusion (from dementia or decreased oxygenation to the brain); decreased visual acuity; hearing impairment; fatigue; and distraction
2. Allow extra time for assessment and care of this patient; make eye contact; address the patient by her last name; ask direct questions; involve a significant other in questioning, if possible; be compassionate; administer high-concentration oxygen; keep the patient warm; monitor vital signs; be prepared to assist with ventilations, if necessary; and transport.
3. Confusion; forgetfulness; lack of money; or not knowing how to get them refilled
4. Yes. Never withhold oxygen from a patient in respiratory distress. Administer high-concentration oxygen via a non-rebreather mask and be prepared to assist with ventilations if necessary.
5. Leave them in place as it helps to form a better seal with the mask.

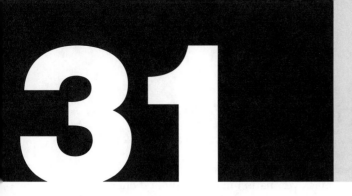

Infants and Children

Reading Assignment: Chapter 31 pages 604–637.

DOT Objectives

• •

Upon successful completion of the EMT-Basic training program, the EMT-Basic should be able to do the following:

- Identify the developmental considerations for the following age groups:
  - infants
  - toddlers
  - preschoolers
  - school-age children
  - adolescents
- Recognize the signs and symptoms of increased respiratory effort in the infant or child.
- Describe differences in anatomy and physiology of the infant, child, and adult patient.
- Differentiate the response of the ill or injured infant or child (age specific) from that of an adult.
- Indicate various causes of respiratory emergencies.
- List the steps in the management of foreign body airway obstruction (Appendix A).
- Summarize emergency medical care strategies for respiratory distress.
- State the usual cause of cardiac arrest in infants and children versus adults.
- List the common causes of seizures in the infant and child patient.
- Describe the management of seizures in the infant and child patient.
- Differentiate between the injury patterns in adults, infants, and children.
- Discuss the field management of the infant and child trauma patient.
- Summarize the indicators of possible child abuse and neglect.
- Describe the medicolegal responsibilities in suspected child abuse.
- Demonstrate the techniques of foreign body airway obstruction removal in the infant and child (see Appendix A).
- Demonstrate the assessment of the infant and child.
- Demonstrate bag-valve-mask artificial ventilations for the infant and child.
- Demonstrate oxygen delivery for the infant and child.

Supplemental Objectives

- Recognize the signs and symptoms of increased respiratory effort in the infant and child.
- List three techniques to accomplish effective bag-valve-mask ventilation in the infant and child.
- List three characteristics of the following diseases: croup, epiglottitis, asthma (reactive airways disease), and bronchiolitis.
- Describe the treatment of an infant or child in status epilepticus.
- Identify the signs and symptoms of an infant or child with meningitis.
- Identify the signs and symptoms of an infant or child with dehydration.
- List the causes of pediatric injuries in the order of most common to least common.
- List three activities that may cause spinal trauma in the pediatric patient.
- List three of the most common types of poisoning in children.
- List five risk factors for child maltreatment.
- List five indicators of child abuse.

Key Terms

1. The period of time immediately preceding a seizure is called the _____.

2. A seizure characterized by a sudden, momentary loss of consciousness is called _____.

3. A condition in which the increased intracranial pressure forces the portion of the brain containing the medulla through the foramen magnum is called _____.

4. An acute viral infection of the lower respiratory tract that occurs primarily in infants under the age of 18 months is called _____.

5. Accumulation of fluid in the brain tissue is called _____.

6. A bacterial infection seen most often in children and characterized by excessive drooling and possible airway obstruction is called _____.

7. A group of neurologic disorders characterized by recurrent episodes of convulsive seizures, sensory disturbances, unusual behavior, loss of consciousness, or all of these is called _____ _____.

8. Inflammation of the stomach and intestines is called _____.

9. The slit-like opening between the vocal cords is called the _____.

10. Another term for croup is _____.

11. A state or quality of being indifferent, apathetic, or sluggish that results from disease is called _____.

12. A disorder of nutrition attributed to an unbalanced, insufficient, or excessive diet, or from impaired absorption or metabolism of food is called _____.

13. Insertion of a needle into the cricothyroid membrane to create a temporary airway opening is called a(n) _____.

Content Review

1. The most common type of EMS call for children 5 to 14 years of age is _____ and for children under the age of 5 years it is _____.

2. EMS calls for children under 2 years of age are usually very serious in nature.
   A. True
   B. False

3. Identify the age for each of the following groups.

   Neonate:

   Young infant:

   Infant:

   Toddler:

   Preschooler:

   School age:

   Adolescent:

4. What are the seven basic components of an effective EMS for children (EMSC) system?

   1)
   2)
   3)
   4)
   5)
   6)
   7)

5. Children represent approximately _____% of all EMS calls.

6. What questions should you ask yourself prior to interacting with a child to help determine the most appropriate approach?

7. Identify the normal range of vital signs for each of the following age groups.

	Pulse	Ventilations	Blood Pressure
Newborn			
Infant			
Toddler			
Preschooler			
School age child			
Adolescent			

8. Approximately 90% of pediatric cardiac arrests start as _____.

9. The best way to prevent pediatric cardiac arrest is _____.

10. The first sign of respiratory distress in an infant is usually _____.

11. Identify the initial signs and symptoms of respiratory distress in infants or children.

12. Identify the signs of increased ventilatory effort in infants or children.

13. Identify the causes of increased heart rates in infants and children.

14. What is the most effective treatment for a slow heart rate in infants and children.

15. Which artery should be assessed in children under the age of 1 year?

16. Which artery should be assessed in an unconscious child older than 1 year of age?

17. The leading cause of shock in children across the world is _____ with dehydration.

18. Severe loss of fluid can lead to _____ shock.

19. Only infants with a soft spot on top of their heads have adequate space to allow for enough intracranial bleeding.
    A. True
    B. False

20. In children with a primary head injury and low blood pressure, the EMT should assume that the cause of low blood pressure is hypovolemia resulting from the head injury.
    A. True
    B. False

21. Identify the causes of shock in children.

22. List the signs and symptoms of shock.

23. If a child suddenly develops respiratory distress with coughing, gagging, stridor, or wheezing, the EMT should suspect _____.

24. List the most common causes of a foreign body airway obstruction in infants and children.

25. Adults can compensate for a serious injury longer than children.
    A. True
    B. False

26. An oropharyngeal airway of proper size should reach from the _____ to the _____.

27. In children, the oropharyngeal airway should be inserted using a tongue blade to depress the tongue.
    A. True
    B. False

28. Low-flow oxygen can be administered to a child by a(n) _____ at _____ L/minute.

29. If a child will not tolerate a face mask, how should the EMT administer oxygen?

30. If effective ventilations do not occur when using a BVM, what should the EMT consider in determining what is wrong or correcting the problem?

31. It is critical to use a BVM system that delivers at least _____ mL of air for full-term infants and children.

32. A neonatal BVM system delivers _____ mL of air.

33. A viral infection with a slow onset that, usually follows an upper respiratory infection and low fever and that causes inflammation of the larynx or vocal cords is called _____.

34. Identify symptoms of croup.

35. How should the EMT care for a patient with croup?

36. Epiglottitis occurs most often in children ages _____.

37. Epiglottitis is caused by bacteria and progresses rapidly.
    A. True
    B. False

38. What is the tripod position and what does it signify?

39. How should the EMT care for a patient with epiglottitis?

40. How should the EMT care for a patient with asthma?

41. Any condition that affects the structure of the cells of the brain may trigger seizures.
    A. True
    B. False

42. List the causes of seizures in infants and children.

43. List the signs and symptoms of meningitis in younger patients.

    Signs:

    Symptoms:

44. List the signs and symptoms of meningitis in the older child.

    Signs:

    Symptoms:

45. List the causes of pediatric injuries from most to least common.

46. The most common cause of death in pediatric patients is _____.

47. What is the most effective way to minimize the secondary brain injury associated with head injury?

48. List the most common types of poisonings that occur in younger children.

49. List the most common types of poisonings that occur in children between school age and adolescence.

50. List a child's individual risk factors for abuse.

51. List family related risk factors for child abuse.

52. List the four major types of child abuse.

    1)
    2)
    3)
    4)

53. Failure to meet a child's basic needs such as food, clothing, shelter, medical care, and safety is called
    _____.

54. List the indicators of possible child abuse.

55. What is the major fear of infants?

56. What is the major fear of toddlers?

57. What is the major fear of preschoolers?

58. What is the major fear of school-age children?

59. What is the major fear of adolescents?

60. Identify the differences between epiglottitis and croup.

61. Identify the differences between asthma and bronchiolitis.

Chapter Quiz

1. All of the following are signs of increased ventilatory effort in the infant or child *except*:
   A. Sternal retractions
   B. Head bobbing
   C. Nasal flaring
   D. Bradypnea

2. A childhood disease, usually caused by a bacterial infection, that has a rapid onset and results in the child drooling while sitting in the "tripod" position is:
   A. Croup
   B. Bronchiolitis
   C. Epiglottitis
   D. Asthma

3. The term "postictal" is associated with which of the following emergencies?
   A. Meningitis
   B. Seizures
   C. Head trauma
   D. Dehydration

4. Major fears of school-age children include all of the following *except:*
   A. Death
   B. Loss of control
   C. Strangers
   D. Bodily injury and/or mutilation

5. Children will present with a particular injury pattern and physiologic response to trauma depending on the child's:
   A. Size
   B. Level of maturation
   C. Overall development
   D. All of the above

6. The EMT should frequently reassess the injured infant or child since they can compensate for a serious injury longer than an adult.
   A. True
   B. False

7. A foreign body airway obstruction should be suspected if an infant or child suddenly develops respiratory distress with coughing, gagging, stridor, or wheezing.
   A. True
   B. False

8. Management strategies specific to respiratory distress or failure include all of the following *except:*
   A. Maintain proficiency in infant and child CPR and techniques for clearing an obstructed airway
   B. Always examine the throat of a child who is complaining of a sore throat and/or difficulty swallowing
   C. Select airway adjuncts based on the size of the patient and the ventilatory support needed
   D. Only use a BVM that delivers at least 450 mL of air to provide the full-term infant or child with an adequate tidal volume

9. Remember to have suction equipment available because pediatric patients are prone to vomiting.
   A. True
   B. False

10. Signs of shock include which of the following?
    A. Altered level of consciousness
    B. Increased ventilatory rate and rapid heart rate
    C. Cool or cold clammy skin and prolonged capillary refill
    D. All of the above

11. Most pediatric patients go into cardiac arrest as a result of ventricular fibrillation.
    A. True
    B. False

12. Causes of seizures in infants and children include:
    A. Abnormal electrical activity in the brain
    B. Elevated body temperature
    C. Hypoxia from head trauma
    D. All of the above

13. _____ is the period immediately preceding a seizure wherein the patient experiences a certain sensation that warns of an impending seizure.
    A. Postictal
    B. Preictal
    C. Aura
    D. Latency

14. In treating a seizure victim, the EMT should use all of the following management techniques *except:*
    A. Gently assist the child to a side-lying position with special consideration given to airway patency
    B. Clear the area from hazardous items that might cause injury during the seizure activity
    C. Insert a wooden tongue depressor into the mouth if teeth are clenched
    D. Consider the use of a nasal airway as an appropriate alternative adjunct

15. Injury patterns in children and adult patients differ due to which of the following factors?
    A. The child is smaller than the adult and is, therefore, prone to a wider range of injuries
    B. In infants and younger children, the head is larger in proportion to the rest of the body
    C. The child's skeleton is not completely calcified and has many active growth centers
    D. All of the above

16. Status epilepticus is a continuous seizure or series of seizures in which the patient does not regain consciousness.
    A. True
    B. False

17. Which of the following is an indicator of child abuse?
    A. Bruises or burns in patterns that suggest intentional infliction
    B. Injuries in various stages of healing
    C. Children under 2 years of age with multiple fractures
    D. All of the above

18. In dealing with suspected child abuse situations, it is important that the EMT:
    A. Be nonjudgmental
    B. Not accuse anyone of child abuse even though it may appear obvious
    C. Carefully document in objective terms exactly what was seen or assessed on the child
    D. All of the above

19. The first sign of respiratory distress in an infant is usually:
    A. A rapid rate of breathing
    B. A decreased pulse rate
    C. A decreased capillary refill time
    D. Increased thirst

Case Scenario

It is 3:00 AM and you are dispatched to a residence for a sick child. En route to the scene, dispatch informs you that the mother called back to say the child is having difficulty breathing and that ALS has been dispatched.

1. What are your immediate thoughts concerning what might be wrong? Identify possible complications for which you should be prepared.

You arrive on location and are directed upstairs to a bedroom where you find a very anxious mother holding her 2-year-old son. You hear the child wheezing from the doorway. The child appears anxious but alert and oriented. His cry is hoarse and you note stridor, nasal flaring, intercostal retractions, and a "barking" cough. The mother states that her son had had a cold, runny nose, and slight fever for the past couple days and that he woke up 1 hour ago with a cough.

2. How should you approach the assessment of this patient?

3. What is most likely wrong with this child? What signs and symptoms led you to this conclusion?

4. How should you care for this patient?

Answer Key

Key Terms
1. Aura
2. Absence
3. Brainstem herniation
4. Bronchiolitis
5. Cerebral edema

6. Epiglottitis
7. Epilepsy
8. Gastroenteritis
9. Glottis
10. Laryngotracheobronchitis
11. Lethargy
12. Malnutrition
13. Needle cricothyrotomy

Content Review

1. Trauma; medical illness
2. True
3. Neonate: birth to 1 month; young infant: 1 to 5 months; infant: 6 to 12 months; toddler: 1 to 3 years; preschooler: 3 to 6 years; school age child: 6 to 12 years; adolescent: 12 to 18 years
4. 1) System description; 2) education; 3) prevention; 4) research and data collection; 5) medical direction and supervision; 6) quality assurance and improvement; and 7) ongoing funding
5. 10
6. What is the child's chronological age? What is the child's level of understanding? Is someone present whom the child knows and/or trusts who can offer reassurance and emotional support? Does anyone know the child's medical history or other pertinent history? Are any special circumstances present (language barriers, physical or mental disability, special equipment, etc.)?
7. Newborn: P = 120 to 160 bpm; VR = 30 to 50; BP = 74 to 100/ 50 to 68 mm Hg
   Infant: P = 80 to 140 bpm; VR = 20 to 30; BP = 84 to 106/ 56 to 70 mm Hg
   Toddler: P = 80 to 130 bpm; VR = 20 to 30; BP = 98 to 106/ 50 to 70 mm Hg
   Preschooler: P = 80 to 120 bpm; VR = 20 to 30; BP = 98 to 112/ 64 to 70 mm Hg
   School age child: P = (60 to 80) to 100 bpm; VR = (12 to 20) - 30; BP = 104 to 124/ 64 to 80 mm Hg
   Adolescent: P = 60 to 100 bpm; VR = 12 to 20; BP = 118 to 132/ 70 to 82 mm Hg
8. Respiratory problems
9. Early identification and intervention of respiratory problems
10. A rapid rate of breathing
11. Rapid breathing; increased ventilatory effort; diminished breath sounds; decreased level of consciousness or response to parents or pain; poor skeletal muscle tone; cyanosis
12. Nasal flaring; intercostal, subcostal, and suprasternal inspiratory retractions; head bobbing; grunting; stridor; or prolonged expiration
13. Hypovolemia; decreased oxygen; anxiety; fever; pain; increased carbon dioxide; and cardiac problems
14. Increased oxygenation
15. Brachial or femoral
16. Carotid
17. Gastroenteritis
18. Hypovolemic
19. True
20. False
21. Hypovolemia (dehydration, blood loss, burns); sepsis (systemic infection); anaphylaxis (life-threatening allergic reaction from insect stings, drug or food allergies); and neurogenic (spinal) shock from spinal cord injury; airway and ventilation difficulties
22. Altered level of consciousness (confusion, irritability, lethargy, sluggishness, coma); increased ventilatory rate; respiratory failure; rapid heart rate; normal blood pressure progressing to low blood pressure; cool, clammy skin; decreased peripheral pulses; prolonged capillary refill time; low urine output; and acidosis; airway and ventilation difficulties
23. A foreign body airway obstruction (FBAO)
24. Hot dogs, balloons, small toys, nuts, grapes, and round candies

25. False
26. Corner of the patient's mouth; angle of the jaw
27. True
28. Nasal cannula; 2 to 4
29. "Blow-by" method—having the child or parent hold the mask in front of the child's face
30. Reposition the head; make sure the mask is snug against the face; lift the jaw; suction the airway; check the bag for damage.
31. 450
32. 250
33. Croup
34. Respiratory stridor, 'barking' cough, and wheezing
35. Administer high-concentration oxygen (cool and humidified if possible); keep the patient as calm as possible; transport in a comfortable position; monitor vital signs; and reassess frequently
36. 3 to 7
37. True
38. Sitting upright and leaning forward on hands with the neck extended forward in an attempt to breathe easier. It indicates respiratory difficulty/distress.
39. *Do not* examine the airway; keep the patient as calm as possible; administer high- concentration humidified oxygen via a mask or "blow-by"; monitor vital signs and pulse rate; do not agitate the child; be prepared to ventilate using a BVM; communicate with the medical director to alert the hospital of ETA; and do not attempt intubation without ALS or ED personnel available to perform cricothyrotomy
40. Administer humidified oxygen; monitor vital signs and pulse rate; communicate with medical director; follow local protocols concerning administration of drugs; be prepared to assist with ventilations or perform CPR if necessary; and transport quickly in a position of comfort.
41. True
42. Hypoxia, head trauma, low blood sugar, tumors, drug toxicity, meningitis, epilepsy of unknown origin, poison ingestion or exposure, or failure to take anticonvulsant medication as prescribed
43. Signs: fever, rash (petechia), dehydration, bulging fontanelle, vomiting, seizures, respiratory distress, and cyanosis
    Symptoms: lethargy; irritability; loss of appetite; poor feeding
44. Those signs and symptoms of meningitis in younger children plus the following: symptoms: pain when extending the legs or moving the hip, pain when flexing the neck, and headaches
45. Falls, vehicular-related trauma, sports-related injury, and assaults
46. Head injury
47. Ventilations and oxygenation
48. Household products, medications, toxic plants, and contaminated foods
49. Alcohol; organic solvents; mind-altering drugs (marijuana, hashish, LSD, PCP); narcotics (heroin, morphine); CNS depressants (barbiturates); and CNS stimulants (amphetamines, cocaine, or crack)
50. Prematurity, prenatal drug exposure, developmental disability, physical disability, chronic illness, or product of multiple birth
51. Alcohol dependency, drug dependency, childhood history of maltreatment, belief in the use of corporal punishment, rigid expectations regarding the child's behavior, negative parental perceptions of the child, unrealistic expectations of the child, a single parent, social isolation, psychological distress, low self-esteem, extreme poverty, or acute and chronic stressors
52. 1) Physical abuse; 2) sexual abuse; 3) emotional or psychological abuse; and 4) neglect
53. Neglect

54. Obvious or suspected fractures in a child under 2 years of age; injuries in various stages of healing, especially burns and bruises; more injuries than normal for the child's age; injuries scattered on many areas of the body; bruise or burn patterns that suggest intentional infliction; suspected increased intracranial pressure in an infant; suspected intra-abdominal trauma in a young child; any injury that does not fit the description of the cause given; an accusation that the child injured himself intentionally; long-standing skin infections; extreme malnutrition; extreme lack of cleanliness; inappropriate clothing for the situation; a child who withdraws from parents; and/or a child who responds inappropriately to the situation (e.g., quiet, distant, or withdrawn)
55. Separation and strangers
56. Separation and loss of control
57. Bodily injury and mutilation, loss of control, the unknown, the dark, and being left alone
58. Loss of control, bodily injury and mutilation, failure to live up to expectations of others, and death
59. Loss of control, altered body image, and separation from peer groups
60. Epiglottitis is caused by a bacterial infection and croup is caused by a viral infection; croup usually occurs during late fall and early winter and epiglottitis has no seasonal preference. Croup occurs in children ages 6 months to 3 years, and epiglottitis occurs in children ages 3 to 7 years. Croup has a slow onset and epiglottitis has a rapid onset. A patient with epiglottitis will sit upright in a "tripod" position, and a patient with croup will either lie down or sit up; a patient with croup will have a "barking" cough and a patient with epiglottitis will not. A patient with epiglottitis will have pain on swallowing causing drooling and a patient with croup will not; and a patient with epiglottitis will have a fever over 104° F and a patient with croup will have a temperature under 104° F.
61. Bronchiolitis occurs between 6 and 18 months of age and asthma occurs at any age. Asthma is more common in winter and spring, and bronchiolitis can occur at any time; bronchiolitis is caused by a virus, asthma is a response to an allergen, exercise, or infection. Drugs will reverse the bronchospasm associated with asthma but may not be effective with bronchiolitis.

Chapter Quiz

1. D	6. A	11. B	16. A
2. C	7. A	12. D	17. D
3. B	8. B	13. C	18. D
4. C	9. A	14. C	19. A
5. D	10. D	15. D	

Case Scenario

1. It may be a respiratory infection, bronchiolitis, croup, epiglottits, a foreign body airway obstruction, or asthma. Complications may include respiratory arrest and cardiac arrest.
2. Keep explanations simple; choose words carefully; let the toddler play with equipment such as your stethoscope; and minimize any separation from his parents.
3. Respiratory difficulty due to croup. This was determined from the age of the child, time of day of the illness, a PMH of a cold and low grade fever, and signs and symptoms including: a barking cough, wheezing, stridor, nasal flaring, and retractions.
4. Administer high-concentration cool and humidified oxygen via blow-by method if the patient will not tolerate a mask; provide support to the parents; allow the mother or father to ride with the child in the ambulance; secure both child and parent on the stretcher; transport to the hospital; and frequently reassess vital signs and for changes or signs of airway obstruction.

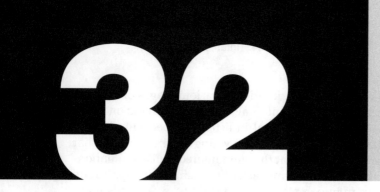

The Patient with Special Needs

Reading Assignment: Chapter 32 pages 638–658.

Supplemental Objectives

- Discuss methods of providing care to patients with special needs.
- Identify developmental considerations for patients with special needs.
- Describe examples of physical and developmental disabilities.
- Identify feelings of the family and/or caregivers in relation to an ill or injured patient with special needs.
- Explain the need for knowledge and skills in treating patients with special needs.
- Discuss the provider's own emotional response to caring for a patient with special needs.
- Develop methods of providing emergency care while appreciating the unique needs of each patient and family.

Key Terms

1. A person who assists another person in carrying out desired wishes is called a(n) _____ _____.

2. A technologic aid used to warn of the cessation of breathing in a premature infant is a(n) _____ _____.

3. A complication of spina bifida in which the brainstem and cerebellum extend down through the foramen magnum into the cervical portion of the vertebrae is called _____ _____.

4. A tube placed in a person's stomach that allows continuous feeding for an extended period of time is called a(n) _____ tube or button.

5. A disability that involves some degree of impaired adaptation in learning, social adjustment, and/or maturation is called a(n) _____ disability.

6. An incision in the colon for the purpose of making a permanent opening between the bowel and the abdominal wall is called a(n) _____.

7. The opposite of acute is _____.

8. A neuromuscular condition in which the patient has difficulty controlling the voluntary muscles due to damage to a portion of the brain is called _____.

9. Another term for reactive airways disease is _____.

10. Paralysis of the lower limbs and trunk is called _____.

11. A disability that involves limitation of mobility is called a(n) _____ disability.

12. The medical term for "water on the brain" or the accumulation of cerebrospinal fluid in the brain is _____.

13. A developmental disability characterized by a lower-than-normal IQ is called _____ _____.

14. The creation of a surgical passage through the abdominal wall into the ileum is called a(n) _____.

15. Paralysis that affects all four extremities is called _____.

16. Prevention of the formation of an immune response is called _____.

17. A developmental anomaly of the CNS in which a hernial sac containing a portion of the spinal cord, its meninges, and cerebrospinal fluid protrudes through a congenital cleft in the vertebral column is called _____.

Content Review

....

1. List the causes of developmental disabilities.

2. List the causes of physical disabilities.

3. People with cerebral palsy are not mentally retarded and may be highly intelligent.
   A. True
   B. False

4. In individuals with severe cerebral palsy, the EMT should assess and monitor the patient's _____ and be prepared for _____.

5. Describe cerebral palsy.

6. The number one disabling birth anomaly in the United States is _____.

7. Cerebral palsy becomes progressively worse as a patient grows.
   A. True
   B. False

8. Describe spina bifida.

9. What is hydrocephalus?

10. What are the signs and symptoms of a blocked shunt?

11. What precautions should the EMT take when performing airway maneuvers on a patient with spina bifida?

12. Allergy to latex products is common in patients with spina bifida.
    A. True
    B. False

13. Patients who require frequent IV medications, repeated blood testing, administration of blood products, or administration of large quantities of fluids, may have a _____ inserted to allow access to a vein without the need for repeated venipunctures.

14. Some patients with seizures who have not responded to medication may have a _____ _____ in place.

15. What considerations should the EMT make when caring for a patient with special needs?

Chapter Quiz

••

1. All of the following are examples of developmental and physical disabilities *except:*
   A. Alzheimer's disease
   B. Mental retardation
   C. Cerebral palsy
   D. Measles

2. The term hemiplegia means paralysis on one half of the body.
   A. True
   B. False

3. All of the following are examples of chronic illness *except:*
   A. Epilepsy
   B. Myocardial infarction
   C. Asthma
   D. Renal failure

4. Asthma is the most common cause of school absences in children.
   A. True
   B. False

5. When dealing with a person who has special needs, life-threatening conditions should be treated before giving consideration to the disability.
   A. True
   B. False

6. Conditions with the potential to interfere with usual growth and development may involve all of the following *except:*
   A. Physical disabilities and developmental disabilities
   B. Chronic illnesses
   C. Forms of technologic support
   D. Acute illnesses

7. Causes of developmental disabilities include all of the following *except:*
   A. Metabolic disorders
   B. Infections
   C. Intracranial hemorrhage
   D. Increased cerebral perfusion

8. Mental retardation is an example of a developmental disability.
   A. True
   B. False

9. Physical disabilities involve some type of limitations of mobility.
   A. True
   B. False

10. Causes of physical disabilities include:
    A. Birth anomalies
    B. Head and spinal cord injuries
    C. Infections
    D. All of the above

11. Most people who have cerebral palsy have a normal level of intelligence.
    A. True
    B. False

12. A person who has cerebral palsy has difficulty controlling the voluntary muscles due to damage to a portion of the:
    A. Brain
    B. Spine
    C. Liver
    D. Heart

13. Individuals who have severe cerebral palsy have a higher risk for:
    A. Kidney infections
    B. Respiratory difficulties
    C. Liver failure
    D. Heart disease

14. In patients who have cerebral palsy, airway obstruction can occur from increased secretions or food.
    A. True
    B. False

15. Spina bifida is the number one disabling birth anomaly in the United States.
    A. True
    B. False

16. Myelomeningocele is the most serious form of spina bifida.
    A. True
    B. False

17. A common occurrence in spina bifida is the presence of hydrocephalus, in which:
    A. Cerebrospinal fluid accumulates in the brain
    B. Lifelong treatment may be required
    C. A shunt is inserted from the brain to another place in the body
    D. All of the above

18. You should perform initial and ongoing assessments on individuals who have special needs using the same method as indicated for patients without these needs.
    A. True
    B. False

19. When dealing with the special needs patient, pertinent questions that should be asked of the patient, parent, or caregiver include:
    A. "Does your child take medications for his or her seizures?"
    B. "What is different today that prompted you to call for an ambulance?"
    C. "Is your child able to take anything by mouth?"
    D. All of the above

20. To determine the patient's level of ability, the EMT should:
    A. Talk with the patient, parent, or caregiver
    B. Direct your questions in a positive light
    C. Realize that the focus is on the patient's abilities instead of their disability
    D. All of the above

Case Scenario

You are dispatched to a residence for a child with seizures. On your arrival, you are directed to a bedroom where you find a 13-year-old female lying in bed. Her parents inform you that she has been deaf and mute since birth. Initial assessment reveals focal motor seizures. You note that the patient has a ventricular shunt in place.

1. List four things you can do to involve the parents in the care of this patient.

2. What are the identified special needs for this patient?

3. How would you care for this patient?

Answer Key

Key Terms
1. Advocate
2. Apnea monitor
3. Arnold-Chiari malformation
4. Gastrostomy
5. Developmental
6. Colostomy
7. Chronic
8. Cerebral palsy
9. Asthma
10. Paraplegia
11. Physical
12. Hydrocephalus
13. Mental retardation
14. Ileostomy
15. Quadriplegia
16. Immunosuppression
17. Myelomeningocele

Content Review
1. Metabolic disorders, infections, intracranial hemorrhage, anoxia (lack of oxygen to the brain), inherited disorders/congenital anomalies, trauma, and any other disorder that damages the brain
2. Birth anomalies (e.g., spina bifida), head and spinal cord injuries, infections resulting in paralysis (e.g. meningitis), and disease processes
3. True
4. Respiratory status; airway obstructions due to increased secretions and/or food
5. A neuromuscular disability with which a person has difficulty controlling the voluntary muscles due to damage of a portion of the brain
6. Spina bifida
7. False
8. A disabling birth anomaly in which the back portion of the vertebrae fails to close and through which the meninges and/or spinal cord may protrude
9. The accumulation of cerebrospinal fluid in the brain—it is a common occurrence in spina bifida and may lead to mental retardation and other neurologic complications, such as seizures, if not treated properly.
10. Increased intracranial pressure, changes in mentation, headaches, vomiting, lethargy, seizures, irritability, and a bulging fontanelle in infants
11. Keep the head and neck in an in-line, neutral position even if trauma is not involved
12. True
13. Central venous access device (VAD)
14. Vagus nerve stimulator (VNS)
15. Focus on the patient's abilities, not on their disabilities; avoid using the word "normal"; develop creative means for communication; communicate in a manner appropriate to the disability; notify the receiving facility of the patient's special needs; treat the patient with the same respect afforded other patients; look for a medical identification bracelet or necklace when assessing patients with special needs; and obtain a list of current medications from a parent or caregiver and ask about side effects.

Chapter Quiz

1. D	6. D	11. A	16. A
2. A	7. D	12. A	17. D
3. B	8. A	13. B	18. A
4. A	9. A	14. A	19. D
5. A	10. D	15. A	20. D

Case Scenario

1. Allow them to stay with the child as much as possible as long as they are emotionally capable to do so; allow the parents to function as your communication link to the patient; involve the parents in the patient's care in whatever way possible; and use the parents as a resource and regard them as experts in their loved one's care.

2. Age, seizure precautions, shunt, communication

3. Ensure and maintain an adequate airway; protect the patient from further injury during any seizure activity; provide high-concentration oxygen; attempt to gain more information about the child's history and any current health concerns; involve the parents in communication and care; continue to reassess the child; provide emotional support to the patient and family; notify the receiving hospital of the patient's needs; talk softly to the child; and try to limit the number of providers touching her.

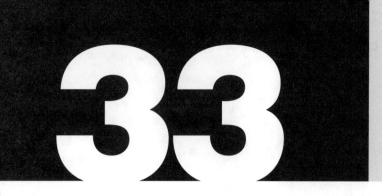

Lifting and Moving Patients

Reading Assignment: Chapter 33 pages 661-685.

DOT Objectives

Upon successful completion of the EMT-Basic training program, the EMT-Basic should be able to do the following:

- Describe body mechanics.
- Discuss guidelines and safety precautions that must be followed when lifting a patient.
- Describe guidelines and safety precautions for carrying patients and equipment.
- Describe the safe lifting of cots and stretchers.
- Describe correct and safe carrying procedures on stairs.
- State the guidelines for reaching, pushing, and pulling.
- Identify seven standard patient carrying devices and their applications.
- State three situations that require the use of an emergency move.
- Describe correct reaching for logrolls.
- Discuss the general considerations of moving patients.
- Working with a partner, prepare each of the following devices for use, transfer a patient to the device, properly position the patient on the device, move the device to the ambulance, and load the patient into the ambulance:
  - Wheeled ambulance stretcher
  - Portable ambulance stretcher
  - Stair chair
  - Scoop stretcher
  - Long spine board
  - Flexible stretcher
- Working with a partner, demonstrate techniques for the transfer of a patient from an ambulance stretcher to the hospital stretcher.

Supplemental Objectives

- Describe time-dependent problems as they relate to trauma patients and medical patients.
- Explain why transport is often the most important intervention in prehospital care.
- List the factors to be considered when assessing the trauma patient for prompt transport.

Key Terms

....

1. A type of move used for patients who are not suspected of having a spinal injury and that uses the patient's arms and legs to move him or her a short distance is called a(n) _____.

2. A type of in-line drag that uses a blanket placed under the patient to pull him or her away from immediate danger is called a(n) _____.

3. The position in which an unconscious patient is placed on his or her side and balanced by the positioning of the arms and legs is the _____ position.

4. A type of in-line drag that uses the patient's arm to provide leverage for dragging the patient away from immediate danger is called a(n) _____.

5. A lift used to move a patient from the ground to a piece of equipment is called the _____
_____.

6. Any move initiated due to immediate danger to a patient and rescuer is called a(n) _____
_____ move.

Content Review

....

1. List the general guidelines for safe lifting.

2. What is the power lift?

3. What is the power grip and why is it used?

4. Always carry a patient head first down the stairs and feet first up the stairs.
   A. True
   B. False

5. What device(s) should be used to move a patient down stairs?

6. List the guidelines to follow when reaching for a patient.

7. List the guidelines to follow when pushing or pulling a patient.

8. What situations would warrant an emergency move?

9. What is the greatest danger of an emergency move?

10. What are the four most common in-line drags?

   1)
   2)
   3)
   4)

11. How do you perform a clothing drag?

12. How do you perform a sheet drag?

13. How do you perform a blanket drag?

14. How do you perform a bent arm drag?

15. Identify some situations in which the EMT should use an urgent move.

16. What are four types of non-urgent moves?

    1)
    2)
    3)
    4)

17. Most ambulance stretchers weigh _____ pounds and are made to hold patients weighing _____ pounds.

18. List the guidelines to follow when loading the ambulance with a two-person stretcher.

19. List the guidelines to follow when loading the ambulance with a one-person stretcher.

20. All stretchers are interchangeable in that a stretcher from one ambulance will fit into another.
    A. True
    B. False

21. List the guidelines to follow for using a scoop stretcher.

22. An unresponsive patient without a suspected spine injury should be placed in what position?

23. An early intervention for a pregnant patient with hypotension is to place her in what position?

Chapter Quiz

• •

1. The best stance for lifting a stretcher is:
   A. Always get as far as possible from the stretcher
   B. Keep your arms and the weight you are lifting 20 inches from your body
   C. Stand with your feet about shoulder's width apart and place one foot slightly in front of the other
   D. Bend at the knees while keeping your feet close together and side by side

2. When lifting, use the back, not the legs.
   A. True
   B. False

3. _____ injuries that result from improper lifting techniques are among the most common causes of injury and disability for prehospital personnel.
   A. Head
   B. Back
   C. Knee
   D. Neck

4. Use a minimum of _____ people to lift, even if a one person stretcher is being used.
   A. One
   B. Two
   C. Three
   D. Four

5. One of the most difficult carries an EMT must perform is to carry a patient _____ up the stairway.
   A. Frontward
   B. Sideways
   C. Backward
   D. Forward

6. Use your _____ muscles when log-rolling a patient.
   A. Hamstring
   B. Shoulder
   C. Gluteal
   D. Quadriceps

7. When pulling a patient, the EMT should keep the line of pull through the _____ of his body by bending the _____.
   A. Center, knees
   B. Center, arms
   C. Medial, back
   D. Periphery, ankles

8. The three categories of moves include all of the following *except:*
   A. Emergency
   B. Urgent
   C. Nonurgent
   D. Rapid

9. A patient should be moved promptly by an emergency move only when there is an immediate danger to the patient or rescuer, including:
   A. Fire or the danger of fire
   B. Danger of explosives or other hazardous materials
   C. An inability to protect the patient from other hazards at the scene
   D. All of the above

10. The motor vehicle collision is an example of a scene that frequently requires a(n) _____ move.
    A. Emergent
    B. Urgent
    C. Nonemergent
    D. Convalescent

11. The majority of moves required for patients are of a nonurgent nature.
    A. True
    B. False

12. The piece of equipment used most often for moving patients is the:
    A. Wheeled stretcher
    B. Stair chair
    C. Stokes basket
    D. Scoop stretcher

13. Stair chairs should *not* be used for patients who are:
    A. Unconscious
    B. Alert
    C. Medical rather than trauma patients
    D. Suspected of having a fractured upper extremity

14. Which piece of equipment would be used to lift and transport a multiple trauma patient?
    A. Flexible stretcher
    B. Stair chair
    C. Long backboard
    D. Scoop stretcher

15. Which of the following is a use of the backboard?
    A. Spinal immobilization
    B. Moving patients
    C. Removing the patient from a vehicle during rapid extrication
    D. All of the above

16. The patient with a suspected spinal injury who is moved with a scoop stretcher should be immediately placed on a long backboard for immobilization.
    A. True
    B. False

17. An unresponsive patient without suspected spinal injury should be placed in what position?
    A. On their back
    B. On their left side
    C. In a prone position
    D. In a seated position

18. A patient with chest pain, chest discomfort, or difficulty breathing should never be walked to the ambulance.
    A. True
    B. False

Case Scenario

You are dispatched to a residence for a sick person. On your arrival you are directed to the basement where you find a 78-year-old female patient sitting on a couch. She states that she started having pains in her stomach that radiated to her shoulder and that she is having a hard time catching her breath. You perform your assessment and treatment and are ready to transport her to the ambulance. The patient insists that she can walk upstairs.

1. Should you allow the patient to walk up the stairs? Why?

2. What device(s) would be appropriate to move the patient from the basement? Why?

Answer Key

Key Terms
1. Extremity lift
2. Blanket drag
3. Recovery
4. Bent arm drag
5. Direct ground lift
6. Emergency

Content Review
1. Consider the weight of the patient together with the weight of the stretcher or other equipment and determine if additional help is needed; know your physical ability and limitations; lift without twisting; position your feet a shoulder's width apart with one foot slightly in front of the other; wear proper boots; communicate clearly and frequently with your partner and with the patient; when lifting use the legs, not the back.

2. Keep your feet flat and a shoulder's width apart; the back is tight and the abdomen muscles lock the lower back in a slight inward curve; distribute the weight to the balls of the feet or just behind, keeping both feet fully in contact with the floor; while standing, keep the back locked in as the upper body comes up before the hips.

3. In the power grip the hands are positioned a minimum of 10 inches apart with the palms face up with palms and fingers in complete contact with the stretcher bar. It is used to get the maximum force from the hands.

4. False

5. Stair chair (if the patient can sit upright); scoop stretcher; canvas stretcher; or long back board (if the patient is unable to sit upright or is unconscious)

6. Keep your back in a locked-in position; when reaching overhead, avoid stretching or over-reaching; avoid twisting when reaching; keep your back straight when leaning over a patient; lean from the hips when reaching; use shoulder muscles to help with log rolls while reaching; avoid reaching more than 15 to 20 inches in front of your body; and avoid situations that require reaching and strenuous effort for more than 1 minute in order to avoid injury.

7. Keep your back in a locked-in position; keep elbows bent with the arms close to the sides; keep the line of pull through the center of your body by bending your knees; keep weight close to your body; push at a level between your waist and shoulders; if weight is below waist level, use a kneeling position when practical; avoid pushing and pulling from an overhead position.

8. Fire or the danger of fire; danger of explosives or other hazardous materials; the inability to protect the patient from other hazards at the scene; further violence erupting on the scene; the inability to gain access to other patients in a vehicle or other location who need life-saving care; or inability to provide care due to patient location or position.

9. Aggravating a spinal injury

10. 1) Clothing drag; 2) sheet drag; 3) blanket drag; and 4) bent arm drag

11. Secure the patient's wrists; clutch the patient's clothing on both sides of the neck to form a support for the head; pull the patient toward you as you back up, watching the patient at all times; be careful not to strangle the patient; the pulling force should be concentrated under the armpit, not the neck.

12. Fold or twist a sheet or large towel lengthwise; place the narrowed sheet across the chest at the level of the armpits; tuck the sheet ends under the armpits and behind the patient's head; grasp the two ends behind the head to form a support and a means for pulling; and pull the patient toward you while observing the patient at all times.

13. Lay a blanket lengthwise beside the patient; kneel on the opposite side of the patient and roll him or her toward you; as the patient lies on his or her side while resting against you, reach across and grab the blanket; tightly tuck half of the blanket lengthwise under the patient and leave the other half lying flat; gently roll the patient onto his or her back; pull the tucked portion of the blanket out from under the patient and wrap it around the body; grasp the blanket under the patient's head to form a support and means for pulling; pull while backing up and while observing the patient at all times.

14. Reach under the patient's armpits from behind and grasp the forearms or wrists, depending on the EMT's hand size; use your arms as a cradle for the patient's head and keep the arms locked in a bent position by your grasp; drag the patient toward you as you walk backward, observing the patient at all times.

15. Extreme weather conditions, hostile or interfering bystanders, environmental conditions such as rapidly rising water, or any factor at the scene that you determine is contributing or may contribute to a decline in the patient's status or risk to the EMT.

16. 1) Extremity lift; 2) direct ground lift; 3) direct carry; or 4) draw sheet method

17. 60 to 80; 400

18. Place the head end of the stretcher close to the bumper of the ambulance and make certain it is locked at the lowest level; with EMTs standing on opposite sides of the stretcher, bend at the knees while keeping backs straight and grasp the lowest bar of the stretcher; position hands at each end of the lowest bar with both palms facing up; on signal, both EMTs stand and move toward the rear

of the ambulance until the front wheels rest on the floor at the back of the ambulance; roll the stretcher forward and guide it into the front of the stretcher catch and lock the foot end into place.

19. With the stretcher in the highest position, place the head end into the rear of the ambulance; one EMT lifts the head end of the stretcher casing the wheels on the head end of the stretcher to contact the floor of the ambulance; the second EMT makes sure that the safety catch on the head of the stretcher engages with the hook on the floor of the ambulance; the second EMT then instructs the EMT at the foot end of the stretcher to pull the wheel adjustment lever on the left foot end of the stretcher; the second EMT then lifts the wheels of the stretcher and the EMT at the foot rolls it forward into the ambulance and secures it in place.

20. False

21. Adjust the length of the scoop stretcher on the ground beside the patient to accommodate the height of the patient; separate the stretcher halves and place one half on each side of the patient making certain not to lift the equipment over the patient; slightly lift the clothing on one side of the patient while another EMT slides one half of the scoop under the patient's side; repeat on the other side; if a spine injury is suspected, another EMT must maintain cervical spine control at all times; lock the head end of the scoop in place, then bring the foot end together until the assembly is locked; if any resistance is met, have an EMT gently lift one side of the patient; attach the padded head support strap if so equipped; secure the patient with at least three straps before lifting

22. The recovery position on his or her left side

23. On her left side

Chapter Quiz

1. C	6. B	11. A	15. D
2. B	7. A	12. A	16. A
3. B	8. D	13. A	17. B
4. B	9. D	14. C	18. A
5. C	10. B		

Case Scenario

1. No. A patient with chest pain or difficulty breathing should never walk on his or her own. The patient may have an unstable gait, and if she loses her balance, she may fall down the stairs. In addition, the walk my cause the patient to exert too much energy and exacerbate the illness.

2. A stair chair would be most appropriate. While a stretcher could be used, it is difficult and strenuous to carry upstairs.

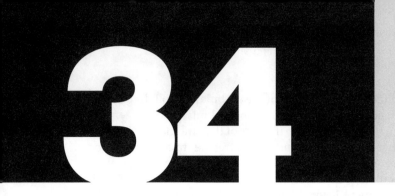

Communications

Reading Assignment: Chapter 34 pages 686–700.

DOT Objectives
···

Upon successful completion of the EMT-Basic training program, the EMT-Basic should be able to do the following:

- List the proper methods for initiation and termination of a radio call.
- State the proper sequence for delivery of patient information.
- Identify the essential components of the verbal report.
- Describe the attributes for increasing the effectiveness and efficiency of verbal communication.
- State the legal aspects to consider in verbal communication.
- Discuss the communication skills that should be used to interact with the patient.
- Discuss the communication skills that should be used to interact with the family members, bystanders, and individuals from other agencies while providing patient care.
- Discuss the difference between skills used to interact with the patient and those used to interact with others.
- List the correct radio procedures in the following phases of a typical call:
  - To the scene
  - At the scene
  - To the medical facility
  - At the medical facility
  - To the station
  - At the station
- Perform a simulated, organized, concise radio transmission.
- Perform an organized, concise patient report that would be given to the staff at a receiving facility.
- Perform a brief, organized report that would be given to an advanced life support (ALS) provider arriving at an incident scene at which the EMT-Basic was already providing care.

Supplemental Objectives
···

- Describe the importance of communication in an EMS system.
- Identify the components of an EMS communication system.
- Describe the various methods that are available to the public to access the EMS system.
- Explain the basic principles of emergency medical dispatch.
- Describe the process for dispatching EMS agencies, including the use of computer-aided dispatch.
- Describe the role of radio communication between the EMT and medical direction.
- Identify the six elements of the "six way" communications model.

- Demonstrate appropriate use of radio communication with the dispatch center in various phases of an ambulance call.

Key Terms

· ·

1. A radio unit that receives a signal from another radio unit and re-broadcasts it boosting the signal strength in the process to overcome dispatcher or geographic obstacles is called a(n) _____ _____.

2. A radio that is operated at a fixed site such as a dispatch center, hospital, or some other location that does not move and transmits at a much higher power than do smaller, portable radios is called a(n) _____.

3. A radio that is mounted on a vehicle and operates off of the vehicle's electrical supply is called a(n) _____.

4. A set of radio frequencies between 150 and 174 MHz that are limited to "line of site" communication because they cannot bend around obstacles or the curve of the earth is called a(n) _____ band.

5. A set of radio frequencies between 32 and 50 MHz that can travel a great distance but are subject to interference is called a(n) _____ band.

6. A set of radio frequencies between 450 and 470 MHz that are almost interference-free but are limited to line of site and travel only short distances is called a(n) _____ band.

7. Computer-controlled radio equipment used in sophisticated communication systems, usually in the 800 MHz range, is called _____ equipment.

8. An approach to deployment of EMS resources (people and vehicles) that seeks to achieve maximum efficiency with minimal sacrifice in quality of care and uses computer modeling techniques to predict EMS call volume and location, thereby allowing systems to position vehicles in the most efficient locations is called _____.

9. An approach to the dispatch function of an EMS system that involves the dispatcher in making decisions about the type and priority of EMS response necessary, providing critical information to responding units while en route, and providing pre-arrival instructions to callers until the EMS units are on the scene is called _____.

10. The transmission of electronic signals over the radio, the most frequent use of which is transmission of an electrocardiogram, is called _____.

Content Review

1. List the equipment or hardware that operates in an EMS communication system.

2. Portable radios provide for a safer workforce due to the EMT's constant link to the dispatch center.
   A. True
   B. False

3. Describe the differences between the following three bands of radio channels.

   VHF low band:

   VHF high band:

   UHF band:

4. VHF low band systems usually work best on their own.
   A. True
   B. False

5. Because of the lack of interference, UHF frequencies most often are used for _____
   _____.

6. Radio waves in the _____ range of frequencies are clean and interference free, using digital radio equipment and numerous repeaters.

7. Describe the advantages and disadvantages of cellular telephones.

   Advantages:

   Disadvantages:

8. The use of AVL devices helps to select the closest resource to respond to an emergency.
   A. True
   B. False

9. Identify the factors that influence the public's access to an EMS system.

10. Describe three methods for accessing the EMS system.

   1)

   2)

   3)

11. The single location where all 9-1-1 calls arrive is called a(n) _____
   _____.

12. Describe the six steps in the communication process.

   1)

   2)

   3)

   4)

   5)

   6)

13. Identify the general principles of radio use.

14. What are the two objectives of communication with the medical director or hospital?

1)

2)

15. List the essential elements and proper sequence of a prehospital care report to the hospital.

16. Identify the essential elements of a verbal report to hospital staff.

17. Identify the essential principles of interpersonal communication.

18. Identify special situations that may create communication challenges.

Chapter Quiz

1. The type of radio installed in the ambulance is called a:
   A. Base station
   B. Mobile unit
   C. Portable unit
   D. Manual unit

2. A device that receives a low-power transmission and re-transmits the signal at higher power is called a:
   A. Remote station
   B. Base station
   C. Repeater
   D. Beeper

3. A radio that is located at a stationary site such as a hospital, mountain top, or public safety agency is called a:
   A. Repeater
   B. Base station
   C. Mobile radio
   D. Portable radio

4. The simplest way to make sure everyone understands what is being said is to:
   A. Communicate in plain English
   B. Use only written communication
   C. Speak softly into the microphone
   D. Speak rapidly in a soft tone

5. All of the following are reasons that prehospital personnel need to communicate with the hospital *except:*
   A. To communicate with a physician
   B. To receive medical direction
   C. To provide the ED with notice of the patient's arrival so preparations can begin
   D. To explain your need to replace supplies used during the call

6. When considering the proper sequence for delivery of patient information, which of the following items should be stated first when giving a report to the hospital?
   A. BP is 140/100
   B. Patient is allergic to penicillin
   C. 65-year-old male
   D. History of asthma

7. Mobile radios are radios that are mounted in vehicles such as ambulances or fire engines and are much less powerful than portable radios.
   A. True
   B. False

8. The center of the communication system is called the _____ and employs a special group of people who receive calls for assistance and dispatch emergency personnel and vehicles.
   A. Dispatch facility
   B. Incident command facility
   C. Command center
   D. Mobile transmitter

9. Public access to an EMS system is influenced by which of the following factors:
   A. Capability of local telephone company equipment
   B. Public service budgets of local and regional governments
   C. Competition within single political jurisdictions over control of public access
   D. All of the above

10. The most common method for accessing the EMS system is the:
    A. Telephone
    B. Roadside call boxes
    C. E 911 system
    D. Repeater

11. General principles of radio use include all of the following *except:*
    A. Make sure the radio is turned on and properly adjusted
    B. Listen to the frequency to make sure there is no other traffic before transmitting
    C. Speak clearly and distinctly
    D. Press the talk switch on the microphone and wait 10 seconds

12. Pre-notification of the patient's arrival can dramatically reduce the time interval between arrival at the emergency department and initiation of definitive treatment.
    A. True
    B. False

13. The essential elements of a radio report to the receiving facility include which of the following?
    A. Identification of the unit and level of provider
    B. Estimated time of arrival (ETA)
    C. Age and sex of the patient
    D. All of the above

14. A brief description of the symptoms of which the patient is complaining is called the:
    A. Chief symptom
    B. Primary complaint
    C. Chief complaint
    D. Diagnosis

15. EMS personnel should notify the dispatcher as soon as the unit leaves the scene with the patient to let the dispatcher know that:
    A. The unit is back in service and ready for another call
    B. Work on the scene is concluded and transport has begun
    C. The patient's condition has improved
    D. All of the above

16. The EMT should notify the receiving hospital of any changes in patient condition or response to treatment en route to the receiving facility.
    A. True
    B. False

17. At the receiving hospital, it is appropriate for the EMT to turn responsibility for a patient over to any of the following individuals *except:*
    A. Physician
    B. Registered nurse
    C. Licensed practical nurse
    D. Admissions clerk

18. General principles of interpersonal communication include all of the following *except:*
    A. Act and speak in a calm and confident manner
    B. Do not look directly at the patient
    C. Speak clearly, slowly, and distinctly
    D. Treat the patient with respect

19. When dealing with hearing-impaired patients, the EMT should:
    A. Always speak clearly with his or her lips clearly visible to the patient
    B. Learn basic sign language to help with communication
    C. Exchange written notes with the patient
    D. All of the above

Case Scenario

· ·

You are dispatched to a residence for a sick person. On your arrival, you are met by a very upset elderly female who informs you that her 76-year-old husband, who has undergone two bypass surgeries in the past 2 years, awoke with severe chest pain 10 minutes ago. He is currently taking Coumadin and has no allergies.

You enter the patient's bedroom and find him sitting up in the bed, clutching his chest. He is sweating profusely and appears anxious. He rates the pain as a 7 on a scale of 1 to 10 and denies experiencing any shortness of breath. His skin is cool and pale. Initial vital signs are: BP, 172/90; VR, 24; and P, 72 and regular. You note no jugular vein distention, and breath sounds are clear and equal bilaterally. You administer high-concentration oxygen via a non-rebreather mask at a rate of 15 L/min and load the patient into the ambulance. You anticipate a travel time of 10 minutes to the hospital.

1. List the proper sequence for delivery of patient information to the receiving hospital.

Skill Sheet #35

•••

RADIO COMMUNICATION – Essential Elements

Start Time: _____

Stop Time: _____   **Date:** _____

Candidate's Name: _____

Evaluator's Name: _____

	Points Possible	Points Awarded
Identify unit and level of provider	1	
Identify estimated time of arrival (ETA) at destination hospital	1	
Identify the age and sex of the patient	1	
Identify the patient's chief complaint, including signs and symptoms and MOI/NOI	1	
Provide a *brief*, pertinent history of the present illness	1	
List any major past illnesses	1	
Identify any medications the patient is currently taking or any allergies that the patient has	1	
Describe the patient's state of responsiveness and alertness	1	
List baseline vital signs	1	
Report any significant findings of the physical examination	1	
Identify emergency medical care given to the patient	1	
Identify any response to emergency medical care initiated	1	
Total:	12	

Critical Criteria

_____ Did not identify pertinent information necessary for the receiving hospital to properly prepare for the patient

_____ Provided confidential information over the air (such as patient's name)

Answer Key

....

Key Terms
1. Repeater
2. Base station
3. Mobile radio
4. VHF high
5. VHF low
6. UHF
7. Digital radio
8. System status management
9. Emergency medical dispatch (EMD)
10. Telemetry

Content Review
1. A base station; mobile two-way radios; portable handheld radios; repeaters; radio frequencies; cellular telephones; automatic vehicle location (AVL) devices; and automatic crash notification (ACN) systems
2. True
3. VHF Low Band: A group of radio frequencies between 32 and 50 MHz that are able to curve and follow the shape of the earth or other obstacles, thus allowing communication over long distances; most susceptible to interference from buildings, electrical equipment, or weather. VHF High Band: A set of radio frequencies between 150 and 174 MHz, with waves that travel in a straight line and do not bend to follow the curve of the earth or around obstacles but are limited to "line of site", and are less susceptible to the interference that bothers low-band communication.
   UHF Band: A set of radio frequencies between 450 and 470 MHz range and are almost interference free, offer some of the cleanest communication frequencies available, but only travel short distances and are limited to "line of site."
4. False
5. Telemetry
6. 800 MHz
7. Advantages: They are relatively inexpensive, highly effective, readily available, usually very small and very portable, and an instant form of mobile communication.
   Disadvantages: There are no protected channels or frequencies for EMS as there are in VHF, UHF, and 800 MHz bands and in many moderate to large scale emergencies, they are almost useless because channels are used up very quickly by the public, other responders, and the news media.
8. True
9. Capability of local telephone company equipment; public service budgets of local and regional governments; formal politics between differing jurisdictions; and competition within a single political jurisdiction over control of public access
10. 1) A 7-digit access number—the most common method for accessing the system; which number to dial is determined by which community the call is made from; if traveling or away from home, a caller would be forced to use a phone book or go through the operator to find help. 2) 9-1-1—a simpler, more efficient and user-friendly method of access using a number that could be used everywhere; the caller need not worry about which number to call; when 9-1-1 is dialed the telephone company computer and switchers route the call to the appropriate dispatch center based on the origin of the call. 3) Enhanced 9-1-1—builds on the original principles of 9-1-1 and adds computer technology so the dispatcher can immediately see the street or billing address of incoming calls based on phone company records.
11. Public safety answering point (PSAP)

12. 1) The sender *thinks* of an idea (what they need to say); 2) the sender *transmits* the message through some type of media (phone, radio); 3) *transfer* of the message occurs through the media (phone lines, radio); 4) the receiver *obtains* the message through a receiver (background noise must be kept to a minimum); 5) the receiver *interprets* the message using his brain, logic, education, etc.; 6) the receiver *confirms* the message, thereby 'closing' the communication loop.

13. Make sure the radio is turned on and properly adjusted; listen to the frequency to make sure there is no other traffic before transmitting; think through the message before pushing the transmit button; press the push-to-talk switch on the microphone and wait for 1 second before speaking; speak clearly and distinctly; use plain English; keep transmissions brief and avoid the use of unnecessary phrases such as "thank you" or "please"; and remember that every word is being transmitted over radio waves, which can be picked up by anyone with a scanner—protect the patient's privacy.

14. 1) It provides the opportunity for EMTs to receive instructions or advice; 2) it notifies the receiving hospital personnel so they can prepare for the patient

15. Unit and level of provider; ETA; age and sex of patient; chief complaint; brief, pertinent history of present illness; major past illnesses; mental status; baseline vital signs; pertinent findings of the physical examination; emergency medical care given; and response to emergency medical care given

16. Identify the EMT and unit; introduce the patient to hospital personnel; summarize the information provided over the radio (chief complaint and pertinent history not previously relayed); give additional interventions made en route; and advise of any significant changes in vital signs or response to interventions noted en route

17. Act and speak in a calm and confident manner; make (and maintain) eye contact with the patient; speak clearly, slowly, and distinctly; treat the patient with respect; use words the patient can understand; be honest and direct with the patient; and be constantly aware of both the patient's and your body language.

18. Hearing and/or speech-impaired patients; non-English speaking patients; children; the elderly

Chapter Quiz

1. B	6. C	11. D	16. A
2. C	7. B	12. A	17. D
3. B	8. A	13. D	18. B
4. A	9. D	14. C	19. D
5. D	10. A	15. B	

Case Scenario

1. *ID unit and level of provider.* ETA is 10 minutes. Inbound with a 76-year-old male patient complaining of severe chest pain, which woke him from sleep 10 minutes prior to EMS arrival and rates a 7 on a scale of 1 to 10. The patient denies shortness of breath and has a history of cardiovascular surgery for which he is on Coumadin. He has no allergies. On physical examination, his skin is cool, pale, and diaphoretic. Vital signs are as follows: BP is 172/90, pulse is 72 and regular, and ventilations are 24 and normal. There is no JVD and lungs are clear and equal bilaterally. Oxygen is being administered at 15 L/min via a non-rebreather mask. *Identify any response to care initiated.*

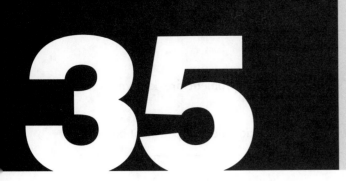

35

Reading Assignment: Chapter 35 pages 701–714.

DOT Objectives

Upon successful completion of the EMT-Basic training program, the EMT-Basic should be able to do the following:

- List, explain, and apply the components of essential patient information in a written report.
- Identify the various divisions of the written report.
- Describe the information required in each section of the prehospital care report and how it should be entered.
- Discuss the legal implications associated with the written report.
- Define the special considerations concerning patient refusal.
- Discuss all state and/or local record and reporting requirements.
- Complete a prehospital care report.

Supplemental Objectives

- State the proper sequence of delivery of patient information.
- Explain the reasons for appropriate documentation and reporting of patient care information.
- Explain the purpose of gathering and reporting information.

Key Terms

1. A form used for making notes during the assessment and history taking process is known as a(n) _____.

2. A diagram of the anterior and posterior view of an anatomic figure located on a prehospital care report is called a(n) _____.

3. One format for a PCR that is completed using an electronic clipboard or mobile data terminal is known as a(n) _____.

4. The official or formal documentation of the physical assessment and care provided to a particular patient is called a(n) _____.

5. Events or complaints associated with the patient's current health problem are known as the _____.

6. The standardized rating system used to evaluate the degree of consciousness impairment based on eye opening, motor response, and verbal response is called the _____ _____.

7. The standardized injury severity index used in pediatric patients is known as the _____ _____.

8. A head-to-toe, hands-on examination is called a(n) _____.

9. The standardized injury severity index that incorporates the GCS and the measurements for the systolic BP and respiratory rate is called the _____.

10. Specific information about the ambulance call that is documented on a PCR such as the ambulance service name and unit number, the location of the call, the response times, and the mileage is known as _____.

11. The presence of a sign or symptoms that helps to substantiate or identify a patient's condition is known as a(n) _____.

12. Any prior or current medical condition, surgery, hospitalization, illness or injury suffered by the patient that might be relative to the patient's current medical condition is known as the _____ _____.

13. The absence of a sign or symptom that helps to substantiate or identify a patient's condition is known as a(n) _____.

Content Review
· ·

1. What is the purpose of proper documentation?

2. A PCR typically has three divisions. What are they?

1)

2)

3)

3. What is the narrative section of a PCR?

4. Proper spelling and general neatness are essential for the PCR in order to convey professionalism.
   A. True
   B. False

5. List the general guidelines and important information to include when completing a PCR.

6. Describe the SOAP method for documentation.

   S:

   O:

   A:

   P:

7. Describe the head-to-toe method of documentation.

8. Describe the chronologic method of documentation.

9. What should you do if you make a mistake while completing the PCR?

10. What should you do if a mistake is discovered following the completion and/or submission of a PCR?

11. What should the EMT include when documenting a patient's refusal of care?

Chapter Quiz

1. The PCR is the official documentation of the physical assessment and treatment of a particular patient.
   A. True
   B. False

2. The patient data includes which of the following?
   A. The patient's name and home address
   B. Date of birth and sex
   C. Age and nature of call
   D. All of the above

3. The narrative section of the PCR is provided for the EMT to document observations at the scene, assessment findings, and care and treatment delivered by the EMS crew.
   A. True
   B. False

4. If a space on the PCR does not apply to the patient, the EMT should:
   A. Mark it N/A
   B. Leave it blank
   C. Print the EMT's initials in the space
   D. Put a question mark in the space

5. The prehospital care report should document the care delivered:
   A. At the scene
   B. En route to the hospital
   C. Prior to arrival of the EMS
   D. All of the above

6. The prehospital care report includes which of the following information:
   A. The patient's name, address, age, and sex
   B. The location of the emergency scene
   C. Findings of the assessment
   D. All of the above

7. Blank spaces in a PCR lead the reader to believe the report is not thorough or complete because information seems to be missing.
   A. True
   B. False

8. Finding that the abdomen is soft and nontender to palpation in a patient complaining of abdominal pain is a:
   A. Pertinent negative
   B. Pertinent positive
   C. Insignificant finding
   D. False finding

9. The head-to-toe method of documentation includes all of the following *except:*
   A. The patient's age, sex, LOC, and initial presentation
   B. Results of the initial and focused assessments
   C. Treatment and care delivered
   D. The name of the family physician

10. Documentation based on the chronologic progress of the call usually begins with the time of arrival on the scene.
    A. True
    B. False

11. If a mistake is made while writing the narrative or on any part of the PCR, the EMT should:
    A. Erase the mistake and continue the report
    B. Mark out the mistake and initial it
    C. Draw a single line through the mistake and initial it
    D. Use correction fluid to cover the mistake and continue the report

12. When a mistake is discovered following the completion and/or submission of the report, the EMT should:
    A. Draw a single line through the error and initial it
    B. Draw a double line through the error and initial it
    C. Add a note with the correct information and initial it
    D. Both A and C

13. In the event that information was omitted from a prehospital care report, the EMT should:
    A. Add a note with the information, current date, and EMT's initials
    B. Not be concerned about the omission
    C. Make the correction on the report
    D. Make a mental note in case the report is later used

14. The EMT must ensure that the patient refusing care is:
    A. Able to make a rational, informed decision
    B. Not under the influence of drugs or alcohol
    C. Not under the effects of an illness or injury
    D. All of the above

15. If a patient refuses care, the patient should be:
    A. Encouraged to accept care
    B. Informed why he needs to go to the hospital
    C. Informed of what may happen if he does not accept care
    D. All of the above

16. When documenting the refusal of care, the EMT should include which of the following in the narrative of the PCR:
    A. Complete patient assessment findings, including vital signs
    B. Care that the EMS crew offered to provide
    C. The fact the patient was advised of possible consequences of refusing care and alternative care options
    D. All of the above

17. The narrative of a prehospital care report can be written using all of the following *except:*
    A. The SOAP method
    B. The head-to-toe method
    C. Chronologic order
    D. The PAOS method

18. The initial S in SOAP refers to:
    A. Treatment delivered by the EMT
    B. What the patient tells the EMT about his condition
    C. What the EMT observes about the patient
    D. The patient's overall condition

19. If the patient continues to refuse care, the EMT should do all of the following *except:*
    A. Have the patient sign a refusal form
    B. Have the form signed by a witness
    C. Contact medical direction (if required by local policy)
    D. Leave the scene immediately

Case Scenario

You and your partner arrive on the scene of an attempted murder. Law enforcement has secured the scene. As you approach the patient, you notice the patient has a gunshot wound in the upper right portion of his back with both entrance and exit wounds. The patient is breathing and has a pulse. You decide that the patient is critical and call for immediate transport.

1. List at least six items that should be documented in the PCR.

Answer Key

Key Terms
1. Field assessment card
2. Injury location chart
3. Computer-based report
4. Patient care report (PCR)
5. History of present illness or injury (HPI)
6. Glasgow coma scale (GCS)
7. Pediatric trauma score (PTS)
8. Physical assessment
9. Revised trauma score (RTS)
10. Run data
11. Pertinent positive
12. Pertinent past medical history (PMH)
13. Pertinent negative

Content Review
1. It provides a record of scene information that may not be available from any other source; provides information for the continuity of patient care from one healthcare provider to another; provides a record of specific prehospital interventions performed or attempted; provides medicolegal evidence; reveals any significant changes in the patient's condition; provides an internal tool for statistics, budgeting, QA/improvement, and education; and reveals problems with record-keeping procedures.
2. 1) Run data; 2) patient data; and 3) narrative
3. It provides for the EMT to document observations at the scene, physical assessment findings, care delivered by the EMS crew, and changes in the patient's condition.
4. True
5. Collect all patient information (name, DOB, sex, age, address, insurance/billing information if necessary); complete all blanks and check all pertinent boxes; begin the narrative by documenting the patient's LOC, age, and how he or she appears initially; document the patient's chief complaint; document HPI, physical assessment findings (including pertinent positives or pertinent negatives), any significant PMH, allergies, and current medication; document interventions, who performed them, and the patient's response or lack of response to the intervention; document vital signs and any orders received from the medical director; attach electrocardiogram documentation (where applicable) with date, time, and patient's name on it; complete the GCS, RTS or Rule of Nines, if required; complete

the injury location chart, if indicated; sign the report and obtain the receiving nurse's or physician's name and/or signature as needed; and leave a copy of the report with the patient's chart.

6. S: Subjective information—what the patient tells the EMT regarding his complaint
   O: Objective information—what the EMT observes about the scene and any obvious patient injuries
   A: Assessment—the EMT's evaluation of the situation, the patient, his or her chief complaint, and findings based on a physical examination
   P: Plan—the plan of action and the care delivered by the EMT

7. Documenting the assessment the way it is performed—head-to-toe; begins with the patient's age, sex, and LOC; how the patient was found initially; then lists the results of the initial assessment and focused history and exam; concluding with interventions and care delivered.

8. Documentation based on the chronologic progress of the call, beginning with the time of arrival on the scene; each entry begins with a time notation.

9. Do not erase or mark out the mistake; simply draw a single line through the error and place your initials beside the line; then write the correct information next to the line.

10. Draw a single line through the error with a different color ink; initial and date the line along with the time and add a note with the correct information; initial it.

11. A complete patient assessment, including vital signs and/or the refusal of assessment; care the EMS crew wished and/or offered to provide to the patient; a statement that the EMT explained to the patient the possible consequences of refusing care, including adverse effects and potential death; the offer of alternative methods for accessing care; and a statement of the crew's willingness to return should the patient's condition change or the patient decide to seek medical attention.

Chapter Quiz

1. A	6. D	11. C	16. D
2. D	7. A	12. D	17. D
3. A	8. A	13. A	18. B
4. A	9. D	14. D	19. D
5. D	10. A	15. D	

Case Scenario

1. Age and gender of the patient; position of the patient on arrival; the patient's LOC at the scene; location of injury; description of the wound; type of weapon used (if readily apparent); treatment provided; vital signs; approximate amount of blood lost; who removed the clothing; who received the clothing (chain of evidence); who received the patient; information provided by the patient; and who was present at the scene. Documentation should only contain objective information, not supposition or conjecture.

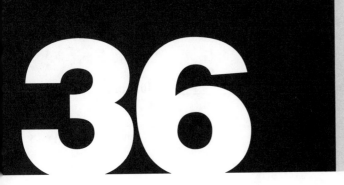

Quality Improvement

Reading Assignment: Chapter 36 pages 715–723.

DOT Objectives

Upon successful completion of the EMT-Basic training program, the EMT-Basic should be able to do the following:

• Define quality improvement and discuss the EMT's role in the process.

Supplemental Objectives

• Define quality assurance and continuous quality improvement.
• Define the terms *prospective evaluation, concurrent evaluation,* and *retrospective evaluation* as they apply to quality assurance.
• Describe four methods used in a continuous quality control program in which an EMT is likely to become involved.

Key Terms

1. A method of quality assurance that involves assessing actual calls with EMTs in order to review the quality of care delivered by the EMS system is called a(n) _____.

2. The quality evaluation tool used after an EMS response has occurred, such as a PCR review, is called a(n) _____ evaluation.

3. A method of continually assessing and improving the care delivered in the EMS system is known as _____.

4. The quality evaluation method used prior to an EMS response (such as skills check off) is called _____.

5. A method of improving a certain aspect or skill of an EMT by providing one-on-one training or coaching is called _____.

6. Ongoing educational experience provided to EMS personnel is called _____ _____.

7. Evaluating the quality of care as it is being given is called _____ evaluation.

Content Review

1. Define quality assurance.

2. How does CQI differ from QA?

3. List some commonly tracked items in EMS systems.

4. Identify and briefly describe the three methods of evaluating quality.

   1)

   2)

   3)

Chapter Quiz

1. An example of a prospective form of quality evaluation would be:
   A. The prehospital care report (PCR) review
   B. The physician riding along with the ambulance crew
   C. Skills check off
   D. On-line medical direction

2. An example of a retrospective form of quality evaluation would be:
   A. Prehospital care report (PCR) review
   B. Physician ride along with the ambulance crew
   C. Skills check off
   D. On-line medical direction

3. Types of evaluation used to measure quality include all of the following *except:*
   A. Retrospective
   B. PCR review
   C. Skill evaluation
   D. Recurrent review

4. Methods of CQI with which the EMT may become involved include which of the following:
   A. Data collection
   B. Case reviews
   C. Continuing education
   D. All of the above

5. Quality assurance is defined as a mix of activities designed to evaluate how well the EMS system and EMTs take care of patients.
   A. True
   B. False

6. Methods of measurement to determine if care is delivered in a timely, efficient, and medically sensible manner include all of the following *except:*
   A. Response times
   B. Patient survival
   C. Skills proficiency
   D. Salaries and benefits

7. Important aspects of QA include evaluating all of the following *except:*
   A. Training
   B. Performance
   C. Patient care
   D. Cross training

8. Continuous quality improvement differs from QA in that it strives to continuously improve how the system takes care of patients.
   A. True
   B. False

9. CQI includes which of the following:
   A. Improving the quality of continuing education
   B. Updating treatment protocols
   C. Skills evaluation and remediation
   D. All of the above

10. Quality assurance measures system or individual performance against a certain standard, whereas CQI uses evaluation to continuously improve the EMS system.
    A. True
    B. False

11. The basic methods available to medical directors for evaluating the quality of EMT performance include all of the following *except:*
    A. Prospective
    B. Concurrent
    C. Retrospective
    D. Preactive

12. Prospective evaluation tools are designed to improve the care delivered by the EMS system:
    A. Prior to responding to a call
    B. While responding to a call
    C. After responding to a call
    D. While delivering patient care

13. The prospective type of evaluation is generally thought to be the most valuable because it allows care to be improved before the emergency call takes place.
    A. True
    B. False

14. Concurrent evaluation in CQI programs includes which of the following:
    A. The direct observation of care delivered by the EMT
    B. A physician providing on-line medical direction
    C. A medical director riding along with the EMT to observe patient care delivered in the field
    D. All of the above

15. Concurrent evaluation is the most useful kind of evaluation to the:
    A. Medical director
    B. Dispatcher
    C. Hospital administrator
    D. ED staff

16. Retrospective evaluation includes methods that are applied:
    A. After the call is completed
    B. While the EMT is responding to the call
    C. Before the EMT completes the call
    D. While the EMT is delivering patient care

17. Retrospective methods of evaluation are the most commonly used because of:
    A. Ease
    B. Cost
    C. Convenience
    D. All of the above

18. Which of the following methods can medical directors use to review what happened after an EMS call?
    A. PCR reviews
    B. Case reviews
    C. Debriefings
    D. All of the above

19. EMTs become involved in the quality improvement loop as:
    A. Data collectors
    B. Valuable participants in the analysis phase
    C. Subjects of change (either in training or individual performance)
    D. All of the above

20. A method that helps the EMT identify the aspects of patient care that are important to the medical director is:
    A. Peer review
    B. Continuing education
    C. Case review
    D. Trends review

Case Scenario

You are the continuing education coordinator for your local ambulance service. You are scheduling the next session and discuss possible topics with fellow EMTs. Your partner suggests a review of patient assessment and vital signs techniques. Others agree that this would be a worthwhile session. You then receive a call for a sick person. Your medical director, Dr. Evans, is also present and elects to take the call with you and your new partner whom you are orienting.

On your arrival you find a 72-year-old female patient complaining of dizziness for the past hour. The patient appears alert and oriented and in no apparent distress. You instruct your partner to take a blood pressure reading. He complies but then asks you to "double check" his reading. The blood pressure you obtain differs significantly from your partner's.

You complete the patient assessment and transport the patient to the hospital without incident. On arrival back at the station, Dr. Evans informs you and your partner that he is very pleased with the quality of care your crew delivered. He then reviews the call and your prehospital care report to see if anything was overlooked or could be improved on. Your partner informs you and Dr. Evans that he seems to have difficulty auscultating a blood pressure in the field. On review, Dr. Evans determines that your partner was overlooking the importance of correct stethoscope placement during blood pressure assessment. Dr. Evans reviews the proper procedure with your partner.

1. What type of quality evaluation methods are being used in this scenario?

2. What benefits would you, your crew, and your medical director receive from the activity described in this scenario?

3. How is patient care improved by the activity described in this scenario?

Answer Key

. . . .

Key Terms
1. Case review
2. Retrospective
3. Continuous quality improvement (CQI)
4. Prospective evaluation
5. Remediation
6. Continuing education
7. Concurrent

Content Review
1. A mix of activities designed to evaluate how well the EMS system and EMTs take care of patients.
2. CQI strives to continuously improve how the system takes care of patients. It examines the performance of all aspects of the EMS system and makes changes to continuously improve the system.
3. Types of calls, response times; on-scene times; patient survival rates; and percentage of extrications done in less than 15 minutes
4. 1) Prospective—quality evaluation method used prior to an EMS response, such as skills check-off; 2) concurrent—evaluating the quality of care as it is being given, such as physician ride-alongs; and 3) retrospective—a quality evaluation tool used after an EMS response has occurred, such as with a PCR review.

Chapter Quiz
1. C	6. D	11. D	16. A
2. A	7. D	12. A	17. D
3. D	8. A	13. A	18. D
4. D	9. D	14. D	19. D
5. A	10. A	15. A	20. C

Case Scenario
1. Quality evaluation methods in this scenario include prospective, concurrent, and retrospective. Identifying and addressing a weakness in an EMT's skills before an EMS call is considered a prospective quality evaluation method. This method is very valuable when the medical director participates because the EMT learns first hand what the physician expects when it comes to patient care, and the physician learns, first hand, the conditions in which the EMT performs skills. Evaluating the EMT skills during patient care is considered a concurrent evaluation method, and reviewing the call is considered a retrospective quality evaluation method.
2. All parties benefit a great deal from this prospective evaluation. The medical director has the opportunity to observe first hand what type of care you and your crew are likely to deliver as well as to evaluate identified weaknesses.
3. Patient care is improved through the application of the prospective, concurrent, and retrospective evaluation methods. EMT skills are evaluated and improved. The physician demonstrates how the EMT can improve care based on evaluation of skills, and this process established a quality improvement loop.

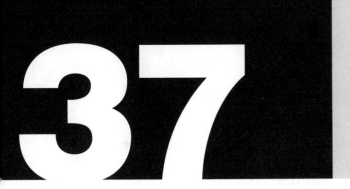

Ambulance Operations

Reading Assignment: Chapter 37 pages 724-741.

DOT Objectives
....

Upon successful completion of the EMT-Basic training program, the EMT-Basic should be able to do the following:

- Identify the medical and non-medical equipment needed to respond to a call.
- List the phases of an ambulance call.
- Describe the general provisions of state laws relating to the operation of an emergency vehicle, including speed, warning lights, sirens, right-of-way, parking, and turning.
- List contributing factors to unsafe driving conditions.
- Describe the considerations that should be given to requests for escorts, following an escort vehicle, and intersections.
- Describe the concept of "due regard for safety of others" while operating an emergency vehicle.
- Identify the essential information for responding to a call.
- Identify factors that may affect response to a call.
- Summarize the importance of preparing the unit for the next response.
- Differentiate among the various methods of moving a patient to the unit based on injury or illness.
- Apply the components of the essential patient information in a written report.
- Identify what is essential for completion of a call.
- Describe how to clean or disinfect items following patient care.

Supplemental Objectives
....

- Explain the rationale for preparing the unit to respond.

Key Terms
....

1. The term used to describe an appropriately trained and qualified driver of an emergency vehicle is

   _____.

2. An ambulance that is a cab and chassis with a modular body mounted on a frame with a walkway between the patient compartment and the driver compartment is a Type _____ ambulance.

3. An ambulance that is a conventional cab and chassis with a modular body (box) without a walkway is a Type _____ ambulance.

4. An ambulance that is essentially a converted van, usually with a raised roof, where the driver's and patient's area form an integral unit is a Type _____ ambulance.

Content Review

1. The federal requirements for ambulances are called _____ standards.

2. What organization developed a variety of requirements concerning ambulances and equipment as they related to the prevention of transmission of infectious diseases?

3. Identify patient lifting and moving equipment that should be carried on the ambulance.

4. What fracture management equipment should be stored on the ambulance?

5. What poisoning treatment supplies should be carried on the ambulance?

6. What safety equipment should be stored on the ambulance?

7. What items should the EMT visually check on the exterior of the ambulance, while the engine is off?

8. What items should the EMT check under the hood of the ambulance, while the engine is off?

9. List the characteristics needed for a good EVO.

10. Identify situations that may affect the response to a call.

11. The EVO should use all warning lights during a response.
    A. True
    B. False

12. The EVO should use the _____ rule when following a vehicle.

13. What is the 4-second rule?

14. Laws concerning the operation of emergency vehicles generally allow the operator leniency with normal traffic laws and traffic control devices as long as visual and audible warning devices are in use and the vehicle is operated with due regard for the safety of others.
    A. True
    B. False

15. The use of an escort, such as a police unit, will allow the ambulance to travel faster to or from a scene and should be used when possible.
    A. True
    B. False

16. List the guidelines which should be followed to make multiple responding units as safe as possible.

17. Where do most crashes involving emergency vehicles occur?

18. What steps should you take if a crash occurs while operating an emergency vehicle?

19. Where should the ambulance be parked at a potentially hazardous scene?

Chapter Quiz

1. The Type I ambulance has:
   A. A conventional cab
   B. A chassis with a modular ambulance body
   C. No passageway between the patient and driver compartments
   D. All of the above

2. The Type II ambulance is essentially a converted van, usually with a raised roof, where the driver and patient areas form an integral unit.
   A. True
   B. False

3. Standards adopted by many state and local jurisdictions for ambulances purchased by the federal government are known as the _____ standards.
   A. OSHA
   B. ICC
   C. KKK
   D. AAA

4. Factors that may dictate different quantities and kinds of equipment carried in the ambulance include all of the following *except:*
   A. Type of service normally delivered in your area
   B. Transport times
   C. Local statutes or regulations
   D. Average age of patients

5. Biohazard disposal bags are an example of equipment that is:
   A. FCC compliant
   B. OSHA compliant
   C. FDA compliant
   D. NIH compliant

6. All of the following are examples of items necessary to monitor a patient's condition *except:*
   A. Sphygmomanometers
   B. Stethoscopes
   C. Flow meters
   D. Thermometers

7. Non-medical equipment includes:
   A. Safety equipment
   B. Equipment used to extricate victims
   C. Comprehensive street maps
   D. All of the above

8. A variety of emergency vehicle driving courses are offered that have been developed by:
   A. Department of Transportation
   B. National Safety Council
   C. Insurance companies
   D. All of the above

9. When preparing to respond to emergency calls, duties of the EMT include all of the following *except:*
   A. Ensuring his partner has prepared the ambulance
   B. Ensuring the unit is in safe operating condition
   C. Assuring the necessary equipment is available
   D. Identifying repairs and maintenance needed

10. Daily vehicle inspection is considered to be part of an EMT's duties.
    A. True
    B. False

11. Seat belts are needed for all occupants of the emergency vehicle.
    A. True
    B. False

12. Which of the following factors may affect response to a call?
    A. An uncooperative motorist
    B. Day of the week
    C. Time of day
    D. All of the above

13. Use of lights and sirens does not exempt an emergency vehicle operator from the requirement to drive with due regard for the safety of others.
    A. True
    B. False

14. A PCR should include which of the following:
    A. Mechanism of injury or illness
    B. Injuries found and treatment initiated
    C. Vital signs
    D. All of the above

15. Essentials for completing a call on arrival at the emergency department include:
    A. Make a verbal report to medical staff
    B. Follow up with a written report of the call
    C. Transfer the patient's effects to medical staff
    D. All of the above

16. When cleaning the ambulance, it is essential that the EMT dispose of biohazards properly.
    A. True
    B. False

Case Scenario

You and your partner are beginning your shift. As the previous crew was leaving, they informed you that one of the units had a near empty tank of gas because they had been too busy to refuel. You and your partner complete the checks of the ambulances and find that the one low in fuel is the only problem area and elect to fill the tank when you go out to lunch.

One hour after your shift begins, you are dispatched to the scene of a multi-victim crash that requires all your units to respond. The location of the incident is 15 miles away from the station and 20 miles from the nearest receiving medical facility. You realize immediately that the unit with the near empty tank cannot be used in this call.

1. What steps should you have taken to prepare your shift prior to the first call?

2. What are you and your partner's responsibilities regarding vehicle checks and maintenance?

Answer Key

Key Terms
1. Emergency Vehicle Operator (EVO)
2. III
3. I
4. II

Content Review
1. KKK-A-1822C
2. Occupational Safety and Health Administration (OSHA)
3. Wheeled stretcher; Reeves stretcher; folding stair chair; scoop stretcher; Stokes stretcher; child safety seat; and backboards
4. Traction splints; padded board splints (various sizes); wire ladder splints (padded); air splint kit; cardboard splints; aluminum splints; vacuum splints; tongue depressors; triangular bandages with safety pins; tape; chemical cold packs; and self-adhering roller gauze
5. Drinking water (changed daily); syrup of ipecac (if approved locally); activated charcoal; paper cups; contact lens remover; irrigation equipment (for flushing eyes); and snake bite kits
6. Heavy fire-resistant coat (turnout gear); leather gloves; goggles or other shatter-resistant eye protection; and a helmet
7. Regular lights; emergency lights; fuel cap; fluid leaks; oil leaks; cooling leaks; tires; lug nuts; wipers; and doors and latches on all compartments
8. Brake fluid (level, color, and smell); oil (level, color, and feel); battery (water level or charge indicators, connection, and mounting); the hood and latch; drive belts; and power steering fluid (level, color, and smell)
9. Adequate vision; adequate hearing; physically fit to perform lifting and moving tasks; ability to work under extreme stress; confident, positive, and realistic; tolerant of the driving of others
10. Day of the week; time of day; weather; detours; railroads; bridges; tunnels; schools and school buses
11. True
12. 3- or 4-second rule
13. It requires that an EVO follow a vehicle at a distance such that an object passed by the first vehicle is passed by the emergency vehicle 4 seconds later.
14. True
15. False
16. If following another emergency vehicle, maintain a distance of at least 500 feet; use a different siren time and/or tone to help other motorists to distinguish multiple units; use radios to coordinate responses to reduce the likelihood of multiple units arriving at the same spot (intersection) simultaneously; and plan alternate routes to reduce conflict
17. At intersections
18. Pull off the road and stop the vehicle as safely as possible; turn off the ignition and turn on the vehicle's four way flashers and other visual warning devices; check for injuries; notify dispatch and request additional resources; if possible and necessary, start triage and management of any injured persons; start the documentation process as soon as possible; follow local procedures (calling the insurance company, etc.); and complete all associated incident reports, forms, etc.
19. Uphill, upwind, and a minimum of 100 feet from the scene

Chapter Quiz

1. D	5. B	9. A	13. A
2. A	6. C	10. A	14. D
3. C	7. D	11. A	15. D
4. D	8. D	12. D	16. A

Case Scenario

1. You should have arranged to immediately fuel the ambulance following your daily inspection.
2. You and your partner both have a duty to check the ambulance and equipment immediately after reporting for duty. While conducting a routine daily inspection, you and your partner should go over the equipment to ensure that everything needed is present and in working condition and make corrections and adjustments as necessary.

Reading Assignment: Chapter 38 pages 742–758.

Supplemental Objectives

Upon successful completion of the EMT-Basic training program, the EMT-Basic student should be able to do the following:

- Discuss the interactions with the following providers:
  - Dispatcher
  - First responder
  - Advanced life support (paramedic)
  - Aeromedical response
  - Child protective services
  - Elder abuse services
  - Managed care organizations
  - Law enforcement agencies (street patrol, criminal investigations, tactical units/SWAT teams)
  - Rescue groups (wilderness search and rescue, urban search and rescue, hazardous materials, ski patrol)
- Identify safety precautions for approaching and loading a patient into an aeromedical helicopter.
- Describe the purpose and procedure for establishing a landing zone.

Key Terms

1. Loading a patient on an aircraft after the rotor systems have completely stopped turning is called a(n) _____.

2. The main body of the aircraft is called the _____.

3. An established location where two emergency vehicles come together is called a(n) _____ _____.

4. The primary set of blades on a helicopter that creates lift for flight is called the _____ _____.

5. An aircraft with wings solidly attached to the main fuselage is called a _____ aircraft.

6. An area established for the aircraft to land is called the _____.

7. Loading a patient on an aircraft when the rotor systems are still turning is called a(n) _____ _____.

8. The manner in which injuries occur is known as the _____.

9. An aircraft with multiple blades that turn at a high speed and create lift as they turn through the air is called a(n) _____ aircraft.

10. The first phase of activating aeromedical support that involves asking that aeromedical services get ready to respond is known as a(n) _____.

11. The downward blast of air created by the main rotor system as the aircraft lands or takes off is known as a(n) _____.

12. The set of rotor blades located at the rear of the fuselage perpendicular to the main rotors is called the _____.

Content Review

....

1. Depending on the aircraft, rotor blades may be _____ feet off the ground.

2. From what direction should the EMT approach a helicopter?

3. What is the most dangerous area of the helicopter?

4. Aeromedical response transportation is an expensive and limited resource that should be used cautiously.
   A. True
   B. False

5. During daylight hours, the main dimensions for a helicopter LZ are _____ and nighttime operations require at least _____.

6. Identify some examples of obstacles that a LZ must not contain.

7. What are some considerations to take into account when setting a landing zone area?

8. Who has absolute say on the appropriateness of a landing zone?

9. When flares are not available, the EMT should point the headlights of the ambulance into the landing area to light the field.
   A. True
   B. False

10. The tail rotor of a helicopter is usually 3 to 6 feet off the ground and spins so fast you cannot see it.
    A. True
    B. False

11. You should always approach the aircraft from the "downhill" side and never carry objects over your head.
    A. True
    B. False

12. Never park a vehicle closer than _____ to the helicopter.

13. Because of limited space in the helicopter, it is important that ground personnel accomplish as much treatment and stabilization as possible on the ground before loading the patient.
    A. True
    B. False

14. The type of police officer EMS providers most commonly interact with are _____ units.

15. It is the job of a _____ to gather evidence and conduct interviews in preparation of a case against a criminal.

16. In most states, a PCR can be shared with law enforcement personnel without the permission of the patient or a court order.
    A. True
    B. False

17. Identify situations in which SWAT units and EMS units may interact at a scene.

18. When it is necessary to transport a police officer for anything other than a minor injury, what should the EMT do with the officer's firearm?

19. Identify guidelines that should be followed to help facilitate conflict resolution.

Chapter Quiz

1. Helicopter rotor blades are usually from 3 to 15 feet off the ground.
   A. True
   B. False

2. Which of the following guidelines can be used to evaluate the need for aeromedical services?
   A. Mechanism of injury
   B. Physical findings
   C. Special situations
   D. All of the above

3. Which of the following physical exam findings does not indicate the need for aeromedical transportation?
   A. Head injury with decreased LOC
   B. Penetrating wound to the chest or abdomen
   C. An airway that needs advanced procedures
   D. Isolated fracture of the radius and ulna with pulses

4. Which of the following circumstances may warrant the use of aeromedical support?
   A. Certain obstetric emergencies with a long ground transport time
   B. Unexpected or complicated premature deliveries with a long transport time
   C. Medical problems that require ALS when none is available by ground
   D. All of the above

5. What are the two phases of activating aeromedical support?
   A. Standby and transport
   B. Standby and respond
   C. Stand down and response
   D. Response and transport

6. An aeromedical team may be asked to respond to a scene when:
   A. The initial call is received from bystanders
   B. When the situation has been identified by on-scene personnel
   C. When first responders state that it sounds like a bad call
   D. When a patient requests air transport

7. What are the minimum landing zone dimensions for helicopters during daylight hours?
   A. 60 ft × 60 ft
   B. 30 ft × 60 ft
   C. 40 ft × 60 ft
   D. 100 ft × 100 ft

8. What are the minimum landing zone dimensions for helicopters during nighttime operations?
   A. 60 ft × 60 ft
   B. 30 ft × 60 ft
   C. 40 ft × 60 ft
   D. 100 ft × 100 ft

9. Which of the following are landing zone hazards?
   A. Wires
   B. Debris
   C. Unmarked towers or poles
   D. All of the above

10. When a landing zone is marked with flares, a flare should be placed in the middle of the zone as a reference point for the pilot.
    A. True
    B. False

11. Bright lights pointed at the landing zone will help the pilot's night vision.
    A. True
    B. False

12. When giving landing instructions to the helicopter pilot, always use references in relationship to the aircraft.
    A. True
    B. False

13. Which of the following is a safety violation when working around a helicopter?
    A. Approaching the helicopter from the rear
    B. Approaching the helicopter from the front
    C. Parking a vehicle 70 feet from the aircraft
    D. Approaching from the downhill side of the aircraft

14. The loading or unloading of a helicopter with the rotor system turning is called a "cool load" and is a very safe procedure.
    A. True
    B. False

15. Which of the following patient care interventions should be performed before loading a patient into the helicopter?
    A. Ensure adequate airway control
    B. Treat life-threatening injuries
    C. Place the patient on oxygen
    D. All of the above

Case Scenario

••

It is a Friday evening and the local high school football game ended 30 minutes ago; traffic is backed up for miles. You and your partner receive a call to a motor vehicle collision involving five vehicles on an interstate approximately 3 miles from the stadium. Based on initial reports from law enforcement officers on the scene, there are multiple injuries and all lanes of traffic are blocked. The local trauma center is 5 miles away by ground. The ALS unit is responding from 20 miles away. Your dispatcher notifies you that a helicopter has been placed on standby.

1. How should you determine the patient transport mode and the necessity for aeromedical response?

2. What types of backup units will you consider summoning to the scene?

3. List at least five considerations regarding the landing zone to be established.

   1)
   2)
   3)
   4)
   5)

4. List at least four considerations regarding preparation of patients for aeromedical transport.

   1)
   2)
   3)
   4)

Answer Key

••

Key Terms
1. Cold load
2. Fuselage
3. Intercept
4. Main rotor
5. Fixed-wing
6. Landing zone (LZ)
7. Hot load

8. Mechanism of injury
9. Rotor-wing
10. Standby request
11. Rotor wash
12. Tail rotor

Content Review
1. 3 to 15
2. From the front in order to be seen by the pilot
3. The tail rotor
4. True
5. 60 feet × 60 feet; 100 feet × 100 feet
6. Wires, debris, vehicles, personnel, trees, and high brush
7. Obstacles; ground condition (firm enough to support the aircraft, lack of rocks, and lack of dry dusty areas); and slope
8. The pilot
9. False
10. True
11. True
12. 50 feet
13. True
14. Street patrol
15. Detective
16. False
17. Hostage situations, barricaded suspects, drug raids, and high-risk warrant service
18. Make sure it is secured by another police officer.
19. If the situation is "too hot to handle," allow for a "cool-down" period; do not escalate the conflict (feed off each other's anger); remain open and objective throughout the discussion; identify the issue or problem and focus on it to the exclusion of extraneous concerns; compromise (there may be more than one appropriate solution); display mutual respect; and forgive, forget, and move on.

Chapter Quiz

1. A	6. B	11. B
2. D	7. A	12. A
3. D	8. D	13. A
4. D	9. D	14. B
5. B	10. B	15. D

Case Scenario
1. From the initial reports of the incident, you realize the seriousness and potential hazards that exist. The determination regarding patient transport mode (ground or aeromedical) is based on: the number of victims; the seriousness of the injuries; the access time to definitive care; and the availability of ALS care.
2. Consider summoning the following backup units: rescue-extrication units; additional ALS units; fire department units; fire police (for traffic control); additional BLS units; aeromedical team(s).
3. Establish a landing zone based on: 1) proximity to the incident; 2) hazards near the scene; 3) weather conditions; 4) the need for a flat area 100 ft × 100 ft (for nighttime operations); and 5) an area free from obstacles (i.e., electrical wires, trees, etc.).
4. To prepare the patient for aeromedical transport: 1) initiate patient care; 2) ensure adequate airway control, breathing and circulation; 3) treat life-threatening injuries; 4) initiate oxygen therapy; 5) immobilize the spine; 6) ensure scene safety; and 7) transfer the patient to air crew properly.

Gaining Access

Reading Assignment: Chapter 39 pages 761–773.

Supplemental Objectives

Upon successful completion of the EMT-Basic training program, the EMT-Basic should be able to do the following:

- Describe the purpose of extrication.
- Describe the role of the EMT-Basic in extrication.
- Identify the personal safety equipment that is required for the EMT-Basic.
- Define fundamental components of extrication.
- State the steps that should be taken to protect the patient during extrication.
- Evaluate various methods of gaining access.
- Distinguish between simple and complex access.
- Differentiate between the various types of rescue operations.
- List ten steps in a rescue plan of action.
- Describe four categories of vehicle rescue situations.

Key Terms

· ·

1. Match the following equipment with their appropriate description.

_____ A heavy bolt driving tool, pneumatically or electrically
powered

_____ A hand tool used for prying and breaking glass

_____ Part of the passive passenger restraint system

_____ A portable hand-operated winch

_____ A hand-operated tool used to cut metal

_____ Piston-like metal shafts operated by air pressure for shoring

_____ A hand tool using compressed air supply to cut metal

_____ A hydraulic power tool consisting of spreader
arms with cutting edges on the inside of the arms

_____ A reinforced part of the interior of a modern automobile door

_____ An extrication tool used for lifting

_____ A metal support used to strengthen the push off point of
a powered hydraulic ram

_____ A lifting maneuver on the front dash of an automobile to
free trapped patients

_____ A hydraulic power tool used to cut metal

_____ A hand tool used to cut steel on chains, locks and other items

_____ Specially cut and/or assembled pieces of wood used to
support raised objects

_____ A tool used to secure objects together

_____ A tool used to break tempered glass for controlled removal

_____ A lifting device designed to mechanically lift a vehicle
that sits high off the ground level

_____ A lifting tool with a piston operated by a manual hydraulic pump

_____ A tool that supports a load by using shafts of wood or
other devices

_____ Hydraulic driven pistons that extend and retract, providing
a lifting capability in a powered hydraulic rescue tool system

_____ An electrically powered unit that moves the blade in an
in-and-out motion to cut metal and wreckage

A. Air chisel
B. Air rescue bags
C. Air restraint bag
D. Base plate
E. Bolt cutter
F. Cargo strap
G. Collision bar
H. Combination tool
I. Come along
J. Cribbing
K. Cutter
L. Dash lift
M. Hacksaw
N. Halligan bar
O. High lift jack
P. Hydraulic jack
Q. Impact wrench
R. Pneumatic struts
S. Reciprocating saw
T. RAMS
U. Shoring
V. Spring load center
punch

2. The area of a passenger vehicle that is used to store or carry items is referred to as a(n) _____
_____.

3. A method of conducting a thorough survey of the incident scene that involves walking in a circle
around the entire scene is called a(n) _____.

4. The term used either to describe the person in control of an emergency scene or to denote the action
of controlling an emergency scene is _____.

5. The safe and efficient removal of unnecessary people from around the vehicles involved in an accident is called _____.

6. A common vehicle rescue term that describes procedures used by rescue personnel to remove trapped
patients is _____.

7. The process of freeing a trapped patient is _____.

8. A method of positioning emergency apparatus at the scene of a vehicle crash such that it provides added protection from traffic is called a(n) _____.

9. An international term used when a rescuer wants other rescuers to make an emergency stop in their activities on the scene is _____.

10. The first hour after an incident, when a traumatized patient has the best chance for recovery if safely delivered to a medical facility is called the _____.

11. Specialized cribbing assemblies made of wood blocks assembled in a stair step configuration and used to stabilize vehicles are called _____.

12. The term for securing a wrecked vehicle in which an injured patient is trapped is called _____ _____.

13. A system of control of the emergency scene that is set up by predetermined procedures for effective control of complex emergency operations is called _____.

14. A type of vehicle crash in which a vehicle drives underneath another vehicle is called _____ _____.

15. A decision process in which problems presented are given priority, usually used in the context of patient handling and treatment of patient's injuries, is called _____.

16. The term that describes the procedure of assessing a vehicle that has been involved in a crash is a(n) _____.

17. Specially designed glass used in automobile windshields that is comprised of layered plate glass separated by clear plastic is called _____.

18. A term that describes a crash in which one vehicle has driven over the top of another vehicle is _____.

19. A term used to describe an accident situation in which the vehicle has come to rest on its roof, with the roof crushed in on the passenger's compartment area, is called a(n) _____ _____.

20. A descriptive term that denotes the action of a rescuer getting to the trapped patient for patient assessment and care is _____.

21. A vehicle design term that is used for the posts that connect the roof of a vehicle to the rest of the body is _____.

22. A small opening made in wreckage that makes room for the insertion of rescue tools to move that wreckage is called a(n) _____.

23. The rolled sheet-metal assemblies on vehicles that attach the roof to the main body of the vehicle are called _____.

Content Review

1. Identify different rescue situations that an EMT may be called to.

2. List the steps involved in a good rescue action plan for most rescue situations.

3. Describe the four categories of vehicle rescue situations.

   1)
   2)
   3)
   4)

4. The EMT should maintain a safe zone of _____ away from side bags, _____ from driver side front bags, and _____ from passenger side front bags.

5. Describe safety precautions to follow when breaking glass.

6. What is the EMT's role in the disentanglement phase of a rescue?

7. What is the first step toward disentangling a patient?

8. Which rescuer is in command of any patient movement action?

9. When should a patient be removed through a cut away roof?

10. When is total immobilization usually achieved?

11. An average extrication time is approximately _____ from the time of the call to the point where the patient is ready for transport.

Chapter Quiz

• •

1. The most common type of entrapment occurs as a result of:
   A. Machinery/industrial accidents
   B. Vehicle collisions
   C. Low-angle confinement
   D. Building collapse

2. At the scene of a MVC, the EMT's primary responsibility is:
   A. Extrication
   B. Scene control
   C. Patient care
   D. Documentation

3. Removal of the wreckage from around the victim so that emergency care can be provided is called:
   A. Disentanglement
   B. Extrication
   C. Evacuation
   D. Shoring

4. _____ involves the actual removal of a patient from the vehicle.
   A. Disentanglement
   B. Entrapment
   C. Extrication
   D. Excavation

5. The EMT's primary responsibility at the scene where one or more victims are trapped is:
   A. Rapid and safe disentanglement and extrication
   B. Providing emergency care while specially trained personnel perform extrication
   C. Traffic control
   D. Triage

6. A type of rescue operation that involves a patient who is trapped in water or in a position in which he or she cannot be reached without crossing a significant body of water is called:
   A. Extrication
   B. Water rescue
   C. Wilderness rescue
   D. Evacuation

7. Water rescue requires the ability of the rescuer to swim and can be attempted routinely by EMTs.
   A. True
   B. False

8. Examples of high-angle rescue include:
   A. A high-rise building under construction
   B. A ski lift or water tower
   C. The ledge of a sheer rock wall
   D. All of the above

9. A cave-in can occur in:
   A. Caves
   B. Construction sites
   C. Utility trenches
   D. All of the above

10. Complex vehicle rescue equipment includes all of the following *except:*
    A. Port-a-powers
    B. Powered hydraulic spreaders and cutters
    C. Hammer
    D. Hydraulic rams

11. During any extrication operation, the primary function of the EMT is to:
    A. Locate victims
    B. Prioritize patients
    C. Treat the victims
    D. All of the above

12. Which of the following is *not* considered appropriate protective equipment for EMT safety?
    A. Turnout gear
    B. A heavy, fire-resistant coat
    C. Heavy tennis shoes
    D. Helmet

13. The best method for stabilizing a vehicle to gain access to the patient is to:
    A. Make sure the car's transmission is in neutral
    B. Place cribbing behind and in front of wheels
    C. Cut the tires
    D. All of the above

14. The process of physically removing the injured patient from within the wreckage is known as the:
    A. Stabilization phase
    B. Extrication phase
    C. Triage phase
    D. Transfer phase

Case Scenario

· ·

You are dispatched to an automobile collision involving a truck and an automobile. En route to the scene, dispatch informs you that there are three persons trapped in the car. On your arrival on the scene, the truck driver is ambulatory.

On initial assessment, you determine that one victim in the car is dead; another entrapped victim is alert, oriented, and positioned so that extrication will not be difficult. The third occupant in the car was ejected and is trapped under the truck and exhibiting agonal breathing.

1. What is the first priority that you and your crew need to consider at this incident?

2. What PPE should you wear at this scene?

3. What initial steps should you take?

4. How will you handle this incident?

Answer Key

1. Q, N, C, I, M, R, A, H, G, B, D, L, K, E, J, F, V, O, P, U, T, S
2. Cargo compartment
3. Circle survey
4. Command
5. Crowd control
6. Extrication
7. Disentanglement
8. Fend-off
9. Freeze
10. Golden hour
11. Step chocks
12. Stabilization
13. Incident command
14. Under ride
15. Triage
16. Circle survey
17. Laminated glass
18. Over ride
19. Pancaked vehicle
20. Patient access
21. Pillars
22. Purchase point
23. Posts

Content Review
1. Building collapse; trench/excavation collapse; confined spaces; low angle/high angle; wilderness; water; machinery or industrial; and vehicles
2. Preparation; response; arrival and size up; stabilization; accessing the patient; disentanglement; removal; transport; securing the scene/preparation for the next call; and post-incident analysis
3. 1) No entrapment—occupants of the vehicle can be readily removed without the use of tools; 2) Light entrapment—minimal use of tools are necessary to remove the patient; 3) Moderate entrapment—one or more occupants are trapped in a way that requires roof and door removal but there is no displacement of the dash or other parts of the car; 4) Heavy entrapment—re-locating the roof and doors
4. 5"; 10"; 15"
5. Always wear proper safety attire including eye, head, foot, and hand protection; and keep your mouth closed.

6. Maintaining patient contact; in-line spinal stabilization; continued critical intervention; and emotional support
7. To provide a more sustained access route so additional patient care can be delivered
8. The rescuer at the patient's head
9. When the patient is critical and not pinned by the wreckage
10. When the patient is secured to a long spine board and his or her head immobilized with a cervical immobilization device
11. 30 minutes

Chapter Quiz

1. B	5. B	9. D	13. B
2. C	6. B	10. C	14. B
3. A	7. B	11. D	
4. C	8. D	12. C	

Case Scenario

1. Your first priority must be to determine that the scene is safe for you and your crew, as well as for other rescuers, and then to size-up the situation
2. You should wear full turnout gear including: gloves, boots, heavy turnout coat; and helmet with eye shield.
3. Assess the damage to the vehicles to determine if additional help will be needed; instruct dispatch to dispatch a rescue unit for extrication of the victims; call for ALS assistance; dispatch additional ambulance units for transport of the patients at the scene; notify the coroner (and law enforcement if not already on the scene) of the deceased victim
4. Ensure scene safety; call for assistance; stabilize the vehicle before entering it to check victims; gain access to the patients; triage patients; and assign resources as they become available for extrication, patient care, and patient transport.

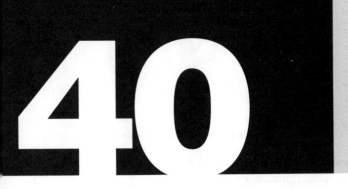

Emergency Preparedness

Reading Assignment: Chapter 40 pages 774–790.

DOT Objectives

Upon successful completion of the EMT-Basic training program, the EMT-Basic should be able to do the following:

- Explain the roles and responsibilities of the EMT in a disaster or multiple-casualty situation.
- Describe the EMT's roles and responsibilities at a hazardous materials incident.
- Describe what the EMT should do if there is reason to believe that there is a hazardous material at the scene.
- Describe the actions that an EMT should take to ensure bystander safety.
- State the role the EMT should perform until appropriately trained personnel arrive at the scene of a hazardous materials situation.
- Break down the steps to approaching a hazardous situation.
- Discuss the various environmental hazards that affect EMS.
- Describe the criteria for a multiple-casualty situation.
- Summarize the components of basic triage.
- Define the role of the EMT in a disaster operation.
- Describe basic concepts of incident management.
- Explain the methods for preventing contamination of self, equipment and facilities.
- Review the local mass casualty incident plan.
- Given a scenario of mass casualty incident, perform triage.

Supplemental Objectives

- Describe the characteristics of a disaster, and differentiate those characteristics from normal operational conditions.
- Identify the importance of disaster planning in disaster preparedness.
- Demonstrate the ability to use the principles of triage in a multiple-casualty situation.
- Define hazardous materials and explain their significance for EMS operations.
- Explain the federal regulations concerning hazardous materials training for emergency responders.
- Review the rules for scene safety, and identify the tools that are available to the EMT for managing a hazardous material situation.

Key Terms

1. Physical components of a community that are necessary for normal, everyday operations, such as roads, bridges, electrical power, and telephone communications are called _____ _____.

2. A term commonly used for any incident involving one or more patients that cannot be handled by the first responding unit(s) to a scene is a(n) _____.

3. A human-made or natural event that involves tremendous damage across a large geographic area is called a(n) _____.

4. Chemical substances that are toxic to humans are called _____.

5. The process of removing hazardous substances from the patient, rescuers, and equipment is called _____.

6. A process of sorting patients based on who should be treated or transported first is called _____.

7. A system or method of managing complex events that involve large amounts of resources (people, equipment, and vehicles) is called the _____.

8. A process of analyzing disasters or mass casualty incidents that are likely to occur in a given community is called _____.

Content Review

1. What are two major activities involved in preplanning for disasters?

   1)
   2)

2. What are three goals of a disaster exercise?

   1)
   2)
   3)

3. Describe situations that would be considered the "highest priority" in triage.

4. Describe situations that would be considered a "second priority" in triage.

5. Describe situations that would be considered the "lowest priority" in triage.

6. Which individuals are "no priority" during triage?

7. The first key step in successfully managing a HazMat response is _____.

8. The most basic level of training for a HazMat is approximately 8 to 12 hours and focuses on recognition and initial management of HazMat incidents.
   A. True
   B. False

9. The EMT is often the first emergency responder to arrive at a HazMat incident and his or her initial actions can make a major difference in lives saved.
   A. True
   B. False

10. What situations should the EMT immediately consider as potentially involving hazardous materials?

11. What methods are in place to identify hazardous materials?

12. A placard is not required until the weight of a substance exceeds a maximum limit, usually _____ pounds.

13. If a placard is not on a vehicle, the EMT is safe to assume a hazardous substance is not being transported.
    A. True
    B. False

14. At an industrial setting, which placard indicates bulk storage of hazardous materials?

15. What information is available on a Materials Safety Data Sheet (MSDS)?

16. When or where are MSDSs required?

17. An EMT should see the MSDS prior to patient contact when there has been an exposure even to a single patient.
    A. True
    B. False

18. An emergency information center that offers assistance 24 hours a day, 7 days a week, 365 days a year, is called _____ and is run by the Chemical Manufacturer's Association.

19. If the EMT approaches the scene of an incident and detects markings indicative of HazMat, what should he or she do?

20. List the priorities for management of a HazMat incident.

Chapter Quiz

1. In general, an MCI exists when an incident has occurred that changes the normal ratio of rescuers and equipment to patients.
   A. True
   B. False

2. Examples of MCI may include:
   A. A hurricane that strikes four states
   B. An airplane crash
   C. A bus crash
   D. All of the above

3. A two-car crash with four serious injuries in a remote rural community may be classified as a multiple-casualty incident
   A. True
   B. False

4. Patients classified as low priority include all of the following *except:*
   A. Minor, painful, swollen, deformed extremities
   B. Minor soft tissue injuries or death
   C. Injuries incompatible with life
   D. Burns or shock

5. Major components of MCI preplanning involve:
   A. Risk assessment
   B. Resource identification
   C. Practice
   D. All of the above

6. A list of resources for an MCI should include:
   A. People
   B. Equipment
   C. Vehicles
   D. All of the above

7. Patients classified as second priority include all of the following *except:*
   A. Back injuries with or without spinal cord damage
   B. Burns without airway problems
   C. Major or multiple bone or joint injuries
   D. Decreased level of consciousness

8. Hazardous material incidents are dangerous for EMS providers because they require a different thought process and approach than do traditional EMS responses.
   A. True
   B. False

9. In what order should priorities of safety be placed at a HazMat scene?
    A. Patient safety, EMT safety, bystander safety
    B. EMT safety, bystander safety, patient safety
    C. Patient safety, bystander safety, EMT safety
    D. Patient safety, EMT safety, bystander safety

10. Which of the following is *not* a high priority patient at an MCI?
    A. One with decreased mental status
    B. One with uncontrolled or severe bleeding
    C. One with injuries incompatible with life
    D. One with airway and breathing difficulties

11. An EMT can prevent becoming contaminated by doing which of the following?
    A. Decontaminating the transport vehicle
    B. Removing and cleaning clothing
    C. Vigorously washing his or her hands
    D. All of the above

12. Triage is the generic term used to describe:
    A. Vehicles used in a disaster response
    B. Systems of sorting or prioritizing patients
    C. EMS response levels
    D. The command sector at an MCI

13. When should the first-arriving EMS personnel start triage?
    A. Immediately on arrival at the MCI
    B. When all sectors have been established
    C. As soon as scene safety has been assured
    D. As soon as all responding personnel have arrived

14. Patients who are still alive, but who have wounds that are obviously fatal, are categorized as:
    A. Highest priority and placed before patients in shock
    B. Urgent priority and placed before heart attack patients
    C. Lowest category and placed immediately ahead of the dead
    D. Second priority and placed after highest priority patients

15. The typical MCI plan calls for:
    A. All high-priority patients to be transported to one hospital
    B. Matching the patients to the hospital's capabilities
    C. All low-priority patients to be transported first
    D. All second priority patients to be transported last

16. Which of the following contributes to the dangers for an EMT at a HazMat incident?
    A. Lack of specific training in the management of HazMat incidents
    B. Being the first emergency responders to arrive at the scene of an incident involving HazMat
    C. Lack of protective equipment necessary to operate in a HazMat environment
    D. All of the above

17. The first/key step in successfully managing a HazMat response is:
    A. Triage
    B. Decontamination
    C. Recognition
    D. Treatment

18. The U.S. Department of Transportation's *Emergency Response Handbook: Guidebook for Hazardous Materials Incidents:*
    A. Provides basic emergency information for known HazMats
    B. Has information corresponding to the 4-digit number on a placard
    C. Should be carried in every emergency response vehicle
    D. All of the above

19. At a HazMat incident, the EMT should wait until victims are extricated and decontaminated by HazMat specialists prior to starting medical treatment.
    A. True
    B. False

20. The method of sorting and prioritizing patients is called:
    A. ICS
    B. MCI
    C. Triage
    D. Identification

Case Scenario

••

You are dispatched to a vehicle collision involving a bus. En route to the scene, you and your partner discuss the probable need for assistance on this call. You note that there are two receiving hospitals in the area—one hospital is located about 12 minutes from the scene and the other, a larger trauma center, is approximately 15 minutes from the scene.

1. What is your initial priority on arrival at the incident?

2. What are your initial tasks on arrival at the scene?

You arrive on location and find a collision between a car and a small transit bus. The bus swerved to miss the car and veered into a telephone pole. After completing the initial triage, you determine that there are eight injured people. Your patient injury list reads as follows:

Patient 1 is the driver of the car—he is entrapped in his vehicle and exhibiting agonal respirations.
Patient 2: is ambulatory with a painful, swollen, deformed extremity.
Patient 3: was a passenger in the car— he was ejected from the vehicle, has obvious head injuries, and is exhibiting abnormal posture.
Patient 4: was the driver of the bus—he has multiple lacerations and is complaining of glass in his eye.
Patient 5: was the passenger in the car—he has been pulled from the vehicle by a bystander and has obvious paradoxical respirations; the patient is conscious.
Patient 6: has an open, painful, swollen, deformed area in his upper right leg.
Patient 7: is crying that she cannot feel her legs.
Patient 8: has burns on the left side of his torso from lying next to the exhaust pipe of the car.

Gasoline spills are obvious and the fire department has been dispatched. The only extrication truck in the area is busy at another site and will not be available for another hour. Dispatch informs you there are four additional ambulance units available, all within 10 minutes of the scene.

3. What additional resources may be needed for this incident?

4. What PPE should you wear for this incident?

5. List, in correct sequence, the patient triage priorities.

6. List at least two scene hazards.

   1)
   2)

7. What considerations are important when determining transport of victims?

Answer Key

Key Terms
1. Infrastructure
2. Mass casualty incident (MCI)
3. Disaster
4. Hazardous materials
5. Decontamination
6. Triage
7. Incident command system (ICS)
8. Risk assessment

Content Review

1. Risk assessment and resource identification
2. 1) Allow participants to actually practice the activities they will be required to perform; 2) allow planners to test the assumptions and guesswork that went into plan development; 3) provide an opportunity to review the positives and negatives of the implementation of the plan
3. Airway and breathing difficulties; uncontrolled or severe bleeding; decreased mental status; severe medical problems (heart attack, stroke, etc.); shock; and severe burns
4. Burns without airway problems; major or multiple bone or joint injury; and back injuries with or without spinal cord damage
5. Minor painful swollen, deformed extremities; and minor soft-tissue injuries
6. Those with injuries incompatible with life and those who are already deceased
7. Recognition
8. True
9. True
10. Any transportation incidents (highway, rails, or air); any response to a fire or incident at an industrial facility; any response to an incident where multiple patients are experiencing similar complaints
11. Placards; and shipping papers, and MSDSs
12. 1000
13. False
14. NFPA 704 placard
15. Specific information about the HazMat, including chemical composition effects on the body, and recommended treatments
16. Commercial and industrial environments are required to maintain MSDSs for all chemicals used or stored in their operations
17. True
18. CHEMTREC
19. Resist the urge to drive right up to the scene and rush in to help victims; identify the substances involved; request assistance from HazMat trained personnel; take the steps necessary to establish response zones around the incident; communicate any relevant information about the identity of the chemical or specifics on the incident to the dispatch center; notify the hospital that a HazMat incident is underway; consider notifying the local poison control center so they can be prepared to provide necessary advice; and wait until victims are extricated and decontaminated by HazMat specialists and then start any medical treatment
20. First priority is for the safety of yourself and other rescuers; second priority is for the safety of innocent bystanders; and third priority is safety of the patient.

Chapter Quiz

1. A	6. D	11. D	16. D
2. D	7. D	12. B	17. C
3. A	8. A	13. C	18. D
4. D	9. B	14. C	19. A
5. D	10. C	15. B	20. C

Case Scenario

1. Scene safety
2. Ensure scene safety (hazards, crowd control, etc.); request assistance as needed; perform an initial assessment; and triage patients
3. Additional BLS units; ALS personnel; fire department for gasoline spill; law enforcement for incident investigation and traffic control; police for traffic and crowd control; fire rescue unit; and aeromedical unit
4. Full turnout gear with gloves, helmet, face shield, boots, and a heavy turnout coat
5. The correct sequence for the patient triage priorities are: highest priority are patients 3 and 5; second priority are patients 4, 6, 7, and 8; lowest priority are patients 1 and 2.
6. Scene hazards include gasoline spills, unstable vehicles, and traffic flow problems.

7. Additional ambulance units and possible aeromedical transport, if available, will be necessary to handle the number of victims at this incident; it is necessary to determine which of the available facilities can accept the high-priority patients; determine the total number of patients that both hospitals can handle; understand that both high-priority patients should be transported to the trauma center that is able to providing definitive care—if the trauma center cannot handle both patients, aeromedical transport should take them to another trauma center (if possible).

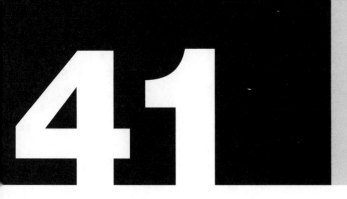

Diving Emergencies

Reading Assignment: Chapter 41 pages 791–805.

Supplemental Objectives

Upon successful completion of the EMT-Basic training program, the EMT-Basic should be able to do the following:

- Explain the mechanics of water, air, and oxygen pressure and how these effects are measured in relationship to the human body.
- Define *Boyle's law* as it relates to pressure and volume relationships for scuba diving injuries.
- Define *Dalton's law of partial pressure* and the effect this has on a scuba diver who is using compressed air.
- Define *barotrauma* as it relates to the human body and how this can affect a scuba diver.
- Describe the pathophysiology and field management of the following barotrauma descent injuries that can be found in a scuba diver: ear, sinus, dental, pulmonary, and mask.
- Describe the pathophysiology and field management of the following barotrauma ascent injuries that can be found in a scuba diver: pneumothorax, hemothorax, pneumomediastinum, air embolism, and subcutaneous emphysema.
- Define *decompression sickness*, and describe how it occurs in a scuba diver and its emergency management.
- Understand the different methods of transfer of patients with barotrauma and other diving injuries.

Key Terms

1. Match the following terms with their description.

_____ Trauma to hollow organs or spaces in the body as a result of significant pressure differences

_____ Air that gets into the blood from a tear in the alveolar capillary membrane

_____ A nitrogen bubble that expands in the vessel as ambient pressure on the diver decreases

_____ An injury that can occur to a scuba diver as they ascend to the water surface at the end of their dive

_____ An injury that can occur to a scuba diver as they descend from the water surface to their dive depth

_____ A condition that can occur to scuba divers as a result of body tissues becoming saturated with nitrogen during a dive on compressed air

_____ A specialized area in which a diver who is suffering from decompression sickness is placed

A. Air embolism
B. Ascent injury
C. Barotrauma
D. Decompression sickness
E. Descent injury
F. Gas embolism
G. Recompression chamber

2. What does the acronym SCUBA stand for?

Content Review

••

1. Oxygen comprises approximately _____% of the air we breathe.

2. Other than oxygen, air is comprised of _____% nitrogen.

3. A 1" × 1" column of air that extends up into the earth's atmosphere exerts a pressure of _____ pounds per square inch on our body at sea level.

4. What does Boyle's law state?

5. What is Dalton's law of partial pressure.

6. Define "bends."

7. A diver without scuba equipment eventually should not be able to use his or her lungs even if they had air available to them because as a diver descends and pressure increases, air space becomes compressed.
   A. True
   B. False

8. What parts of the body contain air spaces that may be affected as a scuba diver makes his or her descent?

9. A scuba diver who has a cold or allergies resulting in congestion of the sinuses or eustachian tubes is at increased risk for a squeeze-type injury resulting in significant pain and/or hemorrhage.
   A. True
   B. False

10. The biggest concern for a scuba diver is a lung expansion injury during _____.

11. What injuries may result from an uncontrolled ascent?

12. Identify two secondary effects of using compressed air for scuba divers?

    1)
    2)

13. If carbon monoxide poisoning is suspected, what question should the EMT ask the diver?

14. Carbon monoxide tends to taste and smell oily or foul.
    A. True
    B. False

15. Identify the signs and symptoms of decompression sickness.

16. How is the "bends" treated?

17. Decompression sickness is always recognizable immediately on surfacing from a dive.
    A. True
    B. False

18. In most cases, symptoms of a gas embolism occur within _____ minutes of surface from a dive.

19. What are the signs and symptoms of gas embolism?

20. Describe the nine steps of the 5-minute neurologic exam.

1)

2)

3)

4)

5)

6)

7)

8)

9)

Chapter Quiz

• •

1. The two major gases in air are oxygen and _____.
   A. Hydrogen
   B. Nitrogen
   C. Helium
   D. Carbon

2. Oxygen comprises _____ % of the air we breathe.
   A. 21
   B. 50
   C. 78
   D. 90

3. A 1" × 1" column of fresh water at a height of _____ feet exerts 14.7 psi on the body.
   A. 15
   B. 33
   C. 34
   D. 100

4. The medical term for a squeeze-type injury is:
   A. AGE
   B. Decompression sickness
   C. A gas embolism
   D. Barotrauma

5. The greatest concern for a scuba diver is:
   A. Lung expansion injury during descent
   B. Lung expansion injury during ascent
   C. Suffocation
   D. Carbon monoxide poisoning

6. All of the following injuries can occur from an uncontrolled ascent *except:*
   A. Pneumothorax
   B. Subcutaneous emphysema
   C. Carbon monoxide poisoning
   D. Air embolism

7. "The bends" is also known as:
   A. Decompression sickness
   B. A gas embolism
   C. Carbon monoxide poisoning
   D. Barotrauma

8. Carbon monoxide poisoning in scuba divers occurs because of all of the following *except*:
   A. The diver's compressor was improperly maintained
   B. The diver went too deep in the water
   C. The air filtration system is contaminated
   D. Exhaust gases are vented too close to fresh air intake during tank filling

9. Decompression sickness is caused by too much _____ absorbed into the body.
   A. Hydrogen
   B. Oxygen
   C. Nitrogen
   D. Carbon

10. Signs and symptoms of decompression sickness includes all of the following *except*:
    A. Skin rash
    B. Paralysis
    C. Pain in joints
    D. Nausea and vomiting

11. Of decompression sickness presentations, 70% occur with divers who were well within the "safe" diving depth limits.
    A. True
    B. False

12. In most cases, symptoms of embolism occur within _____ of surfacing from a dive.
    A. 1 minute
    B. 3 to 5 minutes
    C. 60 minutes
    D. 24 hours

13. Oral fluids should be given to a conscious patient with decompression sickness.
    A. True
    B. False

14. Air density _____ as a diver goes deeper and the amount of nitrogen absorbed by the body

    _____.
    A. Decreases; decreases
    B. Decreases; increases
    C. Increases; increases
    D. Increases; decreases

Case Scenario

●●

You are dispatched to a local lake where a scuba class is being given. You were called by the course instructor who states that the patient had just finished a 50 foot dive.

On arrival on the scene, you find a 26-year-old male patient with an altered level of consciousness. His instructor informs you that when the patient surfaced from the dive, he complained of weakness, dizziness, blurred vision, shortness of breath, and pain in his chest.

1. What is most likely wrong with this patient?

2. Is this condition an ascent or descent injury?

3. What causes this condition?

4. How would you care for this patient?

Answer Key

●●

Key Terms
1. C, A, F, B, E, D, G
2. Self-contained underwater breathing apparatus

Content Review
1. 21
2. 78
3. 14.7
4. As pressure increases, the volume decreases, and as pressure decreases, the volume increases.
5. In a mixture of gases, the pressure exerted by each gas is equal to the pressure it would exert, if it alone occupied the same volume; and the total pressure equals the sum of all the partial pressures in a component gas.
6. A condition in which nitrogen is absorbed and the diver cannot eliminate the nitrogen from the body as fast as pressure decreases; also known as decompression sickness.
7. True
8. The lungs, middle ear, and sinuses
9. True
10. Ascent

11. Pneumothorax, hemothorax, subcutaneous emphysema, and air embolism
12. Carbon monoxide poisoning and decompression sickness
13. If their tank tasted or smelled different
14. True
15. Skin rash, fatigue, pain in joints (especially shoulders and hips), paralysis, and, in more severe cases, unconsciousness
16. Obtain a history of the event, maintain an open airway, administer high-flow oxygen, lay patient in a supine position, and arrange transport to an appropriate facility with a hyperbaric compression chamber.
17. False
18. 3 to 5
19. Fatigue, weakness, dizziness, paralysis or weakness of the extremities or face, visual disturbances, feeling of a blow on chest with progressive worsening, sudden loss of consciousness immediately on or prior to surfacing, bloody frothy sputum, staggering, confusion, uneven gait, convulsions, and cessation of breathing
20. 1) Orientation: Does the diver know his name, age, location, and time? 2) Eyes: Can he or she see clearly (close and far), do his or her eyes follow movement, and are pupils equal and reactive? 3) Face: Are muscles contracted equally during movement and is sensation present and equal everywhere? 4) Hearing: Hold your hand about 2 inches from the diver's ear and rub your fingers and thumb together, move hand closer until the diver hears it. 5) Swallowing reflex: Instruct the diver to swallow and watch her or his "Adam's apple" to make sure it moves up and down. 6) Tongue: Have the diver stick out tongue and see if it is straight. 7) Muscle strength: Have the diver shrug his or her shoulders while you bear down on them to see if strength is equal; check strength of arms and legs. 8) Sensory perception: Sensation should be compared on both sides of the body. 9) Balance and coordination: Have the diver stand up with the feet close together, close eyes and stretch out arms, he or she should be able to move the index finger back and forth rapidly between their nose and your index finger about 18" from the diver's face.

Chapter Quiz

1. B	6. C	11. A
2. A	7. A	12. B
3. C	8. B	13. A
4. D	9. C	14. C
5. B	10. D	

Case Scenario

1. The patient is most likely suffering from a gas embolism.
2. This is an ascent injury.
3. As the diver surfaces, the gas trapped in the lungs expands, rupturing the alveoli and forcing bubbles of gas into the circulatory system, the heart, brain, and body tissues. As the bubbles enlarge and pass into smaller arteries, they reach a point where they can move no further and cut off circulation.
4. Maintain an adequate airway, provide high-flow oxygen, place in a supine position, and transport quickly to the hospital.

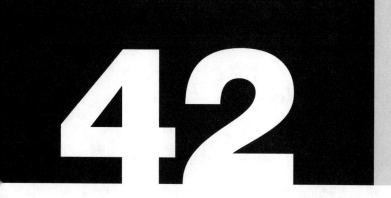

Reading Assignment: Chapter 42 pages 806–824.

Supplemental Objectives

- Define and describe military echelons of care.
- Identify potential threats in a tactical combat situation.
- Identify the stages of care associated with battlefield assessment.
- Describe the threats from biological and chemical weapons.
- Compare and contrast military and civilian mass casualty situations and the conduct of patient triage in these two scenarios.

Key Terms

1. What does MTF stand for?

2. What does BWA stand for?

3. The sorting of casualties into treatment categories is called _____.

4. Noncombat medical transport is termed _____.

5. The U.S. military program that provides non-medical personal education beyond basic first aid is called the _____ program.

6. Nuclear devices, biological agents, and chemical substances are known as _____ _____.

7. What does CASEVAC stand for?

Content Review

1. Describe each of the five levels of care of the U.S. Military Medical System.

   1)

   2)

   3)

   4)

   5)

2. A U.S. Air Force facility with ten holding beds OR enough supplies to perform 50 major surgical cases and ground or air evacuation involves the Echelon of Care _____ .

3. What determines theater evacuation policy or the amount of time that a casualty can remain in theater?

4. Where is definitive care in an Echelon IV facility normally provided?

5. What happens if a patient cannot be returned to duty within a specified time period?

6. What type of care occurs at an Echelon V facility?

7. Where is Echelon of Care V provided?

8. Compare the military and civilian systems of care.

9. Stable patients with serious wounds may bypass intermediate echelons and be sent directly to definitive care, if transport time is short.
   A. True
   B. False

10. _____% of those who die from combat wounds do so on the battlefield before ever reaching a medical treatment facility.

11. What factors interfere with emergency care in the combat setting?

12. When providing emergency care, combat medics and corpsmen must consider the appropriate elements of treatment and _____.

13. Describe the three phases of care that occur with the management of casualties during combat.

    1)

    2)

    3)

14. The term _____ is used to describe phase 3 care during combat missions.

15. The term MEDEVAC is used to describe _____.

16. Management of the airway is temporarily deferred in the "care under fire" phase during a combat mission.
    A. True
    B. False

17. During initial combat rescue in which the casualty may need to be dragged or carried to cover by the rescuer, management of life-threatening extremity hemorrhage may best be accomplished by use of what bleeding control method?

18. When moving a casualty with a penetrating neck or head wound out of a fire fight, immobilization of the cervical spine prior to movement is not necessary.
    A. True
    B. False

19. In the tactical setting, resuscitation of a trauma victim in cardiac arrest should always be attempted providing necessary resources are available.
    A. True
    B. False

20. In what situations should CPR be considered in the tactical setting?

21. If a casualty is unconscious, with spontaneous respirations, and in no respiratory distress, a _____ airway is the airway of choice.

22. List those items that are classified as weapons of mass destruction.

23. Identify those injuries most likely to be encountered in survivors of a nuclear blast.

24. Decontamination should be conducted prior to providing any emergency care.
    A. False
    B. False

25. Describe the components of handling a nuclear incident using the SWIMS acronym.

    S:
    W:
    I:
    M:
    S:

26. What are the four broad categories of biological warfare agents?

    1)
    2)
    3)
    4)

27. Insects purposefully infected with a pathogen in an attempt to propagate the spread of disease as a BWA are called _____.

28. Viruses, bacteria, fungi, and rickettsia, used as a weapons to cause disease in humans and/or animals are called _____.

29. Identify two examples of biologic toxins.

    1)
    2)

30. What are bioregulators?

31. Once disseminated, BWAs degrade quickly.
    A. True
    B. False

32. What is the most effective method of disseminating BWAs?

33. What factors affect dissemination and/or spread of BWAs?

34. How does exposure to Anthrax occur?

35. What nine characteristics determine the usefulness of BWAs?

    1)
    2)
    3)
    4)
    5)
    6)
    7)
    8)
    9)

36. List the five main categories within which chemical agents fall.

    1)
    2)
    3)
    4)
    5)

37. What are the three primary considerations when dealing with biological or chemical warfare agents?

    1)
    2)
    3)

38. What are the effects of nerve agents on the body?

39. Nerve agents can penetrate normal clothing but do not penetrate intact skin.
    A. True
    B. False

40. What are vesicants?

41. What is the appropriate treatment for cyanide poisoning?

42. Lung agents are compounds that cause _____.

43. The most effective decontamination of a liquid chemical agent is that which is performed within _____ after exposure.

44. What steps are taken in decontamination of a chemical agent?

45. What are the three broad categories of patients in the field?

    1)
    2)
    3)

46. What are the three categories of hospital triage and what percentage of patients seen normally fall into each category?

    1)

    2)

    3)

Chapter Quiz

••

1. The first level of care in the military where delayed surgical procedures are performed occur at which level?
   A. Echelon I
   B. Echelon II
   C. Echelon III
   D. Echelon IV

2. The first level of care in the military where transfusion capabilities are first available occur at which level?
   A. Echelon I
   B. Echelon II
   C. Echelon III
   D. Echelon IV

3. The Department of Veteran Affair Hospitals is an example of an Echelon _____ facility.
   A. II
   B. III
   C. IV
   D. V

4. Patients with serious wounds are always treated at an Echelon I facility before evacuation for more definitive care.
   A. True
   B. False

5. Care rendered by a medic or corpsman for an injury that occurs on a mission without hostile fire would occur in what phase of care?
   A. Care under fire
   B. Tactical field care
   C. Combat casualty evacuation care
   D. None of the above

6. Phase 3 of care provided during combat missions is called:
   A. MEDEVAC
   B. CASEVAC
   C. TACEVAC
   D. CCECEVAC

7. The number one cause of preventable death on the battlefield is:
   A. Airway compromise
   B. Infection
   C. Hemorrhage
   D. Hostile fire

8. In the tactical setting, CPR should be considered for which of the following situations associated with cardiac arrest?
   A. Electrocution
   B. Head injury
   C. Abdominal injury
   D. Amputated extremity

9. Which of the following methods of airway control is most appropriate in the tactical setting for an unconscious casualty without respiratory distress?
   A. Oropharyngeal airway
   B. Nasopharyngeal airway
   C. Endotracheal intubation
   D. Cricothyroidotomy

10. Living microorganisms that have the ability to cause disease in humans and/or animals and can cause plant destruction are called:
    A. True biological agents
    B. Biological vectors
    C. Biological toxins
    D. Bioregulators

11. The primary means of exposure to biological warfare agents is:
    A. The GI tract
    B. Skin contact
    C. The respiratory tract
    D. Mucous membranes of the eyes and mouth

12. Which of the following weapons are more toxic weight for weight and provide the largest area coverage?
    A. BWAs
    B. Chemical weapons
    C. Conventional weapons
    D. Nuclear weapons

13. Which of the following methods of exposure to Anthrax is most fatal?
    A. Inhalation
    B. Ingestion
    C. Contact with wounds on skin
    D. All are equally lethal

14. What is the most effective treatment for exposure to nerve agents?
    A. Epinephrine
    B. Oxygenation
    C. Diuretics
    D. Atropine

15. Which of the following is a chemical agent that inhibits the ability of cells to use oxygen and causes death by cellular hypoxemia?
    A. Anthrax
    B. Bacillus
    C. Cyanide
    D. Arsenic

Case Scenario

· ·

You are dispatched to provide assistance at a large-scale incident involving an explosion at a naval base. There are numerous casualties of both military personnel and civilians.

1. En route to the scene, what should be your initial concern?

You arrive on location where you are met by a captain acting as what you would call the Incident Commander. He directs you to the staging area and asks you to assist with the care of the "urgent" level patients. He informs you that the explosion did not involve any nuclear, biological, or chemical agents but that there is a large amount of debris around the scene and that continues to fall from structures.

2. What PPE should you wear at this scene?

3. What are the treatment priorities for the patients you were asked to assist?

4. The care provided at this level would be compared to which phase of military care?

5. Casualties are being transported to a nearby general military hospital with the capability of providing definitive therapy. This facility would be considered what echelon level?

Answer Key

· ·

Key Terms
1. Medical treatment facility
2. Biological warfare agent
3. Triage
4. MEDEVAC
5. Combat lifesaver
6. Weapons of mass destruction
7. Combat casualty evacuation care

Content Review

1. 1) Echelon I is care at the unit level, accomplished by individual soldiers or a trained medic or corpsman and includes care to return the patient to duty or stabilize the patient for evacuation to the next level. 2) Echelon II involves a team of physicians, physician assistants, nurses, and medical technicians capable of basic resuscitation, stabilization, and surgery along with x-ray, pharmacy, temporary holding facilities, limited laboratories, and transfusion capabilities where surgical procedures are limited to emergency procedures to prevent death, loss of limb or bodily function. 3) Echelon III facilities have capabilities normally found in fixed MTFs, are located in lower threat environments, and contain more extensive services and equipment. 4) Echelon IV facilities provide definitive therapy within a theater of operations for patients who can be returned to duty within a set time. 5) Echelon V involves convalescent, restorative, and rehabilitative care.
2. II
3. Enemy threat; type of mission; size of force; air frame availability; and bed occupancy and availability
4. Fleet hospital ship, general hospital, and overseas MTF
5. Evacuation is required, usually to the continental United States.
6. Convalescent, restorative, and rehabilitative care
7. Military hospitals; Department of Veterans Affair hospitals; and civilian hospitals in the United States.
8. The military echeloned medical care system closely matches an integrated trauma system. Echelon I compares to care rendered by paramedics and flight medics; echelon II facilities compare to Level I trauma centers; echelons III and IV provide restorative surgery and medical care provided in acute and intermediate trauma centers; and echelon V provides rehabilitative and support services offered in follow-up phases of care in an integrated trauma system.
9. True
10. 90
11. Darkness, hostile fire, medical equipment limitations, prolonged evacuation times, limited provider experience levels, mission-related command decisions, hostile environments (aquatic, mountain, desert, and jungle settings), and transport of casualties on the battlefield
12. The appropriate time in the continuum of care from battlefield to hospital facility
13. 1) Care under fire: Care rendered at the scene, while the caregiver and casualty are still under hostile fire and with limited equipment. 2) Tactical field care: Care rendered by a medic or corpsman once he and the casualty are no longer under effective hostile fire with equipment still limited to that carried by mission personnel. 3) Combat casualty evacuation care: care rendered once casualty is picked up for transport to higher echelon care and additional equipment and personnel are available.
14. CASEVAC
15. A non-combat medical transport by air force
16. True
17. A temporary tourniquet
18. True
19. False
20. Hypothermia, near-drowning, and electrocution
21. Nasopharyngeal
22. Nuclear devices, biological agents, and chemical substances
23. Thermal burns and trauma complicated by differing degrees of radiologic contamination
24. False
25. S: stop the spill; W: warn others; I: isolate the area; M: minimize contamination; and S: secure ventilation, if in an enclosed building
26. 1) True biological agents; 2) biological vectors; 3) toxins; and 4) bioregulators
27. Biological vectors
28. True biological agents
29. Botulinum and cholera toxins
30. Chemicals that occur naturally, in small amounts within the body, to regulate functions such as heart rate and BP, but may be synthetically derived and when given in altered concentrations, can have a wide variety of adverse effects on the human body

31. True
32. A line source weapon that disseminates the agent from a moving platform such as a spray tank mounted on a vehicle (truck or aircraft) that can disperse large amounts of the agent over a wide area.
33. Atmospheric conditions, high winds, unstable winds, sunlight, rain, and terrain
34. Inhalation, ingestion, and wounds on the skin
35. 1) Infectivity: the ability of the agent to reliably infect humans or animals; 2) Virulence: the ability of the agent to incapacitate or kill target once exposure occurs; 3) Incubation period; 4) Stability: the ability to maintain virulence over time and varying conditions; 5) Environmental persistence; 6) Resistance: the ability to withstand normal medical countermeasures; 7) Protection: the ability of an attacker to protect troops with measures not available to the opponent; 8) Controllability: the ability to predict the extent and nature of the BWA's effect; 9) Producibility
36. 1) Nerve agents, 2) vesicants, 3) cyanide, 4) lung agents, and 5) riot-control agents
37. Contamination avoidance; 2) decontamination; and 3) movement of decontaminated patients from a contaminated to a clean area
38. Involuntary muscle activity; excessive secretion from lacrimal, nasal, salivary, and sweat glands into airways and GI tract; constriction of the muscles of the airway produces bronchoconstriction; and constriction of muscles of the GI tract lead to cramps, vomiting, and diarrhea
39. False
40. A substance that causes burning of the skin with redness and blistering
41. Rapid administration of antidotes; support of circulation as necessary; and administration of oxygen
42. Pulmonary edema
43. 1 minute
44. Remove contaminated clothing; clean skin of residual chemicals; apply large amounts of water under pressure; and use chemical agents that destroy or detoxify the agent (e.g., sodium hypochlorite or undiluted bleach).
45. 1) Agonal (those who are about to die); 2) those who are more scared than wounded; 3) all others
46. 1) "Walking wounded"—injuries that would heal with little or no therapy - comprise 65% of cases; 2) "the expectant"—patients who will probably die no matter what treatment is performed and so are not treated but who are made as comfortable as possible—comprise 10% of all cases; 3) "the priority"—patients who have a meaningful chance at survival with immediate or prompt intervention and treatment—comprise 25% of cases.

Chapter Quiz

1. C	6. B	11. C
2. B	7. C	12. A
3. D	8. A	13. A
4. B	9. B	14. D
5. B	10. A	15. C

Case Scenario

1. Scene safety—were BWAs or WMDs used?
2. Full turnout gear (boots, coats, gloves, pants, and helmet with face shield)
3. Airway management (insert airway and administer oxygen as necessary), assessment of vital signs and major injuries, bleeding control, splinting of any fractures, stabilization and immobilization, and rapid transport based on the injuries found
4. Tactical field care
5. Level IV

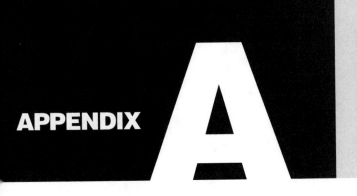

Department of Transportation National Standard Curriculum

Core Cognitive Objectives

Upon completion of the EMT-Basic you should be able to complete the following objectives. Note the date of mastery for each in the following table.

DOT Objective #	Objective	Date Mastered
Module 1: Preparatory **Lesson 1-1: Introduction to Emergency Medical Care**		
1-1.1	Define Emergency Medical Services (EMS) Systems.	
1-1.2	Differentiate the roles and responsibilities of the EMT-Basic from other prehospital care providers.	
1-1.3	Describe the roles and responsibilities related to personal safety.	
1-1.4	Discuss the roles and responsibilities of the EMT-Basic toward the safety of the crew, the patient, and bystanders.	
1-1.5	Define quality improvement and discuss the EMT-Basic's role in the process.	
1-1.6	Define medical direction and discuss the EMT-Basic's role in the process.	
1-1.7	State the specific statutes and regulations in your state regarding the EMS system	
Module 1: Preparatory **Lesson 1-2: The Well-Being of the EMT-Basic**		
1-2.1	List possible emotional reactions that the EMT-Basic may experience when faced with trauma, illness, death, and dying.	
1-2.2	Discuss the possible reactions that a family member may exhibit when confronted with death and dying.	
1-2.3	State the steps in the EMT-Basic's approach to the family confronted with death and dying.	
1-2.4	State the possible reactions that the family of the EMT-Basic may exhibit due to their outside involvement in EMS.	
1-2.5	Recognize the signs and symptoms of critical incident stress.	
1-2.6	State possible steps that the EMT-Basic may take to help reduce/alleviate stress.	
1-2.7	Explain the need to determine scene safety.	
1-2.8	Discuss the importance of body substance isolation (BSI).	
1-2.9	Describe the steps the EMT-Basic should take for personal protection from airborne and bloodborne pathogens.	

DOT Objective #	Objective	Date Mastered
1-2.10	List the personal protective equipment necessary for each of the following situations: - Hazardous materials - Rescue operations - Violent scenes - Crime scenes - Exposure to bloodborne pathogens - Exposure to airborne pathogens	
Module 1: Preparatory Lesson 1-3: Medical/Legal and Ethical Issues		
1-3.1	Define the EMT-Basic scope of practice.	
1-3.2	Discuss the importance of Do Not Resuscitate [DNR] (advance directives) and local or state provisions regarding EMS application.	
1-3.3	Define consent and discuss the methods of obtaining consent.	
1-3.4	Differentiate between expressed and implied consent.	
1-3.5	Explain the role of consent of minors in providing care.	
1-3.6	Discuss the implications for the EMT-Basic in patient refusal of transport.	
1-3.7	Discuss the issues of abandonment, negligence, and battery and their implications to the EMT-Basic.	
1-3.8	State the conditions necessary for the EMT-Basic to have a duty to act.	
1-3.9	Explain the importance, necessity and legality of patient confidentiality.	
1-3.10	Discuss the considerations of the EMT-Basic in issues of organ retrieval.	
1-3.11	Differentiate the actions that an EMT-Basic should take to assist in the preservation of a crime scene.	
1-3.12	State the conditions that require an EMT-Basic to notify local law enforcement officials.	
Module 1: Preparatory Lesson 1-4: The Human Body		
1-4.1	Identify the following topographic terms: medial, lateral, proximal, distal, superior, inferior, anterior, posterior, midline, right and left, mid-clavicular, bilateral, mid-axillary.	
1-4.2	Describe the anatomy and function of the following major body systems: respiratory, circulatory, musculoskeletal, nervous, and endocrine.	
Module 1: Preparatory Lesson 1-5: Baseline Vital Signs and SAMPLE History		
1-5.1	Identify the components of vital signs.	
1-5.2	Describe the methods to obtain a breathing rate.	
1-5.3	Identify the attributes that should be obtained when assessing breathing.	
1-5.4	Differentiate between shallow, labored, and noisy breathing.	
1-5.5	Describe the methods to obtain a pulse rate.	
1-5.6	Identify the information obtained when assessing a patient's pulse.	
1-5.7	Differentiate between a strong, weak, regular, and irregular pulse.	
1-5.8	Describe the methods to assess the skin color, temperature, and condition (capillary refill in infants and children).	
1-5.9	Identify the normal and abnormal skin color.	
1-5.10	Differentiate between pale, blue, red, and yellow skin color.	
1-5.11	Identify the normal and abnormal skin temperature.	

DOT Objective #	Objective	Date Mastered
1-5.12	Differentiate between hot, cool, and cold skin temperature.	
1-5.13	Identify normal and abnormal skin conditions.	
1-5.14	Identify normal and abnormal capillary refill in infants and children.	
1-5.15	Describe the methods used to assess the pupils.	
1-5.16	Identify normal and abnormal pupil size.	
1-5.17	Differentiate between dilated (big) and constricted (small) pupil size.	
1-5.18	Differentiate between reactive and non-reactive pupils and equal and unequal pupils.	
1-5.19	Describe the methods used to assess blood pressure.	
1-5.20	Define systolic pressure.	
1-5.21	Define diastolic pressure.	
1-5.22	Explain the difference between ausculation and palpation for obtaining a blood pressure.	
1-5.23	Identify the components of the SAMPLE history.	
1-5.24	Differentiate between a sign and a symptom.	
1-5.25	State the importance of accurately reporting and recording the baseline vital signs.	
1-5.26	Discuss the need to search for additional medical identification.	

Module 1: Preparatory
Lesson 1-6: Lifting and Moving Patients

1-6.1	Define body mechanics.	
1-6.2	Discuss the guidelines and safety precautions that need to be followed when lifting a patient.	
1-6.3	Describe the safe lifting of cots and stretchers.	
1-6.4	Describe the guidelines and safety precautions for carrying patients and/or equipment.	
1-6.5	Discuss one-handed carrying techniques.	
1-6.6	Describe correct and safe carrying procedures on stairs.	
1-6.7	State the guidelines for reaching and their application.	
1-6.8	Desribe correct reaching for log rolls.	
1-6.9	State the guidelines for pushing and pulling.	
1-6.10	Discuss the general considerations of moving patients.	
1-6.11	State three situations that may require the use of an emergency move.	
1-6.12	Identify the following patient carrying devices: - Wheeled ambulance stretcher - Portable ambulance stretcher - Stair chair - Scoop stretcher - Long spine board - Basket stretcher - Flexible stretcher	

Module 2: Airway
Lesson 2-1: Airway

2-1.1	Name and label the major structures of the respiratory system on a diagram.	
2-1.2	List the signs of adequate breathing.	
2-1.3	List the signs of inadequate breathing.	
2-1.4	Describe the steps in performing the head-tilt chin-lift.	
2-1.5	Relate mechanism of injury to opening the airway.	
2-1.6	Describe the steps in performing the jaw thrust.	

DOT Objective #	Objective	Date Mastered
2-1.7	State the importance of having a suction unit ready for immediate use when providing emergency care.	
2-1.8	Describe the techniques of suctioning.	
2-1.9	Describe how to artificially ventilate a patient with a pocket mask.	
2-1.10	Describe the steps in performing the skill of artificially ventilating a patient with a bag-valve-mask while using the jaw thrust.	
2-1.11	List the parts of a bag-valve-mask system.	
2-1.12	Describe the steps in performing the skill of artificially ventilating a patient with a bag-valve-mask for one and two rescuers.	
2-1.13	Describe the signs of adequate artificial ventilation using the bag-valve-mask.	
2-1.14	Describe the signs of inadequate artificial ventilation using the bag-valve-mask.	
2-1.15	Describe the steps in artificially ventilating a patient with a flow restricted, oxygen-powered ventilation device.	
2-1.16	List the steps in performing the actions taken when providing mouth-to-mouth and mouth-to-stoma artificial ventilation.	
2-1.17	Describe how to measure and insert an oropharyngeal (oral) airway.	
2-1.18	Describe how to measure and insert a nasopharyngeal (nasal) airway.	
2-1.19	Define the components of an oxygen delivery system.	
2-1.20	Identify a nonrebreather face mask and state the oxygen flow requirements needed for its use.	
2-1.21	Describe the indications for using a nasal cannula versus a nonre-breather face mask.	
2-1.22	Identify a nasal cannula and state the flow requirements needed for its use.	
Module 3: Patient Assessment		
Lesson 3-1: Scene Size-Up		
3-1.1	Recognize hazards/potential hazards.	
3-1.2	Describe common hazards found at the scene of a trauma and a medical patient.	
3-1.3	Determine if the scene is safe to enter.	
3-1.4	Discuss common mechanisms of injury/nature of illness.	
3-1.5	Discuss the reason for identifying the total number of patients at the scene.	
3-1.6	Explain the reason for identifying the need for additional help or assistance.	
Module 3: Patient Assessment		
Lesson 3-2: The Initial Assessment		
3-2.1	Summarize the reasons for forming a general impression of the patient.	
3-2.2	Discuss the methods of assessing altered mental status.	
3-2.3	Differentiate between assessing the altered mental status in the adult, child and infant patient.	
3-2.4	Discuss methods of assessing the airway in the adult, child, and infant patient.	
3-2.5	State reasons for management of the cervical spine once the patient has been determine to be a trauma patient.	
3-2.6	Describe methods used for assessing if a patient is breathing.	
3-2.7	State what care should be provided to the adult, child, and infant patient with adequate breathing.	

DOT Objective #	Objective	Date Mastered
3-2.8	State what care should be provided to the adult, child, and infant patient without adequate breathing.	
3-2.9	Differentiate between a patient with adequate and a patient with inadequate breathing.	
3-2.10	Distinguish between methods of assessing breathing in the adult, child and infant patient.	
3-2.11	Compare the methods of providing airway care to the adult, child and infant patient.	
3-2.12	Describe the methods used to obtain a pulse.	
3-2.13	Differentiate between obtaining a pulse in an adult, child and infant patient.	
3-2.14	Discuss the need for assessing the patient for external bleeding.	
3-2.15	Describe normal and abnormal findings when assessing skin color.	
3-2.16	Describe normal and abnormal findings when assessing skin temperature.	
3-2.17	Describe normal and abnormal findings when assessing skin condition.	
3-2.18	Describe normal and abnormal findings when assessing skin capillary refill in the infant and child patient.	
3-2.19	Explain the reason for prioritizing a patient for care and transport.	
Module 3: Patient Assessment Lesson 3-3: The Focused History and Physical Exam—Trauma Patients		
3-3.1	Discuss the reasons for reconsideration concerning the mechanism of injury.	
3-3.2	State the reasons for performing a rapid trauma assessment.	
3-3.3	Recite examples and explain why patients should receive a rapid trauma assessment.	
3-3.4	Describe the areas included in the rapid trauma assessment and discuss what should be evaluated.	
3-3.5	Differentiate when the rapid assessment may be altered in order to provide patient care.	
3-3.6	Discuss the reason for performing a focused history and physical exam.	
Module 3: Patient Assessment Lesson 3-4: The Focused History and Physical Exam—Medical Patient		
3-4.1	Describe the unique needs for assessing an individual with a specific chief complaint with no known prior history	
3-4.2	Differentiate between the history and physical exam that are performed for responsive patients with no known prior history and responsive patients with a known prior history.	
3-4.3	Describe the needs for assessing an individual who is unresponsive.	
3-4.4	Differentiate between the assessment that is performed for a patient who is unresponsive or has an altered mental status and other medical patients requiring assessment.	
Module 3: Patient Assessment Lesson 3-5: Detailed Physical Exam		
3-5.1	Discuss the components of the detailed physical exam.	
3-5.2	State the areas of the body that are evaluated during the detailed physical exam.	
3-5.3	Explain what additional care should be provided while performing the detailed physical exam.	

DOT Objective #	Objective	Date Mastered
3-5.4	Distinguish between the detailed physical exam that is performed on a trauma patient and that of the medical patient.	
Module 3: Patient Assessment		
Lesson 3-6: On-Going Assessment		
3-6.1	Discuss the reasons for repeating the initial assessment as part of the on-going assessment.	
3-6.2	Describe the components of the on-going assessment.	
3-6.3	Describe trending of assessment components.	
Module 3: Patient Assessment		
Lesson 3-7: Communications		
3-7.1	List the proper methods of initiating and terminating a radio call.	
3-7.2	State the proper sequence for delivery of patient information.	
3-7.3	Explain the importance of effective communication of patient information in the verbal report.	
3-7.4	Identify the essential components of the verbal report.	
3-7.5	Describe the attributes for increasing effectiveness and efficiency of verbal communications.	
3-7.6	State legal aspects to consider in verbal communication.	
3-7.7	Discuss the communication skills that should be used to interact with the patient.	
3-7.8	Discuss the communication skills that should be used to interact with the family, bystanders, and individuals from other agencies while providing patient care and the difference between skills used to interact with the patient and those used to interact with others.	
3-7.9	List the correct radio procedures in the following phases of a typical call. - To the scene - At the scene - To the facility - At the facility - To the station - At the station	
Module 3: Patient Assessment		
Lesson 3-8: Documentation		
3-8.1	Explain the components of the written report and list the information that should be included in the written report.	
3-8.2	Identify the various sections of the written report.	
3-8.3	Describe what information is required in each section of the prehospital care report and how it should be entered.	
3-8.4	Define the special considerations concerning patient refusal.	
3-8.5	Describe the legal implications associated with the written report.	
3-8.6	Discuss all state and/or local record and reporting requirements.	
Module 4: Medical/Behavioral Emergencies and Obstetrics/Gynecology		
Lesson 4-1: General Pharmacology		
4-1.1	Identify which medications will be carried on the unit.	
4-1.2	State the medications carried on the unit by the generic name.	
4-1.3	Identify the medications with which the EMT-Basic may assist the patient with administering.	
4-1.4	State the medications the EMT-Basic can assist the patient with by the generic name.	
4-1.5	Discuss the forms in which the medications may be found.	

DOT Objective #	Objective	Date Mastered
Module 4: Medical/Behavioral Emergencies and Obstetrics/Gynecology Lesson 4-2: Respiratory Emergencies		
4-2.1	List the structures and functions of the respiratory system.	
4-2.2	State the signs and symptoms of a patient with breathing difficulty.	
4-2.3	Describe the emergency medical care of the patient with breathing difficulty.	
4-2.4	Recognize the need for medical direction to assist in the emergency medical care of the patient with breathing difficulty.	
4-2.5	Describe the emergency medical care of the patient with breathing distress.	
4-2.6	Establish the relationship between airway management and the patient with breathing difficulty.	
4-2.7	List signs of adequate air exchange.	
4-2.8	State the generic name, medication forms, dose, administration, action, indications and contraindications for the prescribed inhaler.	
4-2.9	Distinguish between the emergency medical care of the infant, child, and adult patient with breathing difficulty.	
4-2.10	Differentiate between upper airway obstruction and lower airway disease in the infant and child patient.	
Module 4: Medical/Behavioral Emergencies and Obstetrics/Gynecology Lesson 4-3: Cardiac Emergencies		
4-3.1	Describe the structure and function of the cardiovascular system.	
4-3.2	Describe the emergency medical care of the patient experiencing chest pain/discomfort.	
4-3.3	List the indications for automated external defibrillation.	
4-3.4	List the contraindications for automated external defibrillation.	
4-3.5	Define the role of the EMT-B in the emergency cardiac care system.	
4-3.6	Explain the impact of age and weight on defibrillation.	
4-3.7	Discuss the position of comfort for patients with various cardiac emergencies.	
4-3.8	Establish the relationship between airway management and the patient with cardiovascular compromise.	
4-3.9	Predict the relationship between the patient experiencing cardiovascular compromise and basic life support.	
4-3.10	Discuss the fundamentals of early defibrillation.	
4-3.11	Explain the rationale for early defibrillation.	
4-3.12	Explain that not all chest pain patients result in cardiac arrest and do not need to be attached to an automated external defibrillator.	
4-3.13	Explain the importance of prehospital ACLS intervention if it is available.	
4-3.14	Explain the importance of urgent transport to a facility with advanced cardiac life support if it is not available in the prehospital setting.	
4-3.15	Discuss the various types of automated external defibrillators.	
4-3.16	Differentiate between the fully automated and the semiautomated defibrillator.	
4-3.17	Discuss the procedures that must be taken into consideration for standard operations of the various types of automated external defibrillators.	
4-3.18	State the reasons for ensuring that the patient is pulseless and apneic when using the automated external defibrillator.	
4-3.19	Discuss the circumstances which may result in inappropriate shocks.	

DOT Objective #	Objective	Date Mastered
4-3.20	Explain the considerations for interruption of CPR, when using the automated external defibrillator.	
4-3.21	Discuss the advantages and disadvantages of automated external defibrillators.	
4-3.22	Summarize the speed of operation of automated external defibrillation.	
4-3.23	Discuss the use of remote defibrillation through adhesive pads.	
4-3.24	Discuss the special considerations for rhythm monitoring.	
4-3.25	List the steps in the operation of the automated external defibrillator.	
4-3.26	Discuss the standard of care that should be used to provide care to a patient with persistent ventricular fibrillation and no available ACLS.	
4-3.27	Discuss the standard of care that should be used to provide care to a patient with ventricular fibrillation and no available ACLS.	
4-3.28	Differentiate between the single rescuer and multi-rescuer care with an automated external defibrillator.	
4-3.29	Explain the reason for pulses not being checked between shocks with an automated external defibrillator.	
4-3.30	Discuss the importance of coordinating ACLS trained providers with personnel using automated external defibrillators.	
4-3.31	Discuss the importance of post-resuscitation care.	
4-3.32	List the components of post-resuscitation care.	
4-3.33	Explain the importance of frequent practice with the automated external defibrillator.	
4-3.34	Discuss the need to complete the Automated Defibrillator: Operator's Shift Checklist.	
4-3.35	Discuss the role of the American Heart Association (AHA) in the use of automated external defibrillation.	
4-3.36	Explain the role medical direction plays in the use of automated external defibrillation.	
4-3.37	State the reasons why a case review should be completed following the use of the automated external defibrillator.	
4-3.38	Discuss the components that should be included in a case review.	
4-3.39	Discuss the goal of quality improvement in automated external defibrillation.	
4-3.40	Recognize the need for medical direction of protocols to assist in the emergency medical care of the patient with chest pain.	
4-3.41	List the indications for the use of nitroglycerin.	
4-3.42	State the contraindications and side effects for the use of nitroglycerin.	
4-3.43	Define the function of all controls on an automated external defibrillator, and describe event documentation and battery defibrillator maintenance	
Module 4: Medical/Behavioral Emergencies and Obstetrics/Gynecology Lesson 4-4: Diabetes/Altered Mental Status		
4-4.1	Identify the patient taking diabetic medications who has altered mental status and the implications of a diabetes history.	
4-4.2	State the steps in the emergency medical care of the patient taking diabetic medicine with an altered mental status and a history of diabetes.	
4-4.3	Establish the relationship between airway management and the patient with altered mental status.	
4-4.4	State the generic and trade names, medication forms, dose, administration, action, and contraindications for oral glucose.	

DOT Objective #	Objective	Date Mastered
4-4.5	Evaluate the need for medical direction in the emergency medical care of the diabetic patient.	
Module 4: Medical/Behavioral Emergencies and Obstetrics/Gynecology Lesson 4-5: Allergies		
4-5.1	Recognize the patient experiencing an allergic reaction.	
4-5.2	Describe the emergency medical care of the patient with an allergic reaction.	
4-5.3	Establish the relationship between the patient with an allergic reaction and airway management.	
4-5.4	Describe the mechanisms of allergic response and the implications for airway management.	
4-5.5	State the generic and trade names, medication forms, dose, administration, action, and contraindications for the epinephrine auto-injector.	
4-5.6	Evaluate the need for medical direction in the emergency medical care of the patient with an allergic reaction.	
4-5.7	Differentiate between the general category of those patients having an allergic reaction and those patients having an allergic reaction and requiring immediate medical care, including immediate use of epinephrine auto-injector.	
Module 4: Medical/Behavioral Emergencies and Obstetrics/Gynecology Lesson 4-6: Poisoning/Overdose		
4-6.1	List various ways that poisons enter the body.	
4-6.2	List signs/symptoms associated with poisoning.	
4-6.3	Discuss the emergency medical care for the patient with possible overdose.	
4-6.4	Describe the steps in the emergency medical care for the patient with suspected poisoning	
4-6.5	Establish the relationship between the patient suffering from poisoning or overdose and airway management.	
4-6.6	State the generic and trade names, indications, contraindications, medication form, dose, administration, actions, side effects and re-assessment strategies for activated charcoal.	
4-6.7	Recognize the need for medical direction in caring for the patient with poisoning or overdose.	
Module 4: Medical/Behavioral Emergencies and Obstetrics/Gynecology Lesson 4-7: Environmental Emergencies		
4-7.1	Describe the various ways that the body loses heat.	
4-7.2	List the signs and symptoms of exposure to cold.	
4-7.3	Explain the steps in providing emergency medical care to a patient exposed to cold.	
4-7.4	List the signs and symptoms of exposure to heat.	
4-7.5	Explain the steps in providing emergency care to a patient exposed to heat.	
4-7.6	Recognize the signs and symptoms of water-related emergencies.	
4-7.7	Describe the complications of near drowning.	
4-7.8	Discuss the emergency medical care of bites and stings.	
Module 4: Medical/Behavioral Emergencies and Obstetrics/Gynecology Lesson 4-8: Behavioral Emergencies		
4-8.1	Define behavioral emergencies.	
4-8.2	Discuss the general factors that may cause an alteration in a patient's behavior.	

DOT Objective #	Objective	Date Mastered
4-8.3	State the various reasons for psychological crises.	
4-8.4	Discuss the characteristics of an individual's behavior that suggests that the patient is at risk for suicide.	
4-8.5	Discuss special medical/legal considerations for managing behavioral emergencies.	
4-8.6	Discuss the special considerations for assessing a patient with behavioral problems.	
4-8.7	Discuss the general principles of an individual's behavior that suggests that he or she is at risk for violence.	
4-8.8	Discuss methods to calm behavioral emergency patients.	
Module 4: Medical/Behavioral Emergencies and Obstetrics/Gynecology		
Lesson 4-9: Obstetrics/Gynecology		
4-9.1	Identify the following structures: uterus, vagina, fetus, placenta, umbilical cord, amniotic sac, perineum.	
4-9.2	Identify and explain the use of the contents of an obstetrics kit	
4-9.3	Identify predelivery emergencies.	
4-9.4	State indications of an imminent delivery	
4-9.5	Differentiate the emergency medical care provided to a patient with predelivery emergencies from a normal delivery.	
4-9.6	State the steps in the predelivery preparation of the mother.	
4-9.7	Establish the relationship between body substance isolation and childbirth.	
4-9.8	State the steps to assist in the delivery.	
4-9.9	Describe care of the baby as the head appears.	
4-9.10	Describe how and when to cut the umbilical cord.	
4-9.11	Discuss the steps in the delivery of the placenta.	
4-9.12	List the steps in the emergency medical care of the mother post-delivery.	
4-9.13	Summarize neonatal resuscitation procedures.	
4-9.14	Describe the procedures for the following abnormal deliveries: breech birth, prolapsed cord, limb presentation.	
4-9.15	Differentiate the special considerations for multiple births.	
4-9.16	Describe special considerations of meconium.	
4-9.17	Describe special considerations of a premature baby.	
4-9.18	Discuss the emergency medical care of a patient with a gynecologic emergency.	
Module 5: Trauma		
Lesson 5-1: Bleeding and Shock		
5-1.1	List the structures and functions of the circulatory system.	
5-1.2	Differentiate between arterial, venous, and capillary bleeding.	
5-1.3	State methods of emergency medical care of external bleeding.	
5-1.4	Establish the relationship between body substance isolation and bleeding.	
5-1.5	Establish the relationship between airway management and the trauma patient.	
5-1.6	Establish the relationship between mechanism of injury and internal bleeding.	
5-1.7	List the signs of internal bleeding.	
5-1.8	List the steps in the emergency medical care of the patient with signs and symptoms of internal bleeding.	
5-1.9	List the signs and symptoms of shock (hypoperfusion).	

DOT Objective #	Objective	Date Mastered
5-1.10	State the steps in the emergency medical care of the patient with signs and symptoms of shock (hypoperfusion).	
Module 5: Trauma Lesson 5-2: Soft Tissue Injuries		
5-2-1	State the major functions of the skin.	
5-2.2	List the layers of the skin.	
5-2.3	Establish the relationship between body substance isolation (BSI) and soft tissue injuries.	
5-2.4	List the types of closed soft tissue injuries.	
5-2.5	Describe the emergency medical care of the patient with a closed soft tissue injury.	
5-2.6	State the types of open soft tissue injuries.	
5-2.7	Describe the emergency medical care of the patient with an open soft tissue injury.	
5-2.8	Discuss the emergency medical care considerations for a patient with a penetrating chest injury.	
5-2.9	State the emergency medical care considerations for a patient with an open wound to the abdomen.	
5-2.10	Differentiate the care of an open wound to the chest from an open wound to the abdomen.	
5-2.11	List the classifications of burns.	
5-2.12	Define superficial burn.	
5-2.13	List the characteristics of a superficial burn.	
5-2.14	Define partial thickness burn.	
5-2.15	List the characteristics of a partial thickness burn.	
5-2.16	Define full thickness burn.	
5-2.17	List the characteristics of a full-thickness burn.	
5-2.18	Describe the emergency medical care of the patient with a superficial burn.	
5-2.19	Describe the emergency medical care of the patient with a partial-thickness burn.	
5-2.20	Describe the emergency medical care of the patient with a full thickness burn.	
5-2.21	List the functions of dressing and bandaging.	
5-2.22	Describe the purpose of a bandage.	
5-2.23	Describe the steps in applying a pressure dressing.	
5-2.24	Establish the relationship between airway management and the patient with chest injury, burns, and blunt and penetrating injuries.	
5-2.25	Describe the effects of improperly applied dressings, splints and tourniquets.	
5-2.26	Describe the emergency medical care of a patient with an impaled object.	
5-2.27	Describe the emergency medical care of a patient with an amputation.	
5-2.28	Describe the emergency care for a chemical burn.	
5-2.29	Describe the emergency care for an electrical burn.	
Module 5: Trauma Lesson 5-3: Musculoskeletal Care		
5-3.1	Describe the functions of the muscular system.	
5-3.2	Describe the functions of the skeletal system.	
5-3.3	List the major bones or bone groupings of the spinal column; the thorax; the upper extremities; the lower extremities.	

DOT Objective #	Objective	Date Mastered
5-3.4	Differentiate between an open and a closed painful, swollen, deformed extremity.	
5-3.5	State the reasons for splinting.	
5-3.6	List the general rules of splinting.	
5-3.7	List the complications of splinting.	
5-3.8	List the emergency medical care for a patient with a painful, swollen, deformed extremity.	
Module 5: Trauma		
Lesson 5-4: Injuries to the Head and Spine		
5-4.1	State the components of the nervous system.	
5-4.2	List the functions of the central nervous system.	
5-4.3	Define the structure of the skeletal system as it relates to the nervous system.	
5-4.4	Relate mechanism of injury to potential injuries of the head and spine.	
5-4.5	Describe the implications of not properly caring for potential spine injuries.	
5-4.6	State the signs and symptoms of a potential spine injury.	
5-4.7	Describe the method of determining if a responsive patient may have a spine injury.	
5-4.8	Relate the airway emergency medical care techniques to the patient with a suspected spine injury.	
5-4.9	Describe how to stabilize the cervical spine.	
5-4.10	Discuss indications for sizing and using a cervical spine immobilization device.	
5-4.11	Establish the relationship between airway management and the patient with head and spine injuries.	
5-4.12	Describe a method for sizing a cervical spine immobilization device.	
5-4.13	Describe how to log roll a patient with a suspected spine injury.	
5-4.14	Describe how to secure a patient to a long spine board.	
5-4.15	List instances when a short spine board should be used.	
5-4.16	Describe how to immobilize a patient using a short spine board.	
5-4.17	Describe the indications for the use of rapid extrication.	
5-4.18	List steps in performing rapid extrication.	
5-4.19	State the circumstances when a helmet should be left on the patient.	
5-4.20	Discuss the circumstances when a helmet should be removed.	
5-4.21	Identify different types of helmets.	
5-4.22	Describe the unique characteristics of sports helmets.	
5-4.23	Explain the preferred methods to remove a helmet.	
5-4.24	Discuss alternative methods for removal of a helmet	
5-4.25	Describe how the patient's head is stabilized to remove the helmet	
5-4.26	Differentiate how the head is stabilized with a helmet compared to without a helmet.	
Module 6: Infants and Children		
6-1.1	Identify the developmental considerations for the following age groups: - Infants - Toddlers - Pre-school children - School age children - Adolescents	

DOT Objective #	Objective	Date Mastered
6-1.2	Describe differences in anatomy and physiology of the infant, child and adult patient.	
6-1.3	Differentiate the response of the ill or injured infant or child (age specific) from that of an adult.	
6-1.4	Indicate various causes of respiratory emergencies.	
6-1.5	Differentiate between respiratory distress and respiratory failure.	
6-1.6	List the steps in the management of foreign body airway obstruction.	
6-1.7	Summarize emergency medical care strategies for respiratory distress and respiratory failure.	
6-1.8	Identify the signs and symptoms of shock (hypoperfusion) in the infant and child patient.	
6-1.9	Describe the methods of determining end organ perfusion in the infant and child patient	
6-1.10	State the usual cause of cardiac arrest in infants and children versus adults.	
6-1.11	List the common causes of seizures in the infant and child patient.	
6-1.12	Describe the management of seizures in the infant and child patient.	
6-1.13	Differentiate between the injury patterns in adults, infants, and children.	
6-1.14	Discuss the field management of the infant and child trauma patient.	
6-1.15	Summarize the indicators of possible child abuse and neglect.	
6-1.16	Describe the medical legal responsibilities in suspected child abuse.	
6-1.17	Recognize the need for EMT-Basic debriefing following a difficult infant or child transport.	
Module 7: Operations		
Lesson 7-1: Ambulance Operations		
7-1.1	Discuss the medical and non-medical equipment needed to respond to a call.	
7-1.2	List the phases of an ambulance call.	
7-1.3	Describe the general provisions of state laws relating to the operation of the ambulance and privileges in any or all of the following categories: - Speed - Warning lights - Sirens - Right-of-way - Parking - Turning	
7-1.4	List contributing factors to unsafe driving conditions.	
7-1.5	Describe the considerations that should be given to: - Requests for escorts. - Following an escort vehicle - Intersections	
7-1.6	Discuss "due regard for safety of all others" while operating an emergency vehicle.	
7-1.7	State what information is essential in order to respond to a call.	
7-1.8	Discuss various situations that may affect response to a call.	
7-1.9	Differentiate between the various methods of moving a patient to the unit based on injury or illness.	
7-1.10	Apply the components of the essential patient information in a written report.	
7-1.11	Summarize the importance of preparing the unit for the next response.	

DOT Objective #	Objective	Date Mastered
7-1.12	Identify what is essential for completion of a call.	
7-1.13	Distinguish among the terms cleaning, disinfection, high-level disinfection, and sterilization.	
7-1.14	Describe how to clean or disinfect items following patient care.	
Module 7: Operations		
Lesson 7-2: Gaining Access		
7-2.1	Describe the purpose of extrication.	
7-2.2	Discuss the role of the EMT-Basic in extrication.	
7-2.3	Identify what equipment for personal safety is required for the EMT-Basic.	
7-2.4	Define the fundamental components of extrication.	
7-2.5	State the steps that should be taken to protect the patient during extrication.	
7-2.6	Evaluate various methods of gaining access to the patient.	
7-2.7	Distinguish between simple and complex access.	
Module 7: Operations		
Lesson 7-3: Overviews		
7-3.1	Explain the EMT-Basic's role during a call involving hazardous materials.	
7-3.2	Describe what the EMT-Basic should do if there is reason to believe that there is a hazard at the scene.	
7-3.3	Describe the actions that an EMT-Basic should take to ensure bystander safety.	
7-3.4	State the role the EMT-Basic should perform until appropriately trained personnel arrive at the scene of a hazardous materials situation.	
7-3.5	Break down the steps to approaching a hazardous situation.	
7-3.6	Discuss the various environmental hazards that affect EMS	
7-3.7	Describe the criteria for a multiple-casualty situation.	
7-3.8	Evaluate the role of the EMT-Basic in the multiple-casualty situation.	
7-3.9	Summarize the components of basic triage.	
7-3.10	Define the role of the EMT-Basic in a disaster operation.	
7-3.11	Describe basic concepts of incident management.	
7-3.12	Explain the methods for preventing contamination of self, equipment and facilities.	
7-3.13	Review the local mass casualty incident plan.	
Module 8: Airway		
Lesson 8-1: Advanced Airway Management		
8-1.1	Identify and describe the airway anatomy in the infant, child, and adult	
8-1.2	Differentiate between the airway anatomy in the infant, child, and adult.	
8-1.3	Explain the pathophysiology of airway compromise.	
8-1.4	Describe the proper use of airway adjuncts.	
8-1.5	Review the use of oxygen therapy in airway management.	
8-1.6	Describe the indications, contraindications, and technique for insertion of nasal gastric tubes.	
8-1.7	Describe how to perform the Sellick maneuver (cricoid pressure).	
8-1.8	Describe the indications for advanced airway management.	
8-1.9	List the equipment required for orotracheal intubation.	
8-1.10	Describe the proper use of the curved blade for orotracheal intubation.	
8-1.11	Describe the proper use of the straight blade for orotracheal intubation.	

DOT Objective #	Objective	Date Mastered
8-1.12	State the reasons for and proper use of the stylet in orotracheal intubation.	
8-1.13	Describe the methods of choosing the appropriate size endotracheal tube in an adult patient.	
8-1.14	State the formula for sizing an infant or child endotracheal tube.	
8-1.15	List complications associated with advanced airway management.	
8-1.16	Define the various alternative methods for sizing the infant and child endotracheal tube.	
8-1.17	Describe the skill of orotracheal intubation in the adult patient.	
8-1.18	Describe the skill of orotracheal intubation in the infant and child patient.	
8-1.19	Describe the skill of confirming endotracheal tube placement in the adult, infant, and child patient.	
8-1.20	State the consequence of and the need to recognize unintentional esophageal intubation.	
8-1.21	Describe the skill of securing the endotracheal tube in the adult, infant, and child patient.	

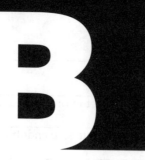

APPENDIX B

Skills Verification Form For Emergency Medical Technicians

STUDENT NAME _____ CLASS NUMBER _____

CLASS LOCATION _____

SKILLS	DATE	INSTR. INIT.
PATIENT ASSESSMENT		
Scene Size-up		
SAMPLE History		
Initial Assessment		
Focused Assessment—Trauma		
Focused Assessment—Medical		
Detailed History & Exam		
Rapid Assessment		
DIAGNOSTIC SIGNS		
Level of Consciousness		
Pulses		
Brachial		
Femoral		
Radial		
Ventilations		
Rate/Depth		
Breath Sounds		
Blood Pressure		
Auscultation		
Palpation		
Pupils		
Skin Color/Temp.		
Capillary Refill (Infant's & Children)		
BLEEDING AND SHOCK		
Amputations		
Bleeding Control		
Dressing & Bandaging		
Head & Face		
Neck		
Torso		
Extremities		
PASG Application		

SKILLS	DATE	INSTR. INIT.
SOFT TISSUE INJURIES		
Abdominal Evisceration		
Blunt Abdominal Injury		
Impaled Objects		
Eyes		
Face		
Chest		
Abdomen		
Extremities		
Lacerations/Incisions/ Abrasions/Avulsions/ Penetrations of:		
Eye		
Head and Face		
Neck		
Torso		
AIRWAY OBSTRUCTION		
Conscious Adult		
Conscious Infant		
Conscious to Unconscious Adult		
Conscious to Unconscious Infant		
Laryngectomies		
Unconscious Adult		
Unconscious Infant		
CARDIAC ARREST		
Single Rescuer		
Adult		
Child		
Infant		
Two Rescuer—Child		

474

SKILLS	DATE	INSTR. INIT.	SKILLS	DATE	INSTR. INIT.
CARDIAC ARREST (cont'd.)			Elbow		
Two Rescuer—Adult			Fingers		
CPR in Transport—Infant			Hand		
			Humerus		
AIRWAY ADJUNCTS			Radius/Ulna		
Nasopharyngeal Airways			Scapula		
Oxygen Equipment			Wrist		
Bag Valve Device			Lower Extremities		
Demand Valve			Ankle		
Nasal Cannulac			Femur		
Non-Rebreather			Fibula/Tibia		
Pocket Mask			Foot		
Rebreather			Hip		
Simple Face Mask			Knee		
Venturi Mask			Pelvis		
Oxygen Setup/Tear Down			Toes		
Suction					
CPR with Airway Adjuncts			**PASG**		
BURNS					
Chemical			**EXTRICATION**		
Electrical			Access		
Light			Through Door		
Radiation			Through Roof		
Thermal			Through Window		
			Disentanglement		
CENTRAL NERVOUS SYSTEM			With Dashboard		
Cervical Collar			With Steering Wheel		
Helmet Removal			With Pedals		
Long Backboard/Straps			Hazard Control		
Short Backboard/Straps			Proper Protective Gear		
KED Device			Vehicle Stabilization		
CID			Rapid Extrication		
Extremities			Patient Extrication		
Wrap Around Backboard					
SUSPECTED FXs & SPLINTING			**CHILDBIRTH**		
Traction Splint			Excessive Bleeding		
Air Splint			Delivery:		
Padded Board Splint			Arm/Leg Presentation		
Sling & Swathe			Breech		
Other			Normal		
Upper Extremities			Prolapsed Cord		
Clavicle			Post Delivery		
			Pre-Delivery		

SKILLS	DATE	INSTR. INIT.	SKILLS	DATE	INSTR. INIT.
			Reeves		
INJURIES TO THE CHEST			Scoop Stretcher		
Flail Chest					
Hemothorax/Pneumothorax			**AMBULANCE OPERATIONS**		
Pericardial Tamponade			Patient Record Form		
Subcutaneous Emphysema			Simulated Radio Report		
Sucking Chest Wound					
Traumatic Asphyxia			**TRIAGE**		
Tension Pneumothorax					
			OVERVIEWS		
PATIENT LIFTING AND MOVING			Use of DOT Guidebook		
Emergency Drag			HazMat		
Log Roll			Recognition of need for ICS		
Two-man Lift					

I verify that the above instructor's initials are those of approved instructors for this program. The presence of the initials signify student familiarization and successful practice with the skill. No guarantee of the future performance is or should be implied by the presence of the initials.

Course Coordinator: _____ Date: _____

Medical Director: _____ Date: _____

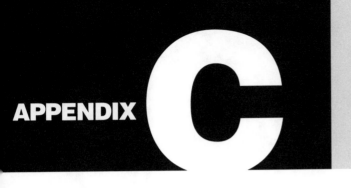

Acronyms and Abbreviations

A

a	before
A	amperes (a measure of electrical current)
AAOS	American Academy of Orthopaedic Surgeons
ABC	Airway, breathing, and circulation
ABG's	arterial blood gases
AC	alternating current
ACEP	American College of Emergency Physicians
ACLS	advanced cardiac life support
ACS	American College of Surgeons
ACT	Advanced Coronary Treatment Foundation
ad inf.	ad infinitum or to infinity
ad lib.	ad libitum or at one's pleasure
AFA	advanced first aid
AFL-CIO	American Federation of Labor and Congress of Industrial Organizations
AHA	American Heart Association, American Hospital Association
aka	also known as
ALS	advanced life support
a.m.	ante meridian or before noon
AM	amplitude modulation
AMA	American Medical Association
AOA	American Osteopathic Association
APO	Army Post Office
ARC	American (National) Red Cross
ARDS	Acute Respiratory Distress Syndrome
ASAP	as soon as possible
ASDH	acute subdural hematoma
ASHBEAMS	American Society of Hospital-Based Emergency Air Medical Services
ASHD	arteriosclerotic heart disease
ATLS	advanced trauma life support
ATS	American Trauma Society
A-V	atrioventricular
avdp.	avoirdupois weight

B

BA	breathing apparatus, blood alcohol, Bachelor of Arts
bbl	Barrel (but nobody seems to know what the second "b" stands for)
BCLS	basic cardiac life support
b.i.d.	twice per day
BLS	basic life support
BOW	bag of waters

Copyright © 2003, by Mosby Inc. All rights reserved.

BP	............blood pressure
BS	............Bachelor of Science

C

$\bar{c}$	............with
Ca	............calcium
C/A	............carcinoma or cancer
CAT	............Computerized axial tomography
cc	............cubic centimeter
C/C	............chief complaint or in supervisors' terms, a chronic complainer
CCRN	............critical care registered nurse
CCU	............critical care unit
CD	............Civil Defense
CE	............continuing education
CEN	............certified emergency nurse
CEU	............continuing education unit
CHF	............congestive heart failure
CHP	............California Highway Patrol (as in ChiPs)
CIM	............Crash Injury Management Course
Cl	............chlorine
CO	............carbon monoxide
CO_2	............carbon dioxide
COPD	............chronic obstructive pulmonary disease
CPR	............cardiopulmonary resuscitation
CSF	............cerebrospinal fluid
CV	............cerebrovascular or cardiovascular
CVA	............cerebrovascular accident (stroke)

D

db	............decibel, a unit or sound volume measurement
DC	............direct current
D/C	............disconnect
DDT	............dichlorodiphenyltrichloroenthane
DEHS	............Division of Emergency Health Services
DEMS	............Division of Emergency Medical Services
DHEW	............Department of Health, Education, and Welfare (U.S.—defunct)
DHHS	............Department of Health and Human Services
DNA	............deoxyribonucleic acid or does not apply
DO	............Doctor of Osteopathy
DOA	............dead on arrival
DOE	............dyspnea on exertion
DOH	............Department of Health
DOT	............Department of Transportation
DPH	............Department of Public Health
Dpx	............duplex (referring to simultaneous radio transmission on coupled frequencies)
DT	............delirium tremens
DTMF	............dual-tone multiple frequency
Dx	............diagnosis or distance

E

ECF	............extended care facility
ECG/EKG	............electrocardiogram
ED	............emergency department
EEG	............electroencephalogram
EENT	............eye, ear, nose, and throat
e.g.	............exempli gratia (for example)
EHSF	............Emergency Health Services Federation
EMA	............Emergency Management Agency
EMD	............electromechanical dissociation
EMRC	............Emergency Medical Resource Center
EMS	............emergency medical services
EMSI	............Emergency Medical Services Institute (southwest PA)
EMSS	............Emergency Medical Services System
EMT	............Emergency Medical Technician
EMT-P	............Emergency Medical Technician - Paramedic
ENA	............Emergency Nurses Association
EOA	............esophageal obturator airway
EOC	............Emergency Operations Center
ER	............emergency room
ERA	............easy rescue attempt
ET	............endo(in)-tracheal (the trachea)
ETA	............estimated time of arrival
et al	............et alii (and others)
etc.	............et cetera (and others)
EVOC	............Emergency Vehicle Operator's Course

F

FAA	............Federal Aviation Administration
FCC	............Federal Communications Commission
FDA	............Food and Drug Administration
FEC	............free-standing emergency center (clinic)
FEMA	............Federal Emergency Management Agency
FM	............frequency modulation
FPO	............Fleet Post Office
FPS	............feet per second
Fx	............fracture
FYI	............for your information

G

GAO	............Government Accounting Office
GC	............gonococcal
GE	............gastroenter(ic), (ology), having to do with the stomach and intestines
GI	............gastrointestinal
gm	............gram
GNP	............Gross National Product
GP	............General Practitioner
GPO	............Government Printing Office
GSA	............General Services Agency

GSW ....gunshot wound
gtt ....drop
GYN ....gynecolog(y), (ical); pertaining to female reproductive system

H

H ....the element hydrogen
HCO_3 ....bicarbonate
H_2CO_3 ....carbonic acid
He ....the element Helium
HORG ....Health Operations Research Group
H+P ....history and physical (examination)
HR ....House of Representatives bill, followed by number; also heart rate
HRPD ....Health Resources Planning and Development
hs ....hour of sleep
HSA ....Health Systems Agency/Health Services Area

I

IAFC/IAFF ....International Association of Fire Chiefs/Fire Fighters
ibid ....in the same place
IC ....intracardiac, into the heart
ICP ....intracranial pressure, pressure in the cranium
ICU ....intensive care unit
id ....(idem) the same
ID ....intradermal, into the skin layers
i.e. ....(id est) that is ...
IM ....intramuscular, into the muscle
IPPB ....intermittent positive-pressure breathing
IQ ....intelligence quotient
IRDS ....Infant Respiratory Distress Syndrome
IU ....Intermediate unit
IV ....intravenous

J

JCAH ....Joint Commission of Accreditation of Hospitals
J.D. ....Juris Doctor, a doctorate in law
jems ....Journal of Emergency Medical Services

K

K+ ....the element potassium, expressed as an electrolyte
kg ....kilogram
KVO ....an IV rate just fast enough to *Keep the Vein Open*

R

R	...........electrical resistance or right-sided
RBBB	...........right bundle branch block, a conduction defect in the heart
RDS	...........respiratory distress syndrome
Rh	...........Rhesus; a blood factor
RLQ	...........right lower quadrant (of the abdomen)
RN	...........Registered Nurse
R/O	...........rule-out
ROM	...........range of motion
ROT	...........rule of thumb
RSVP	...........repondez s'il vous plait, please reply
RTSS	...........radio telephone switches system
RUQ	...........right upper quadrant (of the abdomen)
Rx	...........receive(r) or reception; also treatment

S

$\bar{s}$	...........without
SA	...........sinoatrial
SCUBA	...........self-contained underwater breathing apparatus
SERS	...........special emergency radio service band; a group of radio frequencies designated by the FCC
SIDS	...........sudden infant death syndrome
SOP	...........standard operating procedure or short on planning
SQ	...........subcutaneous
SRO	...........standing-room only
S-T	...........sinus tachycardia; also the portion of the ECG that follows the QRS
STAT	...........right now
SVT	...........supraventricular tach
SX	...........signs or symptoms
SZ	...........seizures

T

TA	...........technical assistance
TB	...........tuberculosis
TC	...........time called, or traffic collision
T+C	...........type and cross-match
TCA	...........tricyclic antidepressant
TIA	...........transient ischemic attack; a minor stroke
t.i.d.	...........three times per day
TKO	...........an IV drip rate just rapid enough *To Keep Open* (the vein)
TSS	...........technical support services or toxic shock syndrome
T-Wave	...........last part of the normal ECG cycle that indicates repolarization of the ventricle
Tx	...........transmit or transmission

U

UHF	...........ultrahigh frequency
URI	...........upper respiratory infection

USO	............United Service Organization
UTI	............urinary tract infection

V

V	............voltage
VASC	............Voluntary Ambulance Service Certification program
VF	............ventricular fibrillation
VHF	............very high frequency
VS	............vital signs
VT	............ventricular tachycardia

W

WHO	............World Health Organization
WNL	............within normal limits

X

Y

y.o.	............years old

Z

ZIP code	............Zone Improvement Plan

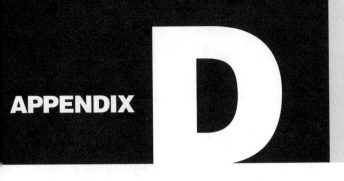

The following charts contain three types of information: 1) signs and symptoms 2) what variations in these signs may indicate; and 3) suggested emergency care procedures. While it is not necessary for the EMT-Basic to identify the specific illness or injury, students should be able to take one sign/symptom (or a combination of signs), state with which problems the EMT may have to deal, and give the emergency care procedure for handling the problems. Students should be able to do this in response to written and oral questions and in simulated patient care situations.

SIGN/SYMPTOM	MAY INDICATE	SUGGESTED EMERGENCY PROCEDURE
LEVEL OF CONSCIOUSNESS		
Alert	Normal brain function	Monitor for change
Stuporous	Impaired brain function	Administer O_2, monitor
Unconscious or comatose	Impaired brain function, possible loss of life processes	Initial assessment, rapid focused assessment, treatment according to signs and symptoms, administer O_2 if indicated, monitor closely and rapid transport to appropriate facility
Change in level of consciousness	Change in level of brain function	Monitor and basic life support as indicated
RESPIRATION		
Smooth and regular	Normal pulmonary function	Monitor
Rapid, frantic, deep	Hyperventilation	Calm patient, instruct patient to breathe slowly, coach breathing.
Deep, sighing	Air Hunger; diabetes	Administer O_2, be prepared to intubate and/or assist with ventilations
Deep, gasping, labored	Airway obstruction, impaired lung function due to injury	Establish and maintain open airway, administer O_2, monitor closely

SIGN/SYMPTOM	MAY INDICATE	SUGGESTED EMERGENCY PROCEDURE
RESPIRATION (Cont'd)		
Chest rales	Pulmonary edema	Administer O_2, place patient in a position of comfort
Rapid, shallow	Shock	Administer O_2, treat for shock, monitor closely
Bright red, frothy blood	Lung damage	Suction, administer O_2
Snoring	Airway obstruction	Establish and maintain an open airway, administer O_2, Monitor
Gurgling	Airway obstruction from liquid matter	Suction, maintain open airway, administer O_2
Paradoxical breathing	Flail chest	Initial assessment, rapid history and focused assessment, immobilize flail segment, administer O_2, monitor closely, be prepared to assist with ventilations
Wheezing on exhalation, use of neck muscles on inhalation	Asthma or severe allergic reaction	Administer O_2, place patient in position of comfort, reassure patient, monitor closely, assist with administration of inhaler or epinephrine auto-injector if indicated
Rapid, shallow ventilations, use of neck muscles in inhalation, pursed lips during exhalation	Emphysema	Airway maintenance, place patient in position of comfort, offer reassurance, administer O_2, monitor closely
Absent	Respiratory arrest	Artificial ventilation, with supplemental O_2, intubate if authorized
PULSE		
60-100 beats/minute, full regular	Normal adult cardiac function	Monitor
Rapid, bounding	Fright, hypertension, insulin shock	Calm patient, administer O_2 if indicated
Rapid, weak, thready	Shock, diabetic coma	Administer O_2, treat for shock, monitor
Irregular, weak	Patient in some life-threatening condition (e.g., severe attack)	Keep patient calm, administer O_2, provide other life support as needed, monitor closely
Absent in one limb	Impaired circulation to that limb (e.g., by bone fracture, clot)	Initial assessment, rapid history and focused assessment, immobilize extremity if fracture is suspected, administer O_2, report observation to ED physician

SIGN/SYMPTOM	MAY INDICATE	SUGGESTED EMERGENCY PROCEDURE
	PULSE (Cont'd)	
Absent in carotid artery	Cardiac arrest	CPR with oxygen until definitive care is available, consider AED and intubation if indicated
	BLOOD COLOR	
Bright red, spurts	Arterial bleeding	Initial assessment, control of external bleeding, rapid history and focused assessment, administer O$_2$ if indicated, estimate amount of blood loss and report to ED
Dark red or maroon, flows steadily	Venous bleeding	Initial assessment, control of external bleeding, rapid history and focused assessment, administer O$_2$ if indicated, estimate amount of blood loss and report to ED
Slow oozing	Capillary bleeding	Initial assessment, control of external bleeding, rapid history and focused assessment, administer O$_2$ if indicated, estimate amount of blood loss and report to ED
	BLOOD PRESSURE	
Diastolic pressure above 90 mm Hg	High blood pressure, stroke, may predispose heart attack	Administer O$_2$, place in position of comfort, offer reassurance, monitor closely
Systolic pressure 80 mm Hg or below	Severe shock (late sign)	Administer O$_2$, treat for shock, monitor closely
Dropping	Shock, warning of deterioration in patient's condition	Administer O$_2$, treat for shock, monitor closely
Absent	A variety of conditions including shock	Check other vital signs, initial assessment and rapid focused history and physical examination, emergency care as indicated if no pulse, begin CPR/AED
Increasing (with decreasing pulse)	Head injury	Check other vital signs, initial assessment and rapid focused history and physical examination, emergency care as indicated

SIGN/SYMPTOM	MAY INDICATE	SUGGESTED EMERGENCY PROCEDURE
MOBILITY		
Present in all extremities	No spinal cord injury	
Impaired in both upper and/or lower extremities	Pressure on spinal cord	Immobilize head, neck, and back
Absent in both extremities	Injury to spinal cord in lower back	Immobilize head, neck, and back
Absent in both upper extremities	Injury to spinal cord in neck	Immobilize head, neck, and back
Absent on one side of body	Stroke, head injury	Basic life support measures as indicated, administer O$_2$, monitor closely
PRESENCE OF PAIN		
General pain present at site of injury	Injury or illness in painful area, probably no spinal damage	Basic life support as indicated, care for underlying condition if possible, monitor
Local pain in extremities	Fracture, occluded artery	Basic life support, immobilize extremity, monitor
Numbness, tingling sensation	Possible spine injury	Basic life support as indicated, head, neck, and spine immobilization
No pain, but obvious injuries	Spinal cord damage, hysteria, shock, excessive use of alcohol or other drugs	Basic life support and emergency care as indicated, head, neck, and spine immobilization
PUPILS		
Pinpoint	Effect on central nervous system, drug use	Initial assessment, rapid history and focused assessment, basic life support as necessary, monitor closely
Dilated	Degree of severe shock, drug use	Initial assessment, rapid history and focused assessment, basic life support as necessary, monitor closely, administer O$_2$
Fixed, not reactive to stimulus	Brain damage	Initial assessment, rapid history and focused assessment, basic life support as necessary, monitor closely, administer O$_2$
Unequal	Head injury, stroke. This should not be used as sole indicator of any condition because 1) personal variation, 2) drugs affecting the pupils, 3) artificial eyes	Initial assessment, rapid history and focused assessment, life support as necessary, monitor closely, administer O$_2$, spinal immobilization as indicated

SIGN/SYMPTOM	MAY INDICATE	SUGGESTED EMERGENCY PROCEDURE
PUPILS (Cont'd)		
Oval as opposed to round	Head injury	Administer O_2, spinal immobilization if indicated
SKIN COLOR		
Blue	Insufficient O_2 for any reason	Initial assessment, rapid history and focused assessment, administer high-flow O_2, monitor closely
Red	High blood pressure, heart attack, hyperventilation, heat stroke	Initial assessment, rapid history and focused assessment, administer high-flow O_2, monitor closely
Cherry red	Carbon monoxide poisoning (Late sign)	Initial assessment, rapid history and focused assessment, administer high-flow O_2, monitor closely
White	Shock, heart attack, fright	Initial assessment, rapid history and focused assessment, administer high-flow O_2, monitor closely, elevate feet and consider PASG use
Yellow	Liver disease, gallbladder disease	Initial assessment, rapid history and focused assessment, administer high-flow O_2, monitor closely, BSI precautions
White, waxy	Frostbite	Initial assessment, rapid history and focused assessment, take indoors, slowly re-warm area as indicated
White, leathery	Burn	Stop burning process, apply dressings, administer O_2 as indicated, monitor
SKIN TEMPERATURE		
Hot, dry	Excessive body heat, as in heat stroke, high fever	Cold packs under arm pits, groin, and/or sides of neck
Cool, clammy	Shock	Keep warm, treat for shock, administer O_2
Cool, moist	Body is losing heat	Keep warm
Cool, dry	Exposure to cold	Keep warm

1. Which of the following scenarios presents the greatest immediate danger for your safety?
   A. a man who appears intoxicated
   B. a verbally abusive female
   C. a man with a knife in his hand
   D. two women shouting at each other

2. You arrive on the scene of a motor vehicle collision. The mechanism of injury suggests a rear end collision. Which of the following injuries would you suspect?
   A. chest injury
   B. neck injury
   C. leg injury
   D. arm injury

3. During your initial assessment of a patient, you discover a leg wound that is bleeding profusely. You determine that the patient is breathing and has a pulse. Your next step should be to:
   A. continue your assessment to locate any additional injuries
   B. hold direct pressure on the wound for 30 seconds, then continue your assessment
   C. administer high-flow oxygen
   D. stop and treat the bleeding immediately

4. You have provided in-line stabilization for a patient who is unconscious following a vehicle rollover. Your next step should be to:
   A. perform a SAMPLE history
   B. take the patient's vital signs
   C. request ALS assistance
   D. open the patient's airway

5. A pulse rate should be determined on an infant by assessing the _____ pulse.
   A. carotid
   B. brachial
   C. radial
   D. femoral

6. The organ that produces insulin is the:
   A. gallbladder
   B. spleen
   C. liver
   D. pancreas

7. You arrive on the location of a patient exhibiting convulsive movements on the floor. Your first action should be to:
   A. insert an oral airway
   B. clear the area to protect the patient
   C. attempt to restrain the patient
   D. insert a bit stick in the patient's mouth

8. You are called to the scene of a 76-year-old female patient who lost her balance and fell off a stool in the kitchen. She is alert and oriented and complaining of pain in her hip. Which of the following assessments is most appropriate for the patient?
   A. rapid trauma assessment with immediate transport
   B. rapid trauma assessment and ongoing assessment
   C. focused physical exam and vital sign assessment
   D. detailed physical exam prior to transporting the patient

9. The phase following a seizure is known as the _____ phase.
   A. postictal
   B. aura
   C. clonic
   D. petit mal

10. While at the scene of a house fire, you are called to attend to a firefighter who was inside the house during a flashover. He is suffering from burns to his chest, abdomen, and the anterior and posterior portions of his left arm. What percentage of BSA does this patient have?
    A. 18%
    B. 22.5%
    C. 27%
    D. 36%

11. While assessing burn injuries, you notice reddened skin with blisters. The patient is complaining of severe pain at the site of the injury. You suspect the patient has what degree of burns?
    A. first
    B. second
    C. third
    D. none of the above

12. You are on standby at a football game one Saturday afternoon in July, when you are called over to a player down. On initial assessment, you find a 16-year-old male patient lying supine on the field, conscious with red, dry skin, constricted pupils, and a pulse of 124 and thready. The coaches state that he "passed out" after the play. What do you suspect is wrong with this patient?
    A. drug overdose
    B. head injury
    C. hyperthermia
    D. diabetic emergency

13. Which of the following medications is most helpful to a patient complaining of chest pain in the pre-hospital environment?
    A. atropine
    B. aspirin
    C. epinephrine
    D. nitroglycerin

14. After completing a rapid physical exam on an unresponsive patient, your next action should be to:
    A. obtain baseline vital signs
    B. perform a focused physical exam
    C. perform a SAMPLE history
    D. obtain a history of the present illness

15. A 26-year-old-female patient is found conscious and alert at the scene of a car rollover. She complains of upper abdominal pain. After establishing scene safety and conducting an initial assessment, your first action should be:
    A. perform in-line stabilization
    B. obtain vital signs
    C. complete a detailed patient assessment
    D. administer high-flow oxygen

16. The AIDS virus is transmitted through contact with which of the following:
    1) Blood
    2) Semen
    3) Urine
    4) Feces
    5) Saliva
       A. 1 only
       B. 1 and 2 only
       C. 1, 2, and 3
       D. all of the above

17. Radios that are mounted in vehicles such as ambulances are called:
    A. portable radios
    B. mobile radios
    C. base radios
    D. cellular radios

18. What is the most appropriate method for managing frostbite?
    A. massaging the part
    B. immersing the part in warm water
    C. applying heat packs to the affected area
    D. packing the affected area in snow

19. You are treating a 17-year-old girl who was injured while playing field hockey. She has a painful, swollen, deformity on her right lower leg. She is obviously upset and as you start to immobilize the leg, she asks you if it will hurt. Which of the following is the best response?
    A. "No, it shouldn't hurt at all"
    B. "It might hurt, but it's no big deal"
    C. "Don't worry, everything will be fine"
    D. "It might hurt a little"

20. You are caring for a 26-year-old female who is deaf and need to determine why she called for the ambulance. What is the best way to communicate with this patient?
    A. Ask dispatch to send an interpreter
    B. Stand so the patient can see your mouth so she can read your lips
    C. Speak very loud in case the patient can hear you
    D. Have a loved one communicate with the patient using notes

21. When giving a verbal report to the hospital en route to the scene, you should:
    A. speak quickly to avoid long air times
    B. only call the hospital if your patient is in severe distress
    C. talk slowly and clearly so the hospital understands
    D. give the total medical history so hospital staff are prepared

22. The primary consideration in an emergency move is protection of the:
    A. face
    B. chest
    C. spine
    D. extremities

23. Which of the following signs indicate inadequate breathing?
    A. a ventilatory rate of 20 breaths per minute
    B. snoring respirations
    C. movement of the diaphragm
    D. bilateral chest expansion

24. You are called to assist a patient complaining of difficulty breathing. On initial assessment of a 72-year-old female patient, you note that her ventilations are 28 and shallow; she is pale and diaphoretic. How should you care for this patient?
    A. intubating the patient
    B. assisting ventilations with a bag-valve-mask
    C. administering high-flow oxygen with a nonrebreather mask
    D. administering oxygen with a venturi mask

25. A severe allergic reaction is called:
    A. psychogenic shock
    B. cardiogenic shock
    C. anaphylactic shock
    D. ventilatory shock

26. What should you do for the patient with an allergic reaction?
    A. Treat the patient for shock and transport immediately
    B. Recommend that the patient take an oral antihistamine
    C. Administer the epinephrine auto-injector stored on the ambulance
    D. Administer oxygen and complete a detailed history

27. How many doses does an epinephrine auto-injector hold?
    A. one
    B. two
    C. three
    D. four

28. Convection is:
    A. heat loss from evaporation
    B. heat loss due to exhalation of warm air
    C. the direct transfer of heat from the body into the environment
    D. heat loss from a current of air or water passing over the body

29. All of the following are signs or symptoms of a patient suffering from hypothermia *except*:
    A. irrational behavior
    B. excessive mucous production
    C. speech difficulties
    D. rapid breathing

30. An EMT-B can legally transport a patient against his or her will if:
    A. the patient's physician requests it
    B. the patient is incoherent
    C. the patient's family requests it
    D. the patient has major injuries

31. You are called to a party where you find a 16-year-old patient who is intoxicated, has ingested LSD, and is vomiting profusely. The patient agrees to treatment but is refusing transport to the hospital. How should you handle this situation?
    A. contact medical direction
    B. leave after advising the patient's legal guardian of the situation
    C. request that the patient sign a release form and leave the scene
    D. stay with patient until he has recovered

32. Your first concern when caring for a patient who has attempted suicide should be:
    A. preserving any evidence at the scene
    B. personal safety
    C. treating life-threatening conditions
    D. the patient's safety

33. The axial skeleton consists of all but one of the following:
    A. neck
    B. lower extremities
    C. trunk
    D. head

34. The five categories of the spine in descending order are:
    A. cervical, lumbar, thoracic, coccyx, sacrum
    B. cervical, thoracic, lumbar, coccyx, sacrum
    C. cervical, thoracic, sacrum, lumbar, coccyx
    D. cervical, thoracic, lumbar, sacrum, coccyx

35. The main artery of the body is the:
    A. aorta
    B. femoral
    C. carotid
    D. brachial

36. When a person swallows, food is guided into the esophagus instead of the trachea by the:
    A. tongue
    B. palate
    C. epiglottis
    D. larynx

37. The cerebrum controls all but one of the following:
    A. memory
    B. sensation
    C. coordination
    D. thought

38. A patient lying flat with his face up would be in which position?
    A. lateral recumbent
    B. semi-Fowlers
    C. prone
    D. supine

39. Stridor is:
    A. unequal breaths
    B. harsh, high-pitched breath sounds
    C. associated with neurogenic hyperventilation
    D. an upper airway obstruction

40. A symptom is:
    A. something you see, hear, or feel
    B. something a patient tells you
    C. assessed after the blood pressure
    D. all of the above

41. Which is not a part of the respiratory system:
    A. larynx
    B. trachea
    C. esophagus
    D. pharynx

42. Clinical death occurs:
    A. after biological death
    B. when breathing and heart action cease
    C. when brain cells are irreversibly damaged
    D. 6 to 10 minutes after respirations cease

43. When delivering artificial ventilation to a 7-year-old, the EMT should ventilate once every _____ seconds.
    A. 2
    B. 3
    C. 4
    D. 5

44. A patient with a suspected spinal injury, the airway should be opened by the _____ method.
    A. head tilt/neck lift
    B. jaw thrust
    C. heat tilt/chin lift
    D. none of the above

45. Oxygen through the nasal cannula should be flowed at the following rate:
    A. 2 to 6 lpm
    B. 1 to 10 lpm
    C. 8 to 12 lpm
    D. 10 to 15 lpm

46. Bag-valve-mask devices:
    A. are preferred for use in children under 12 years
    B. deliver high-concentration oxygen
    C. cannot be used with an endotracheal tube
    D. should be used on medical patients only

47. Which mask is preferred for use with the severely traumatized patient?
    A. nasal cannula
    B. venturi mask
    C. simple face mask
    D. non-rebreather mask

48. CPR should never be interrupted for more than _____ seconds.
    A. 60
    B. 15
    C. 30
    D. 45

49. The heart contracts _____ times per minute in the average healthy infant.
    A. 60 to 80
    B. 80 to 100
    C. 100 to 120
    D. 120 to 140

50. Correct hand placement for CPR in an adult is:
    A. in the middle of the sternum
    B. two fingers below the sternal notch
    C. at the apex of the rib cage
    D. two fingers above the xiphoid process

51. The correct compression rate for two person CPR is:
    A. 60 per minute
    B. 80 per minute
    C. 100 per minute
    D. 120 per minute

52. The best way to relieve an airway obstruction in an infant is to:
    A. turn the baby upside down
    B. use back blows only
    C. use back blows and abdominal thrusts
    D. use back blows and chest thrusts

53. The ventilation to compression ratio for two rescuer CPR on an adult is:
    A. 1 to 5
    B. 1 to 15
    C. 2 to 5
    D. 2 to 15

54. Abnormal lung sound include all of the following *except*:
    A. rales
    B. wheezes
    C. rhonchi
    D. crepitus

55. The EMT-B can treat and transport an unconscious patient through the legal consideration known as:
    A. implied consent
    B. applied consent
    C. immunity consent
    D. triage consent

56. The best legal defense for an EMT is:
    A. upholding Good Samaritan Laws
    B. maintaining malpractice insurance
    C. skillfully rendering required care
    D. maintaining current certification

57. Tendons connect.
    A. bones to bones
    B. muscles to bones
    C. muscles to muscles
    D. ligament to bones

58. With the head being the point of reference, the feet would be:
    A. distal
    B. proximal
    C. posterior
    D. lateral

59. The strongest bone in the body is the:
    A. skull
    B. femur
    C. scapula
    D. tibia

60. The _____ separates the chest from the abdominal cavity.
    A. xiphoid
    B. lungs
    C. stomach
    D. diaphragm

61. The first priority in an emergency is to:
    A. establish and maintain an open airway
    B. check for a pulse
    C. ensure scene safety
    D. obtain consent to treat

62. To suction effectively, an EMT should:
    A. check equipment before using
    B. measure catheter length from earlobe to mouth
    C. apply suction after the catheter is in place
    D. all of the above

63. The left upper quadrant of the abdomen contains the:
    A. gallbladder
    B. spleen
    C. urinary bladder
    D. cecum

64. The major stimulus for respiration is the arterial blood level of:
    A. carbon monoxide
    B. nitrogen
    C. carbon dioxide
    D. oxygen

65. When lifting a loaded stretcher, you should lift with your:
    A. legs bent and back straight
    B. legs straight and back bent
    C. arms only to protect your back
    D. legs and back slightly bent

66. The most effective way for a single EMT to move a patient more than just a few feet is the:
    A. fireman's carry
    B. clothes drag
    C. piggyback carry
    D. blanket drag

67. The most common method of transferring a patient from a cot to the hospital bed is:
    A. direct carry method
    B. three-man carry
    C. slide transfer method
    D. draw/sheet method

68. _____ is a late sign of shock.
    A. thready pulse
    B. vomiting
    C. seizures
    D. low blood pressure

69. A person may be in anaphylactic shock from which preceding event?
    A. sight of a bloody incident
    B. eating berries
    C. heat injury
    D. severe illness

70. Which emergency procedure has priority in treating shock?
    A. preventing loss of body heat
    B. monitoring the patient's LOC
    C. establishing the airway
    D. elevating the lower extremities

71. What type of wound has the greatest risk of infection?
    A. incision
    B. laceration
    C. contusion
    D. puncture

72. Bright red, spurting blood characterizes:
    A. arterial bleeding
    B. venial bleeding
    C. capillary bleeding
    D. none of the above

73. Which of the following is the best method for controlling bleeding and should be applied first?
    A. pressure bandage
    B. pressure point
    C. tourniquet
    D. direct pressure

74. One of the greatest dangers of bleeding from a neck wound is:
    A. shock
    B. an air bubble may be sucked into the wound
    C. you cannot use pressure points
    D. infection

75. Do not try to stop a nosebleed in the case of:
    A. an avulsed eye
    B. fractured skull
    C. fractured jaw
    D. high blood pressure

76. The major objective in treating shock is to:
    A. lower the person's body temperature
    B. improve and/or maintain circulation
    C. help the patient stay conscious
    D. keep the patient's head elevated

77. An EMT should apply traction with a traction splint until:
    A. the limb is noticeably stretched
    B. the patient feels relief
    C. the bone ends realign
    D. the fracture is reduced

78. An EMT can check for spinal cord damage in a conscious patient by:
    A. checking the patient's reflexes at the knees and elbows
    B. asking the patient to speak
    C. asking the patient to read
    D. asking the patient to wiggle their finger and toes

79. Eviscerated organs should be:
    A. replaced within the abdomen
    B. covered with a dry dressing only
    C. covered with a moist, sterile dressing
    D. rinsed thoroughly with copious amounts of sterile water

80. In all chemical burns of the eye:
    A. irrigate with water and vinegar solution
    B. have the victim blink repeatedly to wash the eye
    C. irrigate continuously with water for at least 20 minutes
    D. irrigate the eye with sodium bicarbonate

81. When caring for a patient with a sucking chest wound, the EMT should:
    A. seal the wound with aluminum foil on inhalation and position the patient on the injured side
    B. seal the wound with an occlusive dressing on exhalation and position the patient on the unin-jured side
    C. seal the wound with an occlusive dressing on exhalation and position the patient on the injured side
    D. seal the wound on inhalation and position the patient on the uninjured side

82. In paradoxical movement, a condition associated with flail chest, the loose chest section:
    A. moves in and out with the chest cage as the patient breathes
    B. remains perfectly still while the chest cage moves in and out
    C. moves in the opposite direction from the rest of the chest cage as the patient breathes
    D. none of the above

83. The part of the spine most often injured in a rear end collision is the:
    A. lumbar spine
    B. cervical spine
    C. sacral spine
    D. thoracic spine

84. The exchange of waste products for oxygen occurs in the:
    A. arteries
    B. venules
    C. capillaries
    D. veins

85. An important point for the EMT to remember when splinting a fractured hand is that:
    A. the splint should extend to the elbow
    B. the bandage should be applied loosely
    C. the bandage should never be placed over the fracture site
    D. the hand should be maintained in the position of function

86. In a patient who has sustained brain injury the vital signs reveal:
    A. rising blood pressure and a slow pulse
    B. low blood pressure and signs of shock
    C. vital signs will be near normal
    D. rising blood pressure and a fast but weak pulse

87. The danger of a prolapsed cord is that:
    A. the cord may strangle the baby
    B. the cord may tear during the delivery
    C. the cord may pull the afterbirth free when the baby is delivered
    D. the mother may suffer from significant bleeding

88. Convulsions in a child up to age 2 are generally due to:
    A. epilepsy
    B. fever
    C. hyperglycemia
    D. drowning

89. If a parent and child are both injured, it is generally best if:
    A. the parent and child are transported in separate ambulances
    B. the child is not told of the parent's injuries
    C. the parent is not told of the child's injuries
    D. the parent and child are transported together

90. The most serious threat in status epilepticus is:
    A. lack of oxygen
    B. head injury
    C. swallowing the tongue
    D. dehydration

91. Which of the following symptoms best characterizes a cerebrovascular accident?
    A. normal pupils and drooling
    B. normal pupils, paralysis on one side of the body
    C. unequal pupils and paralysis in both legs
    D. unequal pupils and paralysis on one side of the body

92. A typical sign of drug abuse with narcotics includes:
    A. increased rate of pulse
    B. constricted pupils
    C. increased rate and depth of breathing
    D. dilated pupils

93. You have delivered three shocks to a cardiac arrest patient who remains pulseless. Your next action should be to:
    A. transport the patient immediately
    B. deliver three more shocks
    C. perform CPR for 1 minute
    D. deliver one more shock and then check for a pulse

94. The primary treatment for a patient suffering from carbon monoxide poisoning includes which of the following:
    A. having the patient breathe into a paper bag
    B. administering high-concentration oxygen
    C. administering activated charcoal
    D. administering oral glucose

95. You are caring for a patient who was bitten by a poisonous snake. Treatment for this patient includes all of the following *except*:
    A. keep the patient calm
    B. remove any rings or bracelets
    C. apply light constricting bands above and below the wound
    D. apply ice packs to the wound site

96. The muscular abdominal organ in which the fetus develops is called:
    A. the placenta
    B. the uterus
    C. the birth canal
    D. the amniotic sac

97. Crowning occurs when the:
    A. placenta separates from the uterine wall
    B. umbilical cord presents at the vaginal opening
    C. baby's head presents at the vaginal opening
    D. placenta attaches at an abnormal location

98. Oral suctioniong should not exceed:
    A. 15 seconds
    B. 30 seconds
    C. 45 seconds
    D. 60 seconds

99. Which of the following medications opens the airway passages to help alleviate symptoms of an asthma attack?
    A. nitroglycerin
    B. benzene
    C. ventolin
    D. cortisone

Final Course Self-Evaluation
Answer Sheet

1. _____	26. _____	51. _____	76. _____
2. _____	27. _____	52. _____	77. _____
3. _____	28. _____	53. _____	78. _____
4. _____	29. _____	54. _____	79. _____
5. _____	30. _____	55. _____	80. _____
6. _____	31. _____	56. _____	81. _____
7. _____	32. _____	57. _____	82. _____
8. _____	33. _____	58. _____	83. _____
9. _____	34. _____	59. _____	84. _____
10. _____	35. _____	60. _____	85. _____
11. _____	36. _____	61. _____	86. _____
12. _____	37. _____	62. _____	87. _____
13. _____	38. _____	63. _____	88. _____
14. _____	39. _____	64. _____	89. _____
15. _____	40. _____	65. _____	90. _____
16. _____	41. _____	66. _____	91. _____
17. _____	42. _____	67. _____	92. _____
18. _____	43. _____	68. _____	93. _____
19. _____	44. _____	69. _____	94. _____
20. _____	45. _____	70. _____	95. _____
21. _____	46. _____	71. _____	96. _____
22. _____	47. _____	72. _____	97. _____
23. _____	48. _____	73. _____	98. _____
24. _____	49. _____	74. _____	99. _____
25. _____	50. _____	75. _____	

Final Course Self-Evaluation
Answer Key

1. __C__	26. __A__	51. __C__	76. __B__
2. __B__	27. __A__	52. __C__	77. __B__
3. __D__	28. __D__	53. __D__	78. __D__
4. __D__	29. __B__	54. __D__	79. __C__
5. __B__	30. __B__	55. __A__	80. __C__
6. __D__	31. __A__	56. __C__	81. __C__
7. __B__	32. __B__	57. __B__	82. __C__
8. __C__	33. __B__	58. __B__	83. __B__
9. __A__	34. __D__	59. __B__	84. __C__
10. __C__	35. __A__	60. __D__	85. __D__
11. __B__	36. __C__	61. __C__	86. __A__
12. __C__	37. __C__	62. __D__	87. __A__
13. __D__	38. __D__	63. __B__	88. __B__
14. __A__	39. __B__	64. __C__	89. __D__
15. __A__	40. __B__	65. __A__	90. __A__
16. __B__	41. __C__	66. __D__	91. __D__
17. __B__	42. __B__	67. __D__	92. __B__
18. __B__	43. __C__	68. __D__	93. __C__
19. __D__	44. __B__	69. __B__	94. __B__
20. __B__	45. __A__	70. __C__	95. __D__
21. __C__	46. __B__	71. __D__	96. __B__
22. __C__	47. __D__	72. __A__	97. __C__
23. __B__	48. __C__	73. __D__	98. __A__
24. __B__	49. __C__	74. __B__	99. __C__
25. __C__	50. __D__	75. __B__	